Herbal medicine in paediatrics

translation of a

THAI BOOK OF GENESIS

Best wishes
Jean Mulholland
December 2005

Herbal medicine in paediatrics

translation of a

Thai Book of Genesis

by Jean Mulholland

Faculty of Asian Studies Monographs: New Series No. 14
Faculty of Asian Studies
Australian National University

Published by the Faculty of Asian Studies,
Australian National University, GPO Box
4, Canberra ACT, Australia

Typesetting and layout by Green Words.
Printed by ANU Printery, Acton, ACT.

National Library of Australia
Cataloguing-in-Publication entry

[Phaetthayasaat songkhroh. Vol. 1. English]. Herbal medicine in paediatrics: translation of a Thai book of genesis.

Bibliography.
Includes index.
ISBN 0 7315 0791 6.

1. Pediatrics – Thailand. 2. Herbs – Thailand – Therapeutic use. 3. Medicinal plants. I.Mulholland, Jean, 1926- . II. Australian National University. Faculty of Asian Studies. III. Title. (Series: Faculty of Asian Studies monographs. New series; no. 14).

618.920009593

Distributed for the Faculty of Asian Studies by:
Bibliotech,
Australian National University,
P.O. Box 4,
Canberra 2601
Australia

Acknowledgements

I would like to express my gratitude to all the many people who helped me in this project. In particular, I am deeply indebted to Acharn Wipudh Sobhavong who taught me Thai and led me through the difficult text. I am equally indebted to Professor Vichiara Jirawongse who helped me with medical terms and in revising the translation, and who painstakingly sought out for me the scientific names of most of the natural products used as ingredients in the recipes for medicines. My special thanks go to Dr Tony Diller and Dr Baas Terwiel for their continuing guidance.

Funding between the years 1978-1981 was made available by the History Panel of the Wellcome Trust, London. I thank them for their generous support.

Secretarial and services support was made available for the final preparation for publication by the Ford Foundation through the Child Survival Project, International Population Dynamics Program of the Department of Demography, RSSS, ANU. The final editing and preparation for publication were made possible by the ANU, which invited me to become a Visiting Fellow at the Asian History Centre in the Faculty of Asian Studies for the year 1987-88.

Abbreviations

CS Chote Suvatti. *Fauna of Thailand.* Bangkok: Department of Fisheries, 1950.

DT Dr Dabba Tansubharp, one of the leading traditional doctors practising in Bangkok.

FT Chote Suvatti. *Flora of Thailand.* 2 Vols. Bangkok: Royal Institute, BE 2521 (AD 1978).

HE *Herbal Exhibition of the Fourth Asian Symposium on Medicinal Plants and Spices*. Catalogue. Bangkok. 1980.

JSS *Journal of the Siam Society.*

KP *Krom Paa Mai* (Royal Forest Department). *Chue phan mai haeng prathet Thai. lem 1. Chue phriksasaat-chue phuen mueang* (Siamese plant names. Part 1. Botanical names - local names). Bangkok: Royal Forest Department, BE 2491 (AD 1948).

KPC *Khamphee prathom chindaa.*

KSY *Khamphee sapphakhun yaa.*

LB Laddawan Boonyarattanakornkit, and Thanomjit Supavita. *Chue phuet samun phrai lae prayot* (Names and uses of medicinal plants). Bangkok: Chulalongkorn University, n.d.

LP Leenaa Phuuphattanaaphong. ed. *Samun phrai Thai* (Thai medicinal plants). Vol II. Bangkok: *Krom Paa Mai* (Royal Forest Department). BE 2522 (AD 1979).

Mc McFarland, George Bradley. *Thai-English Dictionary.* Stanford: Stanford University Press, 1944.

MM Mulholland, Jean. *Medicine, Magic and Evil Spirits.* Faculty of Asian Studies Monographs: New Series No. 8. Canberra: Faculty of Asian Studies, Australian National University, 1987.

PB *Pharmaceutical Botany.* Bangkok: Faculty of Pharmaceutical Sciences, Chulalongkorn University, n.d.

PPPT *Photchanaanukrom phaet phesat Thai chabap maattrathaan* (Dictionary of Thai medicine and pharmacy, standard edn.). Bangkok: *Samaakhom phesat lae aayurawet boraan haeng prathet Thai* (Association of Traditional Pharmacy and *Āyurvedic* Medicine of Thailand), BE 2507 (AD 1964).

PP Prasoet Phrommanee, and Parinyaa Uthitchalaanon. eds. *Tamraa phesatchakam Thai phaen boraan* (Text-book of Thai traditional pharmacy). Bangkok: *Samnak phaet phaen boraan Wat Mahathat* (College of Traditional Medicine, Wat Mahathat), BE 2516 (AD 1973).

PT Professor Payom Tantivatana, Head of the Department of Pharmaceutical Botany, Faculty of Pharmaceutical Sciences, Chulalongkorn University, Bangkok.

Skt Sanskrit.

So So Sethaputra. *New Model Thai-English Dictionary.* 2 Vols. 2nd edn. Bangkok: Thai Watana Panich Co Ltd, 1972.

TPS1 *Ngaan nithatsakaan samun phrai khrang thee 1* (The first exhibition of medicinal plants). Bangkok: *Samakhom samun phrai haeng prathet Thai* (Thai Pharmacognosy Society), BE 2518 (AD 1975).

TPS2 The second exhibition of medicinal plants. Bangkok, 1976.

TS Tem Smitinand. ed. *Chue phan mai haeng prathet Thai: chue phriksasaat - chue phuen mueang* (Thai plant names: botanical names - vernacular names). Bangkok: *Krom Paa Mai* (Royal Forest Department), BE 2523 (AD 1980).

VJ Professor Vichiara Jirawongse, President of the Thai Pharmacognosy Society, and formerly Head of the Department of Pharmacognosy, Faculty of Pharmaceutical Sciences, Chulalongkorn University, Bangkok.

WW Phya Winit Wanandorn. *Chue phan mai haeng prathet Thai: chabap chue phuen mueng - chue phriksasaat* (Thai plant names: vernacular names - botanical names). Thai Forest Record No. 1. Bangkok: *Krom Paa Mai* (Royal Forest Department), BE 2503 (AD 1960).

The system of transcription used

This system of transcription is used in preference to the Library of Congress system for two reasons: (1) It is used in an official Thai publication on Thai plant names, Tem Smitinand. ed., *Chue phan mai haeng prathet Thai* (Thai plant names) (Bangkok: 1980) [abbreviation *TS*]. (2) In order to handle the large numbers of drugs and prescriptions in the text, a computer was used, and diacritics could not be included initially.

This system has two unconventional features: (1) It represents the long vowel อี [i:] as 'ee' and (2) does not distinguish between the vowels โอะ [o], โอ [o:] and ออ [ɔ:] which are all transcribed as 'o'.

Consonants	Initial	Final
ก	k	k
ข, ค, ฆ	kh	k
ง	ng	ng
จ, ช, ฌ	ch	t
ฉ	sh	t
ญ	y	n
ด, ฎ, ฑ (some words)	d	t
ต, ฏ	t	t
ถ, ฐ, ท, ฑ, ธ, ฒ	th	t
น, ณ	n	n
บ	b	p
ป	p	p
ผ, พ, ภ	ph	p
ฝ,ฟ	f	p
ม	m	m
ย	y	vowel
ร	r	n
ล, ฬ	l	n
ว	w	vowel
ซ, ทร, ศ, ษ, ส	s	t
ห, ฮ	h	-
ฤ	ri	-
ฤๅ	ree	-

Vowels	
อะ, อั	a
อา	aa
อาย	aai
อาว	aao
แอะ, แอ	ae
แอว	aeo
ใอ, ไอ, อัย, ไอย	ai
อำ	am
เอา	ao
เอ, เอ็	e
อี	ee
เอะ	eh
เอ็ว, เอว	eo
อิ	i
เอีย	ia
เอียะ	iae
เอียว	ieo
อิว	iu
โอะ, โอ, ออ	o
เออะ, เออ, เอิ	oe
เอย	oei
เอาะ	oh
ออย	oi
โอย	ooi
อุ	u
อัว	ua
อัวะ	uae
อวย	uai
อึ, อือ	ue
เอือะ, เอือ	uea
เอือย	uei
อุย	ui
อู	uu

Contents

Preface

This is a translation of a Thai medical text on the diagnosis and treatment of children's diseases.

The Thai '*Book of Genesis*', *Khamphee prathom chindaa (KPC)* or *Tamraa prathom chindaa,* was compiled in 1871, at the instigation of King Chulalongkorn, from earlier texts of unknown origin. Similar texts were in evidence during the seventeenth century and may have been in existence for hundreds of years prior to this.

The name *Book of Genesis* has been chosen because that is what *Khamphee prathom chindaa* means and because that is what it is - a book of genesis - creation, conception, pregnancy and birth, as well as children's diseases. The sub-title *Herbal medicine in paediatrics* has been chosen because that is also what it is about - the treatment of children's diseases with herbal medicine.

KPC is probably the most interesting of a group of 23 medical texts which provide the basic teaching syllabus for the licensing examinations in Thai traditional medicine and pharmacy.

Thai traditional medicine is one of two legally recognised systems of medicine practised in Thailand, the other being Western medicine. This particular form of traditional medicine is known as the Royal tradition, having evolved at the court. The texts were published by the King specifically to enable all Thais to have access to this knowledge. There are numerous variations and other forms of traditional medicine practised in Thailand.

Medical treatment of many kinds is available in Thailand. The practice of Western medicine is spreading from Bangkok and the larger provincial centres to reach increasing numbers of the people, most of whom are rice farmers. Chinese herbalists are found in the cities and most of the smaller towns, but seldom in the villages. Traditional doctors offer treatment in the cities, towns and most, but not all villages, and every village is reported to have at least one spirit doctor or shaman. Faith healers, injection doctors, astrologers and many others offer medical treatment, and domestic or folk medicine is often used.

Even where modern medical facilities are available, it is quite common for Thais of every class and status to turn to the traditional doctors before or after consulting Western trained practitioners.

The reader interested in a detailed analysis of the history and content of *KPC* is referred to the companion volume *Medicine, Magic and Evil Spirits* (*MM*) where the diagnostic and prescribing patterns evident in the text have been examined.

The version of *KPC* used for this translation is found in Volume I of the 1961 edition of *Phaetthayasaat songkhroh* published by the Wat Pho Traditional Medical College Association, Bangkok. This was compared with earlier editions of *Phaetthayasaat songkhroh* and with the 1871 edition of *KPC* compiled by doctors of the court of King Chulalongkorn. Apart from a few major, intentional changes in the 1961 edition, where some sections have been rearranged and some repetition has been deleted, the differences between the 1871 and 1961 editions consist of slight changes in spelling. These differences have no effect on the meaning and content of the text, and have been discussed in the companion volume. The purpose of the translation was to gain an understanding of the theories of medicine and pharmacy which guide the traditional doctor in Thailand in the diagnosis and treatment of disease. It is not a philological study.

The text is written in a form of the Thai language which is no longer in common usage. Consequently no apologies are made for any inadequacies in the translation for which I accept full responsibility. With all its faults it serves the purpose of opening a small window on the practice of herbal medicine in Asia.

If it conveys only the compassion and the concern of the Thai doctors for their children - at a time when no-one, including European doctors had any better answers to the ravages of disease - then this translation will have been worthwhile. Life was so tenuous that a child was not even considered to be human until it had survived the first three days. And in many parts of Thailand these conditions still exist.

KPC is a collection of six books concerning creation, including the recreation of the world at the end of the last era, the divine origin of man, and human reproduction; diseases of infants and children, and their treatment. Each book is reasonably self-contained; some are subdivided into parts. Recipes for medicine are scattered throughout the text in groups.

Books I and VI on the whole appear to be compilations of extracts from other texts. Books II, III and IV, apart from the first few pages of Book II, describe birth *saang* and associated diseases; and Book V is chiefly concerned with parasitic diseases.

Birth *saang* or *saang* of the seven days, is a congenital disease which starts in the womb. It affects all children. None escape. Some are affected all their lives.

Diagnosis is made on the basis of the symptoms of the mother when she is three months pregnant, which point to a particular form of birth *saang*. This, in turn, indicates the day of conception and predicts the same week-day as the day of birth, by which the disease is named.

There are seven kinds of congenital disease or birth *saang*, one for each day of the week. There are several descriptions of each form, mainly collections of symptoms of all kinds likely to occur in children, from skin diseases to dysentery and internal abscesses. Some are illustrated by drawings purporting to show what some of the internal conditions look like. All these diseases are believed to be developments of the original pustule or abscess which developed in the foetus at three months.

Following or during the course of birth *saang* complications set in. Once again, a different name and description is applied to each day of the week. This has been called 'minor' *saang* in this translation. On the whole, some kinds of birth *saang* are more severe than others, but when the combined effects of the birth *saang* and minor *saang* of any one birth day are compared with those of another, it is difficult to distinguish them as far as symptoms are concerned, except for the degree of severity of some forms.

There are certain other diseases associated with each form of congenital disease, a particular variant in each case, as with minor *saang*. These are mouth diseases called *la* and *la-ong*, and a group of diseases which appear to affect the nervous system. These last belong to the class of *lom* or wind diseases and include tetanus. Eventually, after about five years, when this pattern of early childhood diseases has run its course, it is supplanted by severe parasitic infestations also associated with particular kinds of birth *saang* and the effects can continue throughout life.

The inadequacies of this system of classification of diseases in children have not escaped the authors who have offered alternatives such as the interchangeability of some kinds of birth *saang* and the complicating and ensuing diseases.

Outside this complex of diseases, but recognised within the same system, are diseases believed to be caused by spirits. These might be *mae sue, saphan* or various kinds of *paksee.* Also the form of the child, whether *mahatsaruup, athitsaruup, haritaruup* or *manutsaruup,* has its effect on the symptoms that might develop.

In this text, the medical theory based on the Indian *Āyurvedic* system of medicine, relating to disorders of the body elements and the *tridoṣa,* as taught in Thai schools of traditional medicine now, is secondary to the theory of birth *saang* or congenital disease. The greatest occurrence of *Āyurvedic* theory is found amongst the extracts from supplementary texts included in Book VI at the end of *KPC.* Brief passages seem to have been superimposed elsewhere at the beginning or end of already established sections of the text.

While most of the descriptions of diseases in terms of the elements and the humoral theory of *Āyurveda* speak of *saang,* a few attempt to incorporate these foreign ideas with the concept of birth *saang.* Others include references to spirits or relate to the physical appearance of the body, the form. At no time are *Āyurvedic* ideas adapted to explain the diseases associated with birth *saang,* which is understandable since *Āyurveda* reduces most illnesses to three - those resulting in disorders of the *tridoṣa,* wind, bile and mucus.

The text *KPC* stands up on its own without foreign accretions of the elements and the humoral theory. Although *KPC* is a collection of texts, some possibly borrowed material from neighbouring countries, including India, the *Āyurvedic* passages do not sit well within these texts.

There is yet another component in the indigenous medical theory revealed in *KPC* . This is the pragmatic approach to diagnosis. This method has two forms of expression: in simple symptomatic description, and in terms of birth *saang.* It is within this category that we find the rationalisation which overcomes the rigidity of the birth *saang* theory, insisting that the doctor should be careful in his diagnosis of a particular form of birth *saang,* being guided primarily by the symptoms observed in the child rather than its birthday. The uncomplicated diseases of infancy and the minor upsets that occur at the times of change in a baby's development are also described in this straightforward manner, and in *Āyurvedic* terms as well. The effects on the infant of the way it is born and of the quality or quantity of the mother's milk are also described pragmatically.

The treatment of diseases is covered fully in *KPC,* with reference both to the *Āyurvedic* and empirical approaches as well as to the indigenous theory related to congenital birth *saang.* In this text there are only two references to massage. Ritual and incantations are used at times, but most treatment suggested is with medicines administered internally, applied externally or burnt for the purpose of fumigation. The ingredients are of animal, mineral and vegetable origin, most being plant or herbal material.

The use of herbal and other medicaments obtained from natural products has been discussed in detail in *Medicine, Magic and Evil Spirits*. However, it is this volume which contains a complete translation of all the 661 recipes or prescriptions for medicine and the scientific names and other information relating to more than 800 medicinal ingredients used in the recipes.

The identification of the prescription ingredients is not always clear cut and is open to debate in some instances. For this reason, where possible, several sources are given. I am indebted to Professor Vichiara Jirawongse for supplying me with a large number of scientific names of substances named in the text, for which no identification could otherwise be found. Professor Payom Tantivatana was also most helpful in this matter.

One of the main problems in identifying plant names from Thai names is the use of the same name for different plants in different parts of Thailand and, in some cases, different names for the same plant. For these reasons, investigation of prescription ingredients will require study, in the field, of the actual plants used by reputable practitioners in individual cases.

English and scientific names have not been spelt out within the main lists of ingredients. There are many reasons, not the least being the lack of English names and the lack of certainty about some scientific names. But some common simple English names have been given in directions for making up prescriptions and in a few short recipes to add interest.

Prescriptions for medicine are not numbered in *KPC* but have been numbered here for easy reference. The scientific names and other information about the medicinal substances used in the recipes and a few items mentioned in the text itself are listed in Roman alphabetical order in Appendix I.

Bold lettering has been used to indicate names of recipes and words and phrases emphasised by underlining in the Thai text.

ตำราประถมจินดา

นโม ตสฺส ภควโต อรหโต สมฺมาสมฺพุทฺธสฺส.

นมสฺสิตฺวา จ เทวินฺทํ เทวราชสกฺกํ อิว
ชีวกโกมารภจฺจํ โลกนาถํ ตถาคตํ
ปฐมจินฺตารคนฺถํ ภาสิสฺสํ ฉนฺทโสมฺขํ
สงฺเขเปน กิตฺตยิตํ ปุพฺเพ โลกานํ นาถตฺถนฺติ.

แปล (อหํ) อันว่าข้า (นมสฺสิตฺวา) ถวายนมัสการแล้ว (ตถาคตํ) ซึ่งพระศรีสุคตทศพลญาณเจ้า (โลกนาถํ) เป็นที่พึ่งของโลก (จ) อนึ่งโสด (อหํ) อันว่าข้า (อภิวนฺทิตฺวา) ไหว้แล้วโดยพิเศษ (ชีวกโกมารภจฺจํ) ซึ่งชีวกโกมารภัจ แพทย์ผู้ประเสริฐ (เทวราชสกฺกํ อิว) เปรียบดุจสมเด็จอมรินทราธิราชบพิตร (เทวินฺทํ) ผู้มีมหิศรภาพเป็นจอมมกุฎแก่เทพบุตรทั้งหลาย (ภาสิสฺสํ) จักแสดงบัดนี้ (คนฺถํ) ซึ่งพระคัมภีร์แพทย์อันวิเศษ (ปฐมจินฺตารํ) ชื่อประถมจินดา (ฉนฺทโสมฺขํ) อันเป็นหลักเป็นประธานแห่งพระคัมภีร์ฉันทศาสตร์ทั้งปวง (กิตฺตยิตํ) อันพระอาจารย์โกมารภัจแต่งไว้ (ปุพฺเพ) ในกาลก่อน (สงฺเขเปน) โดยสังเขป (นาถตฺถํ) เพื่อจะให้เป็นที่พึ่ง (โลกานํ) แก่สัตว์โลกทั้งหลาย (เอวํ) ด้วยประการดังนี้

(โองการ พินฺทุนาถํ อุปฺปนฺนํ พฺรหฺมา สหมฺปติ นาม อาทิ กปฺเปส อาคโต ปญฺจ ปทุมํ ทิสฺวา นโม พุทฺธาย วนฺทนํ อาจริเยน) อันพระอาจารย์เจ้า กล่าวไว้ในพระคัมภีร์ประถมจินดานี้ ตั้งแต่พรหมปโรหิตเป็นต้นมานั้น ว่าเมื่อจะตั้งแผ่นดินใหม่ครั้งนั้นก็ให้บังเกิดกัลป์พินาศกล่าวคือโลกฉิบหาย ด้วยเพลิงประลัยกัลป์นั้นไหม้ฟ้าแผ่นดิน ภูเขา และเขาพระสุเมรุสิ้นแล้วบังเกิดฝนห่าใหญ่ตกลงมาถึง ๗ วัน ๗ คืน และน้ำท่วมขึ้นไปถึงชั้นพรหมปโรหิตพรหมปโรหิตจึงเล็งลงมาดู ก็เห็นซึ่งดอกอุบล ๕ ดอก ผุดขึ้นมาเหนือน้ำงามหาที่จะอุปมามิได้ ท้าวมหาพรหมจึงบอกแก่พรหมทั้งหลายว่า แผ่นดินใหม่นี้ จะบังเกิดสมเด็จพระพุทธเจ้ามาตรัส ๕ พระองค์ เพราะเห็นดอกอุบลนั้น ๕ ดอก

Tamraa Prathom Chindaa[1]

Book of Genesis
[Book I]

Namo tassa bhagavato arahato sammāsambuddassa
namassitvā ca devindaṃ devarājasakkaṃ iva
jīvakakomārabhaccaṃ lokanāthaṃ tathāgathaṃ
paṭhamacintāraganthaṃ bhāsissaṃ chandasomukhaṃ
saṃkhepen kittayitaṃ pubbe lokānaṃ nāthatthanti

Translation: (*Ahaṃ*) 'I' (*namassitvā*) 'have paid homage' (*tathāgataṃ*) 'to the Lord Buddha' (*lokanāthaṃ*) 'the refuge of all the world' (*ca*) 'and then' (*ahaṃ*) 'I' (*abhivanditvā*) 'made special obeissance' (*jīvakakomārabhaccaṃ*) 'to the honoured doctor Jīvaka Komārabhacca'[2] (*devarājasakkaṃ iva*) 'whose greatness may be compared to that of the illustrious Lord Indra' (*devindaṃ*) 'the greatest of all the kings of the gods.' (*Bhāsissaṃ*) 'Here is' (*ganthaṃ*) 'the special text on medicine' (*paṭhamacintāraṃ*) '*prathom chindaa*' (*chandasomukhaṃ*) 'on which *Khamphee shanthasaat* is based.' (*Kittayitaṃ*) 'It was composed by the master Komārabhacca' (*pubbe*) 'long ago'. (*Saṃkhepen*) 'In brief' (*nāthatthaṃ*) 'so that it may help' (*lokānaṃ*) 'all people' (*evaṃ*) 'it is set out below.'

(*Oṃkāra bindunāthaṃ uppannaṃ brahmā sahaṃpati nāma ādi kappesa āgato pañca padumaṃ disvā namo buddhāya vandanaṃ ācariyena*) In this text, *Phrakhamphee prathom chindaa*, the master explained the origin of man. At the end of the last *kalpa*, before the earth was newly created, the whole world was destroyed by fire. The heavens were consumed by fire, the earth, the mountains and, finally, Mount Sumēru. Then it rained heavily for seven days and seven nights, and the floods rose higher and higher until they reached the level of Phrom Parohit [Brahmā]. Then Brahmā gazed down and saw five lotus blossoms, beautiful beyond compare, rising above the water. So the great Brahmā told all the other brahmas 'On this new earth will be born five Buddhas, because I have seen five lotus blossoms'.

This is what usually happens whenever a sign appears. Mud and water descend for seven days and seven nights as a dense cover, like weeds floating on water, 240,000 *yot* thick. This is explained in *Phrakhamphee chakarawaanlatheep*, but here in *Khamphee prathom chindaa* it is summarised.

When the earth and Mount Sumēru arose, the Lord Isvara invited two *brahmacārī* to come down and taste the sweetness of the earth.[3] Having tasted, they became pregnant and gave birth to twelve children. These twelve children reproduced by stroking each other's abdomen, and their progeny spread out to the four *dvīpa*, and developed different languages. But in this *Jambū Dvīpa* of ours,[4] there is passion, and pregnancy occurs through sexual intercourse. Life thus conceived is called *jalābuja* [born from water]; life born from an egg is called *aṇḍaja* [oviparous]; life conceived from mud is called *saṃsedaja upapātika* [mud-born]; and life conceived by itself is called spontaneous [parthenogenesis]. Of mankind born from the mother's abdomen, women differ from men in two ways. They have a blood gland [menses] and breast milk to feed their children. When mature, a woman's body develops and, before she begins to menstruate, she dreams that a *vidyādhara* comes secretly to admire her and has intercourse with her.[5] From then she has her seasons, such that it is apparent to all, and her breasts develop also.

(*Pañca vidha lohitaṃ hadayaṃ jātaṃ lohitaṃ pittaṃ lohitaṃ mamsaṃ jātaṃ lohitaṃ aṭṭhi jātaṃ pañcavidha lohitaṃ*) Women have five kinds of normal [menstrual] blood. The masters have taken this from *Phrakhamphee mahaachotarat* and inserted it in *Phrakhamphee phrom parohit* for the information of doctors, so that they will completely understand conception and periodic bleeding [menstruation], as follows: *lohitaṃ hadayaṃ jātaṃ* is the first. This is the blood which affects the heart.[6] Then there is blood which affects the gall bladder, blood which affects the flesh, and blood which affects the tendons. *Lohitaṃ aṭṭhi jātaṃ* is the last. This is the blood which affects the bones. Each of these five kinds of menstrual blood produces distinctive symptoms.

Blood which affects the heart can make a woman agitated and excited, and easily provoked to anger. If, at such a time, her lips and the area around her eyes turn blue and the treatment is not successful, she is sure to die.

Menstrual blood which affects the gall bladder and the liver can make her listless, giddy, absent-minded and dull, as if intoxicated, so that she does not know whether it is night or day. She starts in her sleep, trembling with fright; she converses with spirits; and it seems that her *khwan* has eaten up the forest.[7] If it is not understood that all these things are caused by the menstrual blood, as explained, she will die in seven days and, when she is dead, red and blue rings will erupt on her skin.

Blood which affects the flesh makes a woman feel hot inside, her skin gets as red as a ripe *tamlueng* [pillar-box red],[8] she develops a heat rash and feels itchy all over. All these symptoms go when she menstruates.

Blood which affects the tendons can produce pain all over the body, alternate sensations of heat and cold, and severe headache. These symptoms also go at the start of menstruation.

Blood which affects the bones makes them ache, and all the joints are so painful that they feel as though they might come apart. There is severe pain in the waist and back. With menstruation, these disappear.

Doctors should investigate and understand the effects of menstruation. Once the diagnosis has been made, these medicines should be given:

[1] *Phrom phak* [*Brahmā vaktra*, Face of the Brahmā], to rid her completely of foul blood; then

[2] the blood tonic called *Kamlang raatchasee* [Strength of a lion]; followed by

[3] a tonic for the elements, to restore them to normal.[9]

Then the [menstrual] blood will be in perfect condition and the woman will be able to conceive normally and assume her role of motherhood.

There is also a type of woman who usually has good blood, whether she has a husband or not; but sometimes her face, hands and feet are pale, and she has a pain in her back and waist. This is because the blood is dry and stuck to the backbone. It is probably *ritseeduang*.[10]

Another kind of woman has dry blood which forms a lump as large as a hen's egg. This lodges in the supra-pubic region or in the chest or rolls around in the abdomen, sometimes causing flatulence, diarrhoea or abdominal pain and chest pain so severe that it seems as if she will die.

Doctors should be familiar with what has been described above, because if it is not cured this might develop into *ritseeduang haeng*.[11]

Then there is the virgin who reaches puberty, or even twenty or thirty years of age without menstruating. She will do so once she has a husband.

These female characteristics were evident even in those early days.

Phrom parohit ends here

The masters have taken this section from *Khamphee roknithaan*, and summarised it here in *Phrakhamphee prathom chindaa* for the information of doctors.

When life is conceived by the parents, it is made complete by the combination of the four elements, comprising twenty elements of earth, twelve of water, four of fire and six of wind. Life originates from the normal union of the blood of the parents, that is, from the element water, in that the mother's blood gland causes conception to occur.

At the time of conception, they say that [the embryo] is the finest particle, so fine, it could be compared to the size of the particle of oil which remains on the tip of a single hair of a yak after the hair has been dipped in clear sesame oil then whipped in the air seven times. But, having been conceived in the mother's womb, it can become liquified more than seven times a day, it is so difficult to retain.

After seven days, first a cell is formed from the blood. It is called *chaya phet*, and the mother has one period of watery menstruation. If this does not occur, she might have an unusual dream and then she knows she is pregnant.

When the pregnancy has lasted seven days without miscarriage, the blood becomes thicker, like water which has been used to wash meat. After another seven days it becomes flesh. After another seven days it assumes the form of a snake's egg. After another seven days it divides into the five branches [*pañca sākhā*], that is, the head, two hands and two feet. After a further seven days the hair on the head, the body hair, nails and teeth are formed, in that order.

When the pregnancy has lasted for a month and twelve days, the blood is formed and it rotates [towards the centre] like the eye of a peacock [feather]. At the heart is the receptacle of knowledge. If [the foetus] is female, the revolutions are to the left; if it is male, they are to the right.[12] But this is not visible.

After three months, the blood divides to conform to the five branches. After four months, all the 32 parts [important organs] of the body have been formed. The eyes and the forehead come first, then everything else in order. After five months, the mind and the five senses,[13] as well as the form, have developed and then [the foetus] is conscious and can feel heat and cold. Then whenever the mother eats something hot-and-spicy, the foetus will be distressed and restless and push and shove.

Next comes the ability to feel pleasure and pain. The foetus in the womb endures pain and suffering and is tortured just like the creatures in hell. It sits on its heels, hugging its knees, holding its clenched fists up under its chin, turns its face towards the mother's spine and its back towards her navel and sits like a baby monkey in the hollow of a tree.

It sits on top of the digested food. The undigested food is above its head, and the juices from the undigested food filter down and are absorbed rapidly through the crown of the head [fontanelle] of the foetus in the womb, because the crown of the head is open. So whenever the mother eats, the baby can eat its mother's food and be content. If the mother does not eat, the baby gets no nourishment, so it becomes distressed and restless and agitated, and struggles and squirms.[14]

Here, in *Khamphee prathom chindaa* the masters also include the essence of what is said in *Khamphee chaturaariyasat* about the treatment of the diseases of pregnancy.

If the mother craves for fishy tasting food, they say that that life came from hell; if she craves for sour and bitter food, it came from snow-covered forest; if she craves for honey, sugarcane juice and sugar, it came down from heaven to be born as a human being; if she craves for fruit, it came from an animal; if she craves for clay, it came from Brahmā; if she craves for things which are hot-and-spicy, it came from a human being.

It is normal in this world for the mother to have such cravings and this makes the baby in the womb sick.

Once the baby is completely formed physically, and has the five senses and the 32 parts, it thinks: 'My mother is very kind. She has taken the utmost care of me. When I am born, I will be able to show her my gratitude.' This has always been the normal custom of Bodhisattvas.[15]

Phrakhamphee prathom chindaa, Book I, Part 2 [sic], abridged, on conception, prenatal care, miscarriage, pregnancy and birth, ends here.

End of Part 1.

Puna ca paraṃ māturakkhipatiṭṭhitaṃ jīvakakomārohaṃ ābhataṃ thāne idaṃ sutaṃ isi etthavacanassa mahātherato ahosīti, (*puna ca paraṃ*). In other words: (*Ahaṃ*) 'I' (*jīvakakomāro*) 'Jīvaka Komārabhacca' (*sutaṃ*) 'learnt' (*mahātherato*) 'from the house of the great *thera* Tamyae;[16] (*abhataṃ*) (*patiṭṭhitaṃ*) 'and made a permanent record [of what I learnt]' (*mātugabbharakkhamhi*) 'here in *Khamphee khanpharaksaa*.' (*Etthavacane*) 'In Part 1' (*assa mahātherassa*) 'of the work of the great *thera* ' (*iti*) 'the following explanation is given of Rogāmṛtindra who was Jīvaka Komārabhacca's teacher.'

This is a summary of the teaching of the doctor who was the adopted son of a prince and a pupil of Mṛtindra, who was known as Rogāmṛtindra [doctor conqueror of death], because he was blessed by the great god Brahmā, so that the people he treated would not die. But, if someone's time to die had come, no matter where Rogāmṛtindra was, he could not be seen. He had a collection of magical formulae, and knew the properties of all medicinal plants. This was due to his great merit. Wherever he went, each tree and medicinal plant would cry out and tell him 'My name is "so and so"; I can cure "such and such" disease of mankind'. They shouted to him all over the forest, but only he could hear. That is how he was able to make medicine, and he compiled texts of his medicines so that they could be passed down from one doctor to another from the time of the first Buddha, Phra Kakkusantha, to the time of our Lord Buddha, Phra Khodom.[17]

If anyone wants to study medicine, he should first study the text called *Sapphakhun*. If he wants to be a paediatrician, he should first become proficient in these three basic texts: *Apphayasantaa, Prathom chindaa* and *Mahaachotarat*, then study the other texts.

Puna ca paraṃ[18] This is a continuation of the summary of the teaching on conception of the great *thera* Tamyae. *Tumhe passathimaṃ lokasmi sattapaṭisandhikaṃ mātugabbhaṃ tividhaṃ temāsaṃ kumāramātaro bālahagilāniyo tiṭṭhanti.* When a life has come to be conceived in a mother's womb, it [the embryo] becomes liquefied seven times a day for seven days, and it is not certain, at this stage, whether or not life has definitely begun. After fifteen days it is certain and it is obvious to all. If anyone wishes to know the date of conception, they can know by observing the mother's condition when she is three months pregnant, and estimating the date by counting back.

When a mother has been pregnant for three months, and she becomes very constipated, has spasms of the hands and feet, is thin and yellow, cannot walk far, has pain in the supra-pubic area and lower abdomen, severe pain in the iliac region, and craves for sweet things; and the sole of her left foot is red, then the baby will be a girl. If the sole of the right foot is red, it will be a boy. In either case, it should be realized that the child was conceived on a Sunday, and will be born on a Sunday,[19] because *saang phloeng*[20] is the main illness of such a child, and it presents itself in this way in the mother.

When a mother has been pregnant for three months, and she has headaches, painful breasts, a craving for sweet things, muscular fatigue in both arms, blurred vision, difficulty in hearing, is dazed and dry retches, the doctor who observes this should be aware that the child was conceived on a Monday, and will be born on a Monday, because *saang nam*[21] is the main illness of such a child, and it presents itself in this way in the mother.

When a mother has been pregnant for three months, and she has gastric pain, dizziness, swelling of the backs of the hands and of the legs from the feet up to the iliac region, general fatigue and muscular pain, insomnia and pustules the size of maize kernels on the palate, it should be realized that the child was conceived on a Tuesday, and will be born on a Tuesday, because *saang daeng*[22] is the main illness of such a child, and it presents itself in this way in the mother.

When a mother has been pregnant for three months, and she has gastric pain, vomiting, swelling of the legs and feet and pain in the iliac region; and she finds the taste of food bitter; and around the anus and urethra small raised spots erupt, then become inflamed and suppurating sores; it should be realized that the child was conceived on a Wednesday, and will be born on a Wednesday, because *saang sako*[23] is the main illness of such a child, and it presents itself in this way in the mother.

When a mother has been pregnant for three months, and she has inflamed pustules in the mouth and on the tongue, so that she is unable to take hot-and-spicy food for six months; and the sores spread out to the sides of the tongue and to the palate, then crack like clay in a dry field; and if she swallows her saliva, she passes mucus and blood in the stools and has diarrhoea until the time of delivery; it should be realized that the child was conceived on a Thursday, and will be born on a Thursday, because *saang wua*[24] is the main illness of such a child, and it presents itself in this way in the mother.

When a mother has been pregnant for three months, and she has a very itchy rash like heat rash, an inflamed, suppurating eruption around the anus and urethra, pain in the supra-pubic area, hips and lumbar region on both sides, with difficulty in urinating[25] and at six months she has gastric pain; and at eight or nine months, continuing until delivery,[26] swollen hands and feet; it should be realized that the child was conceived on a Friday, and will be born on a Friday, because *saang chaang*[27] is the main illness of such a child, and it presents itself in this way in the mother.

When a mother has been pregnant for three months, and she has constipation, relieved once every two or three days; a craving for raw and undercooked fish and meat; is restless; and spots like a heat rash erupt at the nipples, break and suppurate; and at six months she has diarrhoea, with mucus and blood-stained faeces; pain at the waist; is always hungry, and craves for sweet and sour flavours, and strong salads,[28] up to the time of delivery; it should be realized that the child was conceived on a Saturday and will be born on a Saturday, because *saang khamooi*[29] is the main illness of such a child, and it presents itself in this way in the mother.

End of signs of conception, summarised for doctors.

Puna ca paraṃ Here we will deal with prenatal care, according to the teaching, as follows. When a woman has been pregnant for fifteen days or a month, it is obvious to all from her appearance that she is pregnant, because the tendons which cross her chest have become blue, her nipples have become darker and there are small spots around the nipples. In short, the doctor will know from this that the woman is pregnant.

If a woman is one month pregnant and she develops *khai ram phe ram phat*[30] with symptoms of vomiting, abdominal colic, severe nausea and delirium, as if possessed by a spirit, the doctor will not know whether it is *sannibaat*,[31] but it will affect the foetus. He should first treat it in the traditional manner. They made a five-cornered tray *[bat]*[32]. Then they rolled a ball of dough on the [woman's] abdomen, reciting this mantra seven times:[33] (*om dhijūbhūbha savāha*). Then they took the ball of dough and moulded it into shapes: a woman, a mountain, a chicken and a horse. Then they took seven kinds of fruit and seven kinds of flowers and strewed some husked rice amongst the offering of fruit. Then they offered it and took it to the South-East. They did this [each day] for three days, then she was better. If not, they prepared medicine from this recipe:

[4]	*chan hom*[34]	
	hua [bua] phuean	flowers
	bua luang	root
	khaao nieo kanyaa	

Mix these 4 items and prepare pills to be taken mixed with cow's milk.[35]

If that was ineffective, they gave her:

[5] roast beef, popped rice and black, gluten rice mixed with honey.

If this medicine made her feel hot, they prepared:

[6]	*sai yoi*	leaves

yaa phraek	leaves
phrommi	leaves
tamlueng	leaves
din prasiu khaao	

These 5 items to be mixed together and taken or applied mixed with water used to wash rice. It has been used a great deal.

If a woman is two months pregnant, and she has chills daily at regular intervals, insomnia, loss of appetite, is dull and listless or has any illness, whether regular or intermittent, first treat this in the traditional manner. They made a round tray. Then they rolled a ball of dough on the abdomen, reciting this mantra seven times: (*om amara hi jivanatiye savāha*). Then they took the ball of dough and moulded a cat from it. Then they took three kinds of vegetables, three kinds of fruit and three kinds of flowers, and scattered cooked rice on the base of the leaf blade [of the tray], and sprayed perfumed powder and essence on the tray. Then they took it to the East. If she did not recover, they prepared medicine from this recipe:

[7]	*bua luang*	pollen
	chong konlanee	flowers
	haeo muu	rhizome
	thian dam	
	krachap bok	

To be taken mixed with water used to wash rice.

If that was ineffective:

[8]	*bua luang*	root
	bua phuean	root
	haeo	raw
	krachap	raw
	phak waen	leaves

Add a little fresh ginger. To be taken mixed with dew or cow's milk to relieve abdominal pain and flatulence.

And this application:

[9]	*bai naat*	
	phok phaai	leaves
	phak hai	root
	khanun lamut	seeds
	din so phong	

To be applied mixed with water used to wash rice. This will be effective. It is very potent, and is recommended.

If a woman is three months pregnant, and she is ill with diarrhoea, vomiting, colicky pain both back and front and cannot eat or sleep, be careful as she might miscarry. First treat this in the traditional manner. They made a three-cornered tray, then they rolled a ball of dough mixed with mung beans on the abdomen, reciting this mantra seven times: (*om siddhi sā makāreti debina vā ahaṃ ijā kānaṃ mārehiehi* [repeated] *āgacchanti kāmehine*). Then they took the ball of dough, and moulded from it the shapes of a woman and a rabbit. Then they made a heap of cooked rice like a termite mound, and put liquor [*lao*] and rice in the tray, cow's milk, three kinds of vegetables and three kinds of flowers; and smeared perfumed paste on the tray and sprinkled essence on it, then took it to the West. They did this [each day] for three days, and succeeded in making her better. If not, they prepared medicine from this recipe:

[10]	*khai nao*	sap
	mamuang	sap
	kradom	

To be taken mixed with hot water.

If she was not better, they gave her a mixture of:

[11] popped rice and black, gluten rice with cow's milk and applied this lotion:

[12]	*krachap bok*	root
	bua luang	juvenile leaves
	kho	fresh dung
	chan hom	
	proh hom	
	yaa phraek	
	faek hom	
	ching chaa chaalee	vine

Mix with water used to wash rice. This is an excellent lotion.

Whenever a woman who is four months pregnant has fever due to mucus which causes problems; fainting, sweating and bleeding; and these four symptoms occur together, it is called *sannibaat.* First treat it in the traditional manner. They made a four-cornered tray then they rolled a ball of dough on the abdomen, reciting this mantra seven times: (*om he he hotiṭha hotiṭha heyanaheyana om pakkhasaṃ sābhatāva pasayunna sanā rihe*). Then they moulded the shapes of a vulture, a green snake and two people from the ball of dough. And they took two kinds of fruit and two kinds of vegetables and placed mango leaves under the tray, then took it to the North-West. They did this [each day] for three days, then she recovered. If not, they prepared this medicine:

[13]	*kot khamao*	
	bua luang	pollen
	khat mon	root
	chong konlanee	flowers

To be taken mixed with cow's milk.

If ineffective:

[14]	*sattabongkot*	flowers
	kot kraduuk	
	bua luang	root
	krachap bok	
	chan hom	
	khat mon	root
	haeo muu	rhizome
	matuum	root
	phak chee	fruit

	khing	fresh

Mix together equal parts of these 10 items.[36] Reduce to 1/3 volume by boiling.[37] To be taken in conjunction with this application:

[15]	*salon [salot] nam*	root
	yaa naang	root
	thong laang naam	root
	phum riang baan	root
	phum riang paa	
	chan daeng	
	chan khaao	
	phung do	root
	tamlueng	root
	fak khaao	root
	bua luang	pollen
	din prasiu	
	din so phong	

Grind equal parts of these 12 items to a fine powder and prepare pills to be taken or applied mixed with water used to wash rice. Excellent medicine to comfort and safeguard the foetus.

When a woman has been pregnant for five months, and she is sick with diarrhoea and vomiting, sharp pains in the chest and back, or any illness of pregnancy; first treat it in the traditional way. They made a five-cornered tray, and rolled a ball of dough on the abdomen, reciting this mantra seven times: (*santipakkhā apattanā santipādā avañcanā mātāpitā ca nikkhantā jātaveda patikkama patikkamantu bhūtānisohaṃ namo bhagavato namo sattannaṃ sammāsaṃ buddhānanti*). Then they modelled the ball of dough into the figure of a woman, and offered it, with five flowers, strong salads, liquor, cooked rice and dried meat, then took it to a big tree in the South-West. They did this [each day] for three days, then she was better. If not, they prepared medicine from this recipe for her to take:

[16]	*bua phuean*	flowers
	bunnaak	flowers
	mamuang	sap

To be taken mixed with cow's milk, to treat diarrhoea and rectal haemorrhage, and for abdominal colic.

If this was ineffective:

[17]	*bua bok*	leaves
	thian dam	
	khamin	powder
	puun daeng	

To be taken mixed with alcohol [*suraa*], to treat rectal and urethral haemorrhage.

And this application for muscular stiffness and fatigue:

[18]	*samun waeng*	bark
	plao noi	root

sakhaan
son thet
Equal parts to be ground together and mixed with lime water. To be applied wherever there is muscular pain, except to the abdomen, as this is dangerous for the foetus.

If a woman who has been pregnant for seven [six] months has pain in the shins, legs and iliac region, anal and urethral itch, and often faints; even if an offering of *sia krabaan* is made,[38] she gets no relief. Even so, the traditional method is tried first. They made a four-cornered tray, with two tiers, and rolled a ball of dough on the abdomen, reciting this *gāthā* seven times:[39] (*aggohamasmi lokasminti bhavatilokitilokassa sannibhabbhadma hiri gabbhapamuñcanti*). And they made from the ball of dough, a cow, a horse and a chicken; and they took some lime-juice and sesame oil; seven kinds of vegetables, seven kinds of fruit, seven kinds of flowers and seven kinds of sweets; and they placed popped rice on the base of the leaf blade, and liquor, and sprinkled perfumed powder and essence on the tray, and offered it and sent it to the South-West. They did this [each day] for three days. If she was not yet better, they prepared this medicine for her to take:

[19]	*som saa*	kernels
	sakae	bark
	chan daeng	
	chan khaao	
	chong konlanee	flowers

Equal parts to be ground together, to be taken mixed with cow's milk.

If that was ineffective, they prepared a milder remedy, because the foetus is sufficiently developed and has the five branches and the 32 parts [i.e. the body is fully formed]:

[20]	*khon thee song [so]*	roasted fruit	
	waan nam		
	thian dam		
	thian khaao		
	mahaa hing		
	proh hom		
	haeo muu	rhizome	
	boraphet		
	bua luang	pollen	
	bunnaak	flowers	
	opchoei thet		
	en	fruit	
	ngoh	bark	
	cha-em thet		
	phak chee	fruit	2 *salueng* of each[40]
	phrik Thai	11 seeds [peppercorns]	

Prepare pills from these 16 items to be taken mixed with cow's milk. This is very good, and has been used often.

Then apply:

[21]	*thong laang naam*	leaves
	khanun lamut	leaves
	yaa naang	leaves
	bai naat	
	phekaa	leaves
	waan nam	leaves
	yaa phraek	leaves
	khamin oi	

Equal parts of these 8 items to be ground together and made into pills, to be applied mixed with water used to wash rice. Excellent for all disorders of pregnancy.

When a woman has been pregnant for seven months and is sick and has diarrhoea, vomits blood and feels hot inside, first treat her in the traditional way. They made a four cornered tray, with two tiers, and rolled a ball of dough on her abdomen, reciting this mantra seven times: (*om namassāmi namo ca sugato paccuppannā pañcabuddhā pana om simahāsi.* When I have given birth, I will make an offering to the spirits [*devatā*][41] in the process of transmigration: *om siddhikālamahāsiddhikāla savāha*). Then they moulded the ball of dough that had been rolled over the abdomen into the forms of a tiger and a vulture. They placed white, husked rice at the base of the leaf blade and offered it, with red and white sandalwood, three kinds of vegetables, popped rice, and flowers, then took it to the West. She recovered after this was done [each day] for three days.

When a woman is eight months pregnant and gets sick, it does not matter, because the foetus is sufficiently mature and the time of birth is near. If she has *khai ram phe ram phat*, first treat her in the traditional way. They made a round tray, and rolled a ball of dough on the abdomen, repeating this *gāthā* seven times: (*sabbedevā pisāceva ālavakādayopica khaggaṃtālapattaṃ disvā sabbe yakkhā palāyanti*). From the dough, they moulded the form of a horse. They scattered white, husked rice on the base of the leaf [of the tray], placed on the tray two kinds of vegetables and two kinds of flowers, with mango leaves underneath and, after sprinkling it with fragrant powder and essence, offered it before placing it near a large tree in the North-Eastern direction. If she was not better after this had been done [each day] for three days, they prepared this medicine:

[22]	*phak kaat*	seeds
	bua luang	root
	khaao nieo kanyaa	

To be taken mixed with water used to wash rice, or river water.

If this was ineffective:

[23]	*chaa phluu*	root
	kraphang hom	root
	krachap bok	root
	bua luang	root
	haeo muu	rhizome
	boraphet	
	chan daeng	

chan khaao	
matuum	almost ripe
khamin oi	
sadaao	33 leaf stalks

Mix together equal parts of these 11 items and reduce to 1/3 volume by boiling. To be taken.

And this application:

[24]	*mong*	root
	lamduan	root
	sai yoi	root
	yaa phraek	root
	tamlueng	root
	fak khaao	root
	din prasiu khaao	

Equal parts of these 7 items to be made into pills to be mixed with water used to wash rice. To be applied.

If a woman is nine months pregnant and is sick, it is still necessary to take care of the foetus, but it is already mature. So, if she is ill, it will affect only the mother, unless she has cholera [*ahiwaatok rok*]. Even so, if she has a severe abscess [*fee ek*] which bursts, the foetus will be lost before the mother. It this is not the case, the mother must make obeissance to Khun Sai. All this depends on whatever merit the foetus chances to have. If there is any reason to do so, first treat this in the traditional way. They made a round tray of nine tiers, just like a *bat phraket*.[42] They then rolled a ball of dough on the abdomen, reciting this *gāthā*: (*thero pāpimate aṃgapaccaṃgāni ahaṃ passāmi kimaṃgaṃ pana sakala sarīraṃnikkhama lahupāpima*), made the incantation according to the day, then sprinkled holy water, repeating this *gāthā* eight times: (*santi pakkhā apattanā santi pādā avañcanā mātāpitā ca nikkhantā jātavedapaṭikkama saha sacce kate mayhaṃmahāpajjalito sikhī vajjesi solasa karisāni udakaṃ patvā yathā sikhi saccena mesamo natthi esā me sacca pāramīti*). Then they moulded from the ball of dough the forms of a lion, a vulture, and a garuda. They took seven kinds of salad and seven kinds of flowers, and placed mango leaves underneath, then sprinkled the tray with perfumed paste and essence, and made the offering then took it to the South-East. They did this [each day] for three days, and she was better. If not, they prepared medicine from this recipe for her to take:

[25]	*lahung daeng*	root
	ngiu	sap
	khing	fresh

To be taken mixed with dew.

If she was not yet recovered:

[26] *kot khamao*
kot chiang
kot hua bua
kot phung plaa
thian dam

thian daeng	
thian khaao	
thian khaao plueak	
thian yaowa phaanee	
sattabut	flowers
bua khom	flowers
bua phuean	flowers
lin chong	flowers
chong konlanee	flowers
phak chee lom	fruit
phak chee laa	fruit
faek hom	
kradom	flowers
boraphet	
khamin oi	
khamin khruea	
krachap bok	
khee lek	heartwood

Mix together equal parts of these 23 items, and reduce to 1/3 volume by boiling. To be taken.

And this application for muscular fatigue:

[27]	*khee lek*	leaves
	phak khet	leaves
	nam tao	leaves
	bai ngoen bai thong	
	yaa naang	leaves
	din prasiu khaao	
	din so phong	

Equal parts of these 8 items to be made into pills, to be mixed with water used to wash rice or fresh jasmine flower water. To be applied. This has long been used very effectively to treat general fatigue and muscular pain.

If a woman is ten months pregnant, and if she is a high class woman and a *devatā* has descended to be conceived in her womb, and she suffers from any illness of pregnancy, first treat it in the traditional manner. They made a round, three tiered tray, rolled a ball of dough on her abdomen, and recited this *gāthā*: (*yatohaṃ bhagini ariyāya jātiyā jāto nābhijānāmi sañcicca pāṇaṃjīvitā voropetā tena saccena sotthi te hotu sotthi gabbhassa jātiyā jāto nābhiyaṃ samphassānaṃ paṭighātāya abyāpajjhaparamatāyāti*). Then they shaped the ball of dough into the forms of a lion, a garuda and a vulture. They prepared seven kinds of vegetables and meat and fish dishes and sprinkled the tray with perfumed powder and essence. Then they lit a candle and made the offering, repeating this *gāthā* according to the day:

(*pūratthimasmi disābhāge santidevā mahiddhikā tepitumeha anurakkhantu ārogeyana sukhena ca bhavatu sabba buddhā nubhāvena sadā sotthī bhavantu te;*

maṃgalaṃ rakkhantu sabbadevatā sabba dhammā nubhāvena nubhāvena sadā sotthī bhavantu te;

saṃghā nubhāvena sadā sotthī bhavantu te).

Having made the offering they then took it to the East. When they had done this [each day] for three days, she recovered. If she was still not well, they prepared this medicine for her to take:

[28]	*bua phuean*	flowers
	cha-em thet	
	maak song	
	chan daeng	
	chan khaao	

Excellent taken mixed with cow's milk or aromatic water.

And this application:

[29]	*chan daeng*	
	chan khaao	
	chueak khao muak daeng	
	chueak khao muak khaao	
	chaluut	
	opchoei thet	
	khondok	
	son	
	sak	
	krak khee	
	praduu	heartwood
	khai nao	bark
	masaang	bark
	san phraa naang ae	bark
	sattabut	flowers
	bua phuean	flowers
	bua khom	flowers
	lin chong	flowers
	phikun	flowers
	bunnaak	flowers
	saaraphee	flowers
	mali son	flowers
	mali laa	flowers

Equal parts of these 23 items to be made into pills, to be taken or applied, mixed with jasmine flower water. There is no doubt that this medicine, taken or applied, will relieve all disorders of pregnancy, from the first to the tenth month.

(End of description of prenatal care, summarised for doctors.)

Puna ca paraṃ This is a summary of the features of abnormal pregnancy. *Puna ca paraṃ yā itthī gabbhamādhāreyya tejosamuṭṭhānaṃ kāmavitakkaṃ uppannaṃ udaraṃ napaṭisandhikaṃ vitantarāyaṃ sattā hontīti. (Yā itthī)* 'If a woman' (*ādhāreyya*) 'who is' (*gabbhaṃ*) 'pregnant' (*uppannaṃ*) 'with child' (*kāmavitakkaṃ*) 'thinks too much about sensual matters' (*tejosamuṭṭhanaṃ*) 'because she is too passionate,' (*satta*) 'beings' (*napaṭisandhikaṃ*) 'which cannot be reborn'[43] (*vitantarāyam*) 'face many dangers' (*honti*) 'as a result' (*iti*) 'of this'.

(*Yā itthī*) 'A woman who eats food that she should not eat' (*vitakkādikaṃ*) 'such as hot-and-spicy food' (*suvitādisaṃ*) 'or food that causes diarrhoea, for example' (*nānāvisaṃ*) 'or takes harmful medicine' (*āposamuṭṭhānaṃ*) 'indicating a disorder of the element water' (*tassa puggalassa*) 'in that being [the foetus],' (*kappavināsaṃ*) '[will miscarry]. Just as the fire at the end of a *kalpa* destroys the world, this destroys the life which has come to be reborn' (*imasmi gabbhe*) 'in this woman's womb' (*naṭhitaṃ*) 'and it cannot be reborn' (*iti*) 'therefore.'

(*Apica*) 'Moreover' (*yā itthī*) 'a woman' (*dosacittaṃ*) 'who is often bad-tempered' (*turitaturitaṃ*) 'who runs quickly back and forth' (*kadācikodhakkhaṇaṃ*) 'and sometimes when she is angry throws herself down' (*pahāriyaṃ*) 'and hurts' (*attānaṃ*) 'herself [will miscarry].'

(*Apica*) 'Moreover' (*kharādiyā*) 'a woman who has a foul mouth (*adosakaṃ*) 'and uses bad language' (*paribhāsanaṃ*) 'and abuses' (*sāmikaṃ*) 'her husband' (*aññajanaṃ vā*) 'and others' (*parakappadosaṃ*) 'will be punished by those people, who will hit her and hurt her' (*udaraṃ*) 'and her baby' (*patti*) 'will be lost' (*iti*) 'because of this.'

(*Apica*) 'Moreover' (*yānārī*) 'a woman' (*dhāreyya*) 'who is' (*gabbhaṃ*) 'pregnant' (*amanussovā*) 'who is harmed by spirits' (*naṭhito*) 'will miscarry' (*sātraguṇenavā*) 'or if she is the victim of a magic spell' (*puttaṃ*) 'the child' (*imasmi gabbhe*) 'in her womb' (*pattanteva*) 'will be lost' (*evaṃ*) 'because of this.'

(End of summary of the four types of abnormal pregnancy)

Puna ca paraṃ Next we will discuss pregnancy in general, as follows: If a woman pregnant for from three to ten months has not responded to treatment recommended prior to this for any of the illnesses already described, prepare this medicine:

[30]	*kot so*	
	kot khamao	
	kot hua bua	
	kot chiang	
	kot kaan phraao	
	thian dam	
	thian daeng	
	thian khaao	
	thian yaowa phaanee	
	thian sattabut	
	sattabut	flowers
	bua phuean	flowers
	bua khom	flowers
	lin chong	flowers
	chong konlanee	flowers

		krisanaa	
		kralam phak	
		chaluut	
		khondok	
		chan daeng	
		chan khaao	
		son	
		krak khee	
		thep thaaro	
		samun waeng	
		opchoei thet	
		saam sip	root

Mix together equal parts of these 27 items. Reduce to 1/3 volume by boiling. To be taken. This is very good for absolutely any disorder of pregnancy from beginning to end.

Also:

	[31]	*khee lek*	heartwood
		sadao	heartwood
		son	heartwood
		chan daeng	
		chan khaao	
		yaa naang	root
		makhaam pom	fruit
		kradom	fruit
		boraphet	
		matuum	almost ripe fruit
		haeo muu	rhizome
		raatcha phrik	pods
		sadao	33 leaf stalks

Equal parts, 13 items. Reduce to 1/3 volume by boiling. To be taken to treat all disorders and diseases of pregnancy which cause pain, diarrhoea, vomiting blood, and blood poisoning. [Give this] even if it causes delivery of the dead foetus. This medicine has often been used to treat blood poisoning that makes the woman feel hot and cold and agitated.

For haemorrhage of pregnancy:

[32] *saan som*
phrik Thai
faang
khanthatsakon
Reduce to 1/3 volume by boiling. To be taken.

Also:

[33] *kluai mai*
khaao tit naa taphon

saan som

Add a little pepper, mix with *nam mangua* and take an amount the size of a Chinese date fruit [about the size of a cherry].

If a pregnant woman haemorrhages from the rectum or urethra:

[34]	*khing*	dried	
	cha-em		
	son thet	heartwood	

To be taken mixed with alcohol.

Also:

[35]	*maduea din*	bark	
	chaa phluu	root	
	kluai teep	root	

Three parts mixed with one part of honey to be taken in the morning.

Also:

[36]	*khamin oi*		
	phlai		
	phak chee lom	fruit	

To be taken mixed with cow's urine.

If this is ineffective:

[37]	*mamuang khan*	bark	
	phayom	bark	(3 pieces)
	thung theng	root	

Reduce to 1/3 volume by boiling. One cupful to be taken.

For diarrhoea [*bit*] during pregnancy:

[38]	*bua luang*	pollen	
	thap thim	almost ripe fruit	
	makhaam	bark	
	khrang		

To be taken mixed with hot water.

If this is ineffective:

[39]	*chan hom*	3 fruits	
	thalaai maak dip	a piece 30 inches long.	

To be taken mixed with alcohol.

If ineffective:

[40]	*bit*	[a number of] fruit equal to the age [of the patient]	
	lek bit chai long thee mai sak	sawdust obtained after boring 3 holes in a piece of teak wood	
	bit khlaai ok ao khui	fine particles produced by boring into the hide of a buffalo	
	benyakaanee	galls	
	makok	kernels	

Equal parts reduced to 1/3 volume by boiling. To be taken.

If ineffective:

[41] *mamuang kalon* 5 kernels
son
sak
krak khee
krisanaa
chan koh [kroh] fruit
benyakaanee galls
palong bark
Equal parts. Reduce to 1/3 volume by boiling. Dilute with lime water and boil. To be taken.

[42] **Mahaa udom** *to treat diarrhoea*
khrang
benyakaanee galls
see siat thet
chan mai takhian
khamin oi
chan seeds
Reduce equal parts of these items to a fine powder, place the powder inside a pomegranate and cook on a slow fire. Prepare pills to be taken mixed with lime water and honey. This has been found to be very effective.

If a woman pregnant for three to four months has diarrhoea [*bit*] or diarrhoea with severe pain, mucus and blood:

[43] Grind *makok* fruit to a pulp and boil with the jaws of [a] serpent-headed fish. To be taken.

If a woman pregnant four months has diarrhoea, with severe pain, mucus and blood, prepare this:

[44] *chan daeng*
chan khaao
waan keep raet
waan rong thong
sang karanee
neraphuusee
chan seeds
chan arils
benyakaanee galls
Equal parts of each ingredient. Mix with *tabuun* fruit, the same quantity as the total of the other ingredients. Prepare pills. To be taken mixed with the juice of *phlap cheen* fruit.

[45] ***Kumaan raksaa***
thian thang 5
benyakaanee galls
chan seeds
chan arils

	neraphuusee		
	saaraphat phit	fruit	
	waan keep raet		
	waan rong thong		
	chang thang 2		
	krathin daeng		
	khrai khruea	root	
	tabuun	fruit	
	san phraa naang ae		3 parts
	talum phuk	fruit	4 parts
	tumkaa daeng		5 parts

29 items.[44] Prepare pills to be taken mixed with *nam chan* to treat diarrhoea; also used as an intestinal astringent; to protect the foetus in the womb; and to treat women's disorders; *atisaan*[45] and disorders of pregnancy.

If a pregnant woman haemorrhages or passes pus or mucus with blood:

[46]	*thao yaai mom*	root
	son	

1 *baht*[46] of each

Equal parts to be boiled with a solution of equal parts of alcohol and water. To be taken.

If a woman has been pregnant for seven or eight months and the foetus has not quickened:

[47]	*haeo*	raw
	krachap	raw
	bua luang	pollen
	chong konlanee	flowers
	rak son	root
	saam sip	root
	thian khaao plueak	
	khanthatsakon	

Equal parts, 8 items. Prepare pills to be taken mixed with cow's milk. Then the foetus will quicken.

Another:

[48]	*haeo*	raw
	krachap	raw
	cha-em thet	
	yaa klet hoi yai	
	sadao	bark

Equal parts, 5 items, to be taken mixed with cow's milk. Then the foetus will quicken.

Another:

[49]	*chong konlanee*	flowers
	bua luang	flowers

khanaak root
cha-em thet
khanthatsakon
Equal parts, 5 items, to be taken mixed with cow's milk, then the baby will be normal.

If a woman who has been pregnant from one to two or three months is constipated and has abdominal colic or epigastric pain:

[50] *bencha kradom*
khee lek heartwood
Reduce to 1/3 volume by boiling. To be taken. Then the foetus will not be in any danger.

If a woman who has been pregnant for four or five months is constipated or has diarrhoea:

[51] *thao khan* ripe fruit
Discard the flesh and place the seeds in a cloth. Pound to a powder, then soak overnight in water. Boil until cooked, together with fresh whole *hoi khong*, including the shell. One teacupful to be taken.

If a woman who has been pregnant for six or seven months is constipated and has severe abdominal pain:

[52] *phlai*
salot leaves 1 *baht* of each
khing fresh 2 *salueng*
Reduce to 1/3 volume by boiling. Before it is taken, add
phrik Thai 9 peppercorns
krathiam 3 cloves
kluea 3 crystals
chan hom
A little of this is to be taken, then it is to be used as an application after the addition of powdered mature betel leaves. This is very effective.

If a woman has been pregnant for eight, nine or ten months and is constipated or has diarrhoea:

[53] *bua nam thang 5* flowers
champaa flowers
kradang ngaa flowers
1 *baht* of each of these 7 ingredients.
tree katuk
mahaa hing
cha-em thet
1 baht of each
Prepare pills to be taken mixed with honey, hot water or sugar-cane juice, to which Borneo camphor has been added. This is very good.

When the pregnancy is almost at term, the foetus becomes very restless. This is probably because the mother has eaten something irritating, such as hot food or hot-and-spicy food. To soothe the foetus, give the mother medicine called

[54] ***Klom naang non*** to be taken [see no. 451]

At any time during pregnancy from the first to the tenth month, to protect the foetus from danger and harm, such as injury from poisons from the mother, for example, from snakebite, smallpox or one of the five kinds of internal abscesses which might develop in a pregnant woman at any stage - there are many dangers, as has been explained - prepare the medicine called *Klom kumaan* to be taken in the hope of counteracting any harm which might befall the foetus.

[55] ***Klom kumaan***

thian thang 5	
kot thang 5	
bua thang 5	pollen
khrai khruea	root
sang karanee	
chaluut	
khondok	
cha-em thet	
nam prasaan thong	
chan thang 2	
krisanaa	
kralam phak	
matuum	skin of under-ripe fruit
chamot	
phimsen	

2 *salueng* of each of these 32 items

Prepare pills using aromatic water as excipient. To treat restlessness, this is to be taken mixed with aromatic water, civet or musk and a little Borneo camphor. To treat listlessness, to be taken mixed with a triturate of eagle wood in water. To treat mucus and blood, to be taken mixed with cork wood bark sap and a little opium. To treat diarrhoea, to be taken mixed with *nam kluai teep.* To treat mucus in the throat, to be taken mixed with *nam mawaeng khruea.* To treat heat [a raised temperature], to be taken or applied mixed with aromatic water. Whatever is the matter, this is an excellent remedy to protect the foetus.

If a pregnant woman is almost at term and the foetus moves about restlessly and the mother feels very hot in the abdomen:

[56] Mix bark of the bael tree with lime water and apply all over the abdomen [by rubbing with the fingertips]. This will calm the baby, then it will settle down.

If the mother has a difficult labour, give her this medicine:

[57] *khamin oi* 4 pieces sliced like this: 

	samo thet	9 fruits
	samo Thai	9 fruits
	samo phiphek	9 fruits
	thao wan priang	3 pieces each 10 inches long
	makaa	a handful of leaves[47]

Hold the breath and trim the ends. Mix together and reduce to 1/3 volume by boiling. To be taken. If she takes this 2 or 3 times, then the child will be born easily.

If the birth is delayed:

[58] Take the first faeces from a new born calf and mix with powdered leaves from the Indian cork tree. Apply to the soles of the mother's feet. After the baby is born, quickly wash off the preparation which was applied to the feet. If this is not washed off, the mother's intestines will be damaged and protrude. This medicine is to induce labour [to make the uterus contract to its normal position][48] and has been used often.

Medicine to make the uterus contract:

[59]	*mayom tua phuu*	root
	som poi	root
	makhaam khee maeo	root
	khanun	leaves
	samae thale	sap

Reduce to 1/3 volume by boiling. To be taken. Very effective in causing the uterus to contract. It has been used often.

To expel a retained placenta:

[60]	*faai daeng*	7 leafy tips of new shoots
	phrik Thai	7 peppercorns
	khing	7 pieces
	krathiam	7 cloves

To be taken mixed with alcohol. This has been used often as a very effective preparation to expel the retained placenta.

If the foetus dies in the womb:

[61]	*kluai taanee*	decayed rootstock
	fak khieo	fruit
	phak waen	

Equal parts of each ingredient. Apply as a poultice to the lower abdomen for a few minutes, and the dead foetus will be expelled. A very effective remedy to expel a dead foetus.

To treat a woman who faints and becomes unconscious [literally, motionless and silent, temporarily deaf and blind], and has lockjaw and a stiff tongue, prepare this snuff:

[62]	*phrik Thai*	just ripened seeds
	khai fak	shell
	dee plee	
	bia tua phuu	calcined

	bai naat		
	thian dam		
	nam prasaan thong		
	maaraa	nest	
	cha-em		
	khaa	dried	
	opchoei thet		
	1 *baht* of each		
	kaan phluu		2 *salueng*
	khing	dried	1 *baht*
	phimsen		
	malaeng muum	33 dead carcasses	

Powder these 15 ingredients, mix with musk and a little Borneo camphor and reduce to a very fine powder for use as a snuff. To treat *lom uthonsunthonwaat, lom waataphak*, and *lom waayonaowanaaree*, and the sorts of *lom* which occur in women during and after pregnancy. And to treat the harmful effects of *lohit tee khuen*,[49] such as *peesaat*[50] entering the body. This recipe is called *Thanuu kaaka*.[51] Just as the crow is afraid of the arrow, so the *lom lohit*[52] and *peesaat* are afraid of this medicine.

If a pregnant woman has abdominal colic, vomiting, diarrhoea or heavy perspiration whether caused by *lom uthonwaat* or cholera [*puang lom*]:

[63]	*thep thaaro*		
	plaa chon	burnt scales	
	phluang	baked leaves	
	khat mon	root	
	chan	seeds	
	khing	fresh	
	krathiam	whole bulb	
	2 *salueng* of each of these		
	phimsen		1 *baht*

Prepare pills from these 9 ingredients to be taken mixed with *nam luuk chaak*.

An application for heavy perspiration:

[64]	*puu thale*	claws
	thua phuu	fruit
	din so phong	
	matuum	skin of under-ripe fruit
	proh hom	
	waan nam	
	phimsen	

Equal parts, 7 items. Prepare pills to make a very good lotion to treat coldness of the body [to warm].

End of section on treatment of the pregnant mother.

Tasmi aparabhāge kumārapaṭisandhikaṃ dasamāsesu pakatiyā anantarāyena ekavāto nāma kammajjavāto nikkhepo hotipattasīse utthāyāti. (Tasmi khaṇe) 'When' (*kumāre*) 'a baby' (*paṭisandhikaṃ*) 'conceived' (*mātugabbhaṃ*) 'in the mother's womb' (*aparabhāge*) 'has developed' (*anantarāyena*) 'without mishap' (*pakatiyā*) 'normally' (*udare*) 'in the womb' (*yāva dasamāse*) 'from the time of conception to the tenth month' (*ekavāto*) 'one of the [elements] of wind' (*kammajjavāto*) 'called *kammatchawaat* (*nikkhepo*) 'blows strongly in the tendons and muscles which bind the baby' (*pattasīse*) 'so that they move and make the head turn down.' (*Nakkhattanikkhamaṃ*) 'At the auspicious time, the baby will be born.'

(The beginning of this section is in Pāli. For those who may not understand, it is translated here into Thai.) [sic]

After the baby is born, it completely forgets its thoughts of repaying its mother's kindness, because it is so shocked and convulsed with fear by the force of *lom kammatchawaat* buffeting and pushing it. The shock and fright can be compared to that of a person who falls from a place the height of one hundred people, and the pain can be compared to that of a very large elephant driven out through a very narrow passage. The elephant is compelled to go on, as it is unable to protest, through its great fear of the elephant keeper and the mahout. The pain is beyond description. This is why new-born babies get sick, because the doctor and the mid-wife push with all their might. Since the baby's bones and tendons are still weak, they are pushed out of place.

They say that babies like this are ordinary people. When the Lord Buddha was in his mother's womb, he did not have to endure pain and suffering like ordinary people. He was not turned upside down by *lom kammatchawaat* and terrified, so that he trembled and shook. He sat, facing out towards his royal mother's abdomen, in a state of tranquility and composure, like a monk giving a sermon - and when the sermon was finished, he came down.[53]

Here in *Khamphee prathom chindaa*, the masters say that a doctor who is to care for babies should examine an infant when it is first born, when it has been turned upside down by *lom kammatchawaat* and frightened, tossed about and rolled around; when it beats its hands and feet and tears the umbilical cord so that it is completely broken. The blood in the mother's womb and in the torn cord then scatters about in the womb, and some of it enters the baby's mouth and some of it comes out through the mother's vagina.

This is why the doctor should know that if a baby is born face down and crying, it will vomit [a clot of] blood about the size of a hen's egg from its mouth. If this happens, it will be easy to rear. It will not have much sickness and will not have *taan* and *saang* until grown up;[54] and if it does get sick, the doctors will be able to care for it easily.

If a baby is born face up, when it starts to cry the blood in its mouth gets into its throat and stomach. They say that such a baby will be difficult to rear. It will have a lot of sickness, such as *khamao*,[55] and *taan* and *saang*. As it grows up, it will have scabies and boils and these will cause *taan* and *saang*, hardening and enlargement of the spleen, diarrhoea, abdominal distension and dropsy and five kinds of internal abscesses, all because of the foul blood that it swallowed. It will be a sickly child, as described.

If a baby is born facing sideways, to the right or to the left, some of the blood in its mouth will drop out and some will be swallowed. This child will be neither easy nor difficult to rear - somewhere in between. Any dangerous diseases that it gets will not be severe.

If an infant fails to cry at birth, whether it is born face up or face down or facing sideways, whether to the right or to the left, but it is still breathing, it is made to cry by turning its face down. If it still does not cry, do not let the mid-wife take the baby. Blow shallot and *proh* or *phlai* on to [the baby's body]. If it starts to cry, the blood will come out of its mouth, then it will not have to cope with sickness, as explained.

If the birth is extremely difficult, so that it is obstructed for any reason - sometimes the obstetrician or mid-wife does not know when the baby is due; or they do not know how to manage, and maltreat the baby by pushing and pulling with great force while there is an obstruction and the child's neck is twisted sideways and sprained; or if it falls on to the floor; as the child grows up it usually has boils on its chin and in the groin and a series of boils at the base of its neck. And these three [groups of] boils may recur during childhood, or at fifteen, twenty or thirty years of age, and cause *fee en*, *fee prakhamroi* and *fee khanthamaalaa*,[56] which are the result of the beating and bruising caused at birth.

If you want to know whether a baby will be easy or difficult to rear, examine it when it is seven days old. If you notice at the upper chest a red mark, about the size of a Chinese date leaf [oval shaped and about 1" across] and the colour of bruised [petals] of white lotus and *tabaek*, sometimes the colour of candle smoke; that baby will be difficult to rear. If the mark is the colour of a new earthen pot [*mo mai* - terracotta], it will be moderately easy; and if it is the colour of a new earthen pot [*mo mai on* - a pot made of clay which is a lighter biscuit colour], it will be very easy to rear.

When a baby is three days old, look at the abdomen between the navel and the chest. If you see a patch about the size of a Chinese date or a tamarind leaf, beware of *lom sunthonwaat*. Even if you do manage to get rid of this, in the end, in three weeks time - 21 days - the baby will be sick.

If you want to treat this, give medicine to make it better. If you give a laxative to disperse the accumulation of mucus in the abdomen, the child will recover. If it does not work and the amount of mucus increases, doctors should know that in three weeks - 21 days - the baby will no longer be alive. And if an infant has thick mucus in the right side of the chest, as explained previously, the eyes roll back and it rejects food and milk, vomits, and has yellow stools and urine, this is *lom waataphak*. If the collection of mucus remains, it will make the baby pale and emaciated. If the quantity of mucus increases it will cause diarrhoea, flatulence and convulsions [literally, spasms of the hands and feet and the eyes roll back] and the child will be dull and listless and fatigued, and have shallow breathing and will vomit and will be unable to eat or drink. For every child like this who lives, two will die. If the baby has a high temperature at regular intervals and convulsions and is like this,[57] it will die. There is no alternative.

If a baby seven, eleven, fifteen or twenty one days old is blue around the eyes, starts in its sleep, has convulsions, a stiff back, flatulence, stiff tongue and lockjaw, they say it is *lom sunthonwaat* and *lom waataphak* and *saphan fai.*[58] All these occur because the baby swallowed a clot of blood from its mother at birth. It is predicted that out of ten babies so afflicted, one will live and nine will die. Do not doubt it!

After a child is born, normal changes in its early development cause vomiting and diarrhoea and other illnesses on seven occasions. These are:

- When it learns to hold up its head, because the tendons move and *saang* then affects the infant.[59]
- When the baby learns how to turn its body to lie face down [on its stomach] and the muscles move.[60]
- When it learns how to sit up, the bones of the spine are partially dislocated, so *saang* occurs.
- When the baby learns how to crawl, it gets sick because the hips and knees change their positions.
- When the milk teeth erupt, this makes the baby sick.
- Mild vomiting is brought on when the child takes its first steps, because the 300 bones are disturbed and all the tendons move.
- When the child can stand up and walk, because the intestines, abdomen, liver and lungs are shaken up, and the vomiting is severe, so be careful.

This is absolutely normal for everybody without exception, and the reason for the promulgation of the therapeutic uses of medicines that are given to babies each month to settle their stomachs and counteract the vomiting, *taan* and *saang* which occur naturally as explained.

When a child is one month old they give:

[65]	*kaphrao*	leaves
	saniat	leaves
	taan mon	leaves
	boraphet	

To be taken mixed with river water. This is very good to soothe the stomach and prevent vomiting in infants during their first month.

Babies two months old:

[66]	*khon thee so*	leaves
	sadao	leaves
	phak khuang	leaves
	khop chanaang daeng	leaves
	boraphet	

To be taken mixed with hot water as a stomach mixture to prevent vomiting during the second month. Excellent.

Babies three months old:

[67]	*sawaat*	leaves
	khop chanaang khaao	leaves
	kaphang hom	leaves
	boraphet	

To be taken mixed with hot water as a potent stomach mixture to prevent vomiting during the third month.

Babies four months old:

[68]	*phak krashet*	
	thap thim	leaves
	taan mon	leaves
	saniat	leaves
	boraphet	

To be taken mixed with hot water. A very good stomach mixture to prevent vomiting during the fourth month.

Babies five months old:

[69]	*phak khraat*	leaves
	yaa tai bai	leaves
	krathuep yot	leaves
	kraphang hom	leaves
	boraphet	

To be taken mixed with hot water as a stomach mixture to prevent vomiting during the fifth month. This is extremely effective.

Babies six months old:

[70]	*faai daeng*	leaves
	krathum naa	leaves
	khop chanaang daeng	leaves
	bai naat	

Prepare pills to be taken mixed with hot water. An excellent stomach mixture to prevent vomiting during the sixth month.

Babies seven months old:

[71]	*nom phichit*	leaves
	maklam khruea	leaves
	samo phiphek	leaves
	khamin oi	
	boraphet	

Prepare pills to be taken mixed with hot water. This is very good as a stomach mixture to prevent vomiting during the seventh month.

Babies eight months old:

[72]	*maduea*	leaves
	phimsen	leaves
	phlai	
	khamin oi	

Prepare pills to be taken mixed with hot water. An excellent stomach mixture to prevent vomiting during the eighth month.

Babies nine months old:

[73]	*makhwit*	juvenile leaves
	sakae	leaves
	phlai	

	khamin oi		
	boraphet		

Prepare pills to be taken mixed with hot water. A potent stomach mixture to prevent vomiting during the ninth month.

Babies ten months old:

[74]	*khon thee so*	leaves	
	khon thee khamao	leaves	
	khamin oi		

Prepare pills to be taken with hot water as a stomach mixture to prevent vomiting during the tenth month. Very effective.

Babies eleven months old:

[75]	*saniat*	leaves	
	phak khraat	leaves	
	peep	leaves	
	rangap	leaves	
	khee kaa daeng	leaves	
	khee kaa khaao	leaves	
	khok kra-om	leaves	
	khee lek	leaves	
	sadao	leaves	
	phlai		
	kathue		
	tree katuk		

Prepare pills to be taken mixed with hot water. A very good stomach mixture to prevent vomiting during the eleventh month.

Babies twelve months old:

[76]	*thian*	leaves	a handful
	khamin oi		
	boraphet		
	prakham kai	leaves	
	bai naat		
	khon thee so	leaves	
	tree katuk		
	phlai		
	khing		
	kaarabuun		
	phak kaat	seeds	
	krathiam		
	hom		
	saan som		
	din prasiu khaao		

Prepare pills to be taken mixed with hot water. Without doubt, this is an excellent stomach mixture to treat vomiting in infants twelve months old.

If a baby has hiccoughs as a result of vomiting:

[77] Popped rice and salt to be taken mixed with citron fruit juice.

If a baby vomits and has a cold or diarrhoea:

[78] 7 spider carcasses, scorched peacock tail feathers and a mixture of 3 parts buttermilk and 1 part water, to be given mixed with hot water.

If a baby vomits and has diarrhoea:

[79]

matuum	under-ripe fruit
phak sian phee	
khon thee so	leaves

Reduce to 1/3 volume by boiling. To be taken.

If a baby vomits for any reason:

[80] Boil a piece of tamarind bark, about 10 inches long, with sugar-cane juice until reduced to 1/3 volume. To be taken.

If an infant has severe diarrhoea:

[81] Measure the distance from the navel to the toes. Then measure the same length of a tamarind tree, from the base up. Take this piece of wood, and play a trick by turning it upside down and cutting shavings upwards and away from the body, beyond the end of the piece of wood. Then give 7 peppercorns, 7 pieces of ginger and 7 cloves of garlic, mixed with alcohol. This is very effective.

Prescriptions to treat children who are difficult to rear

To treat children who are difficult to rear:

[82] Mix together flowers of the candelabra bush with zedoary rhizome, and powder the child's body. This is excellent.

Also:

[83]

phlai	3 pieces
phrik Thai	3 peppercorns

Mix together, then say these powerful words: (*Sabbedevāpīsāceva alavakādayopica khaggaṃtāla pattaṃdisvā sabbeyakkhā palāyanti*). Then spray the crown of the infant's head with the medicine by squirting it from the mouth. Powder the armpits and the lower abdomen, then prepare this medicine and tie the wrists to prevent all kinds of *taan* and *saang*.[61]

[84]

yaa phan nguu daeng	roots and aerial parts, dug up at midday[62]
waan nam daeng	
khop chanaang daeng	
kot so	

Mix together and mould into the form of a string of rosary beads,[63] then dry them in the sun. Next, repeat these powerful words eighteen times: (*Kalayage etc. palāyanti*). Then tie the child's wrists and it will be easy to rear. This is very effective against all sickness.

Also to apply to the crown of the head:

[85]

nguu hao	cast off skin

	malaeng mum	cast off skin
	phlai	
	khamin oi	

Powder the crown of the child's head and also the mother's nipples. This is very good.

Also, to be applied to the child's body to prevent any illness, *khai apphikaat* or *opakkamikaaphaat*:[64]

[86]	*makhwit*	leaves
	nguu hao	cast off skin
	hom daeng	
	saap raeng	
	men	quills
	phlai dam	
	phlai lueang	

Prepare a stick to be mixed with cow's milk and applied to the child's body to clear up all harmful effects and blemishes.

Medicine to prevent all diseases

[87]	***Winaatsaphit***	
	nam tao	leaves
	bai naat	
	phak khet	leaves
	rangap	leaves
	samee	leaves
	khamin oi	
	phrik	
	khing	
	bia tua phuu	3 calcined shells
	malaeng mum	3 carcasses
	maaraa	burnt nest
	lamphan [possibly *lamphan haang muu*]	

Prepare a stick.

When both [sic] these prescriptions have been dispensed, recite this incantation seven times: (*Viddhagāmo mahārājā kumbhandayakkho mahārājā vā bhūtapīsācadevanubhāvena kumāre ca surāgaṇā bhūtapīsācayakkhagaṇā devā āgacchantu ehi ehi*). Then powder the baby's body all over, and it will be protected from all harm.

End of brief description of child-birth.

Here are all the recipes to protect children.

To cleanse the intestines to prevent the occurrence of *saang*:

[88]	*sawaat*	leaves
	khon thee so	leaves
	kaphrao	leaves
	matuum	leaves

	Equal parts of each	
	salot	leaves, an amount equal to the whole

First steam all these leaves, then add *khamin oi* and *phlai.* Prepare a stick to be taken mixed with alcohol, in doses according to the strength of the child. If a good bowel motion is required, then use leaf juice of sacred basil.

Then prepare this medicine to cleanse outside the intestines [*nok lam sai*], to be taken next:

[89]	*khrai hom*	leaves
	sawaat	leaves
	kaphrao	leaves
	ching cho	leaves

Take a cup of juice from the crushed leaves of each ingredient, then boil down until thick. Stir in 1 *salueng* of aloes, and make into pills the size of the seed kernel of Job's tears. To be taken, mixed with hot water, by any child from one month to seven years of age, the dose depending on the strength of the child. This will build him up and give him a beautiful complexion, and he will grow nice and plump and throw off all diseases.

But diseases occurring outside the intestines cause clumps of fibrous membranes to develop, and [lumps like] egg plant seeds are found in the mucus or the blood, resulting in aches and pains and fever [*khai sabat ron*]. This prescription is very effective in such cases. Then prepare the following medicine to be taken next:

[90]	*khamin oi*	
	benyakaanee	galls
	sawaat	leaves
	sakae	leafy tips of new shoots
	faai daeng	leaves
	thian	leaves
	thap thim	leaves

Equal parts of each. Add an amount of sacred basil leaves equivalent to the whole. Prepare pills [or a stick] to be taken in doses according to the strength of the child. If the aches and pains are severe, add some python's bile and they will go.

Then prepare the medicine called *Prasa kaphrao* to be taken next:

[91]	***Prasa kaphrao***	
	taan dam	
	taan khamooi	fruit
	san phraa naang ae	bark
	khrai khruea	
	takhop	bark
	phlai	
	khamin oi	

yaa tai bai
samo thang 3
chan thang 2
thian yaowa phaanee
nam prasaan thong
saan som

Equal parts of each. Add an amount of sacred basil equal to the whole. Prepare pills from these 17 ingredients using alcohol as excipient. When it is to be taken, add some python's bile and Borneo camphor. To be taken to treat the poison of *taan* and *saang*; to improve the fire element; and to regulate the pulse. If this is given to the child regularly each day, it will improve his appetite. To expel flatus when the child's abdomen is distended, mix with leaf sap of sacred basil. If there is mucus and blood in the stools, mix with a triturate of dracaena and sandalwood in water; if the child has a regular fever [fever at the same time each day] mix with ink nut fruit juice; if unconsciousness results from the increasing effects of *saang*, mix with bile from the soft-shelled turtle. When this potent medicine is given, the child will recover.

[92] ***Bencha taan***[65]

taan mon	root	
taan sian	root	
taan dam	root	
taan khamooi	root	
taan tanot	root	
chan thang 2		
khrai khruea		
san phraa naang ae	bark	
phitsanaat		
1 *baht* of each		
chan	seeds	2 *salueng*

11 items. Prepare a stick. If to be taken in the morning, add python's bile. If to be taken at midday, mix with aromatic water. If to be taken in the evening, mix with *nam chan*. To reduce the temperature, it can be used as a lotion. To expel flatus, first divide the medicine into halves, then steam nickernut leaves and croton leaves and mix with an equal quantity of the medicine prepared first. To be taken mixed with a triturate of tamarind fruit pulp in water. This will give great relief.

Wise doctors follow this text and use whichever treatment is appropriate to protect children from disease.

Children's medicine to relieve morning flatulence:

[93]	*khon thee so*	leaves
	kaphrao	leaves
	phak khraat	leaves

phak sian phee	leaves	
taan mon	leaves	
chan	seeds	
chan	arils	
krawaan		
kaan phluu		
mahaa hing		
yaa dam		
phrik		
khing		
dee plee		
rong thong		

Take equal parts of these 16 ingredients and powder finely. Prepare pills, using *nam khaa* as excipient. To be taken mixed with hot water. Excellent to relieve morning flatulence in children.

Medicine to treat flatulence in children:

[94]

yaa dam		
taan mon	leaves	
sawaat	leaves	
chum het	leaves	
2 *salueng* of each		
thian khaao		
krawaan		
kaan phluu		
chan	seeds	
chan	arils	
1 *salueng* of each		
neraphuusee		
dee plee		
yaa tai bai		
1 *salueng* of each		
mahaa hing		1 *baht*
kraphrao	leaves	2 *baht*

Reduce these 14 ingredients to a fine powder and prepare pills the size of kapok seeds, using *nam khaa* as excipient. One pill to be given to a month old infant, otherwise, the dose to be calculated according to age. [Probably to be given mixed with some kind of liquid.]

[95] ***Thang khuen thang long***

phrik Thai
khing
dee plee
krathiam
nam prasaan thong
1 *salueng* of each

cha-em		
mahaa hing		
yaang pho		
1 *baht* of each		
kluea sinthao		1 *fueang*[66]
makruut	[fruit] skin	2 *baht* , 2 *salueng*
kraphrao	leaves	1 *tamlueng,*[67] 1 *baht,* 1 *salueng,* 1 *fueang*

Powder together these 10 ingredients. Prepare pills the size of peppercorns, using alcohol as excipient. To be taken according to strength, mixed with hot water or the leaf sap of sacred basil. This is a tried and true remedy for flatulence or diarrhoea.

Abdominal application to expel flatus:

[96]	*yaa dam*	
	mahaa hing	
	rong thong	
	raatcha phrik	pods
	makhaam piak	
	phlai	
	khamin oi	
	nam prasaan thong	

Mix together, warm over a fire, and apply to the stomach. Extremely good.

To treat *la* and all forms of *saang* which cause diarrhoea and flatulence:[68]

[97]	*phak hom naam*	both aerial parts and roots
	yaa phan nguu daeng	both aerial parts and roots

Roast these two ingredients until dry [almost burnt], then mix with lime water. Prepare a stick. To use as a mouthpaint, mix with lime water and add Borneo camphor if required. This has been tried.

Infants' throat paint to bring up mucus from the throat and chest

[98]	*kammathan daeng*	
	manaao	seeds
	krathiam	
	mayong paa	root
	nam prasaan thong	
	chorakhe	bile

Equal parts of these 6 ingredients to be made into a stick, to be used mixed with lime juice, to paint the child's throat so that he will bring up the mucus from the chest. This prescription has been used. There is no doubt about its efficacy.

To treat the *lom* associated with the seven kinds of *saang* of the seven days, such as *lom sunthonwaat*, arising in the abdomen or lower abdomen, causing first, abdominal pain and flatulence, then diarrhoea and drowsiness, convulsions, with spasms of the hands and feet, and a blue abdomen and face.

[99]	*phimsen*		
	kaarabuun		
	makruut	[fruit] skin	
	1 *baht* of each		
	mahaa hing		2 *baht*
	bai naat		
	krathiam		
	phrik Thai		
	khing		
	1 *tamlueng* of each		

These 8 items to be finely powdered and made into pills, to be taken mixed with lime juice, to treat piercing gastric pain, *lom irin* and all kinds of *lom* associated with *saang.*

First, to treat *lom sunthonwaat,* and the *lom* of the *saang* of each of the seven days:

[100]	*phrik Thai*		
	khing		
	dee plee		
	krathiam		
	waan nam		
	makruut	[fruit] skin	
	phlai		
	mahaa hing		
	yaa dam		
	kaarabuun		1 *baht* of each
	kaphrao	leaves, an amount equal to the whole	

These 11 items to be ground finely and made into pills to be taken mixed with kaffir lime juice. To treat flatulence, lime water may be used. Then add *chetta phang khee* and apply to the abdomen. This is very potent.

Also:

[101]	*samo Thai*	
	samo phiphek	
	makhaam pom	
	1 *salueng* of each	
	horaphaa	fruit
	phak chee	fruit
	see siat	
	chan	seeds
	chan	arils
	krawaan	
	kaan phluu	
	chan thet	
	2 *salueng* of each	

benyakaanee	galls	3 *salueng*

These 12 items to be finely ground and made into pills to be taken mixed with lime water, to which are added some snake's bile, opium and long turmeric. To treat *lom* which causes severe diarrhoea.

And a decoction:

[102] *yaa luuk khlao*

thaeng thuai	bark
thian	leaves
thap thim	leaves
kathue	
phlai	
khaa	
khamin oi	
hom	bulb

Equal parts of these 9 items to be boiled with a mixture of equal parts of alcohol and river water until reduced to 1/3 volume. To be taken. An excellent remedy.

To treat *saang daeng* if it affects the liver, causing diarrhoea with blood for four to five days, then a severe cough, with yellow eyes and pain at regular intervals, then the liver hangs down below the ribs on the right side:[69]

[103]	benyakaanee	galls	1 part
	krathiam		2 parts
	faang sen		3 parts

Prepare pills to be taken, according to strength [of the patient], mixed with lime water.

Poultice to apply to the ribs to make the liver contract:

[104] *no mai*
khamao lek
puun khaao a small quantity

Mix together and apply as a poultice for three days and if not completely contracted:

[105] *tree phalaa*
makhaam pom

aai nieo	root
lep mue naang	root
khai nao	bark
haeo muu	rhizome
matuum	under-ripe fruit
raatcha phrik	pods
bua luang	pollen
bunnaak	flowers
yaa dam	
saan som	

1 *baht* of each

thian dam		
thian khaao		
nam prasaan thong		
2 *salueng* of each		
khee kaa daeng	half of one fruit	
boraphet	3 inches [of stem]	
khamin oi	3 pieces	
kaphrao	leaves	3 *tamlueng*, 3 *baht*, 2 *salueng*

Boil with a mixture of 1 part alcohol with 2 parts of river water. Reduce to 1/3 volume. To be taken. This mixture has been used. There is no doubt about its efficacy.

Here ends the brief discussion on postnatal care.

Phrakhamphee prathom chindaa, Book I, Part 3, abridged, on newborn babies, burying the placenta, and lying by the fire.[70]

Puna ca paraṃ Next the masters discuss newborn babies, from the first day to the first month, when they are still by the fire.

[After delivery] while she is lying by the fire, the mother faces many dangers. She has blood disorders, such as *lohit tee khuen* [see note 49], and eventually, she is unable to sleep by the fire. In that case, the infant is not permitted to take her milk, because it is harmful, it is too raw, and blood and serum are mixed with the milk. The baby will get sick if it is allowed to have her milk, as has been explained.

During the time spent lying by the fire, when *khamao* develops in the infant, if it goes down to the heart and chest this will make the mouth as purple as jambolan fruit, as if it has been smeared with a mixture of vermilion paint and the [black] sap of the Burmese lacquer tree. Then the *saang* will go down to the stomach, affecting the liver. At some time from two or three days up to one or two months after [the mother and child] have left the fire, the *khamao* disappears and when it has gone *saang* develops, because all the 307 blood vessels of the mother gather together at the nipples, and when the baby is fed, the *saang* enters and makes the child sick.

During the time spent lying by the fire, some women come to no harm, but even so, their blood is not normal. That kind of woman is called *benchasatree*, and her main illness is caused by parasites which feed in the heart, the liver, the lungs, abdomen and breasts. These five kinds of parasites cause dryness in the chest. The bodies of the parasites are as white as ivory coloured milk and they have pointed black mouths. Infants who are fed with this milk will develop parasitic diseases. Doctors should take note!

Puna ca paraṃ The masters next describe the burial of the placenta. Do not bury the placenta while the infant is only one, two or three days old, because *phraai* and *kumphan* will smell it and come and eat it;[71] and having eaten it, will take possession of the mother, and later will be a danger to her. The placenta may be buried from the seventh day up to the first month.

When the placenta is to be buried, pay homage to the spirits [*devatā*] of the pathways with an offering of fragrant powder and essence, popped rice, flowers, fragrant woods - aloes wood, sandalwood - and candles, and make a vow promising them a thank-offering. Also, pay homage to the tree spirits, the spirits of the land and all the gods, before burying it according to this text.

During the fourth, fifth and sixth months, the placenta should be buried in the South-West, then the child will have power. It is forbidden to bury it in the South because it will be dangerous for the child.

During the seventh, eighth and ninth months, the placenta should be buried in the East and North-West, then the child will be good and will prosper. It is forbidden to bury it in the South-East and South-West because it will be dangerous for the child.

During the tenth, eleventh and twelfth months, the placenta should be buried in the North-East and South, then the child will be a leader. It is forbidden to bury it in the North-West because it will be dangerous for the child.

During the first, second and third months, the placenta should be buried in the South-East and West. The child will then be a good child and a happy one, and will come to no harm. It is forbidden to bury the placenta in the North-West and North-East because it will be dangerous for the child.

If anyone does not know what is in this text and buries the placenta in a forbidden direction, then both mother and child are certain to meet with misfortune.[72]

Apica Furthermore, if a child is born with the placenta [and cord] wrapped two or three or four or five times around the body crosswise [under one arm and over the shoulder], the placenta should be roasted on the fire until it is dry and crisp, then ground and sprinkled on the baby's food for it to eat. Then the baby will not whine or cry or come to any harm and will not have any sickness until it has grown up, and it will have more merit than others.

Apica Furthermore, if a baby is born with the placenta [cord] wound around its neck or body, the placenta should be put in a pot of 1000 cowrie shell capacity, speared with an iron rod and roasted over a fire until it is dried, then ground and sprinkled on the baby's food. The child will not, then, cry at all, will be wiser than others and will have a beautiful figure. If you want the child to be charming, stick resin on the mouth of the pot containing the placenta and bury the pot at the foot of a big tree standing in the middle of a place where many people gather and pass by. Then cover it completely with thorny plants of many kinds for all to see and the child will have the confidence of all and, without a doubt, will have the greatest charm.

Apica Furthermore, whether or not the placenta is wrapped around the baby's neck, do what was done in the past. If it is a girl, to ensure that she becomes what her parents would like her to be, put [a symbol of] that in the pot with the placenta and bury the pot in the direction already mentioned, then the child will be as desired. If it is a boy and the parents want him to be fearless and strong, and knowledgeable in the three *vedas* or whatever they wish,[73] put [a symbol of] that object in the pot with the placenta and bury the pot in the direction already mentioned, then the child will grow up as the parents would like him to be.

Anyone burying a placenta should bury it in the direction given, at the same time consecrating it by reciting this *gāthā* three times, while sprinkling water on the pot: (*ime kumārā vasantithāne atthabhavāmihaṃ anekajātisatasahassu tattha tattha tattha mā daliddo bhavāmihaṃ*). Then chant this *gāthā* three times: (*bhavatu sabbamaṃgalaṃ rakkhantu sabbadevatā sabbabuddhā sabbadhammā sabbasaṃghānubhāvena sadā sotthī bhavantu te*). Then cover the pot with earth; then take a branch of the tree appropriate to the year of the child's birth, as mentioned in *Tamraa phrommachaat*, and ram the branch into the mouth of the hole where the pot containing the placenta is buried; then sprinkle water on the branch, at the same time reciting this *gāthā* three times: (*santi pakkhā apattanā santi pādā avañcanā mātā pitā ca nikkhantā jātavedapaṭikkama saha sacce kate mayhaṃ mahāpajjalito sikhī vajjesi solasa karcīsāni udakaṃ patvā yathā sikhī saccena me samo natthi esā me saccaparamīti*). After sprinkling water, chant this *gāthā* three times: (*sabba buddhānubhāvena sabba dhammānubhāvena sabba saṃghānubhāvena buddha, dhamma, saṃgha, ratanaṃ tiṇṇaṃ ratanānaṃ ānubhāvena caturāsītisahassa dhammakkhandhānubhāvena piṭakatyayānubhāvena jinasāvakānubhāvena sabbe te rogā sabbe te bhayā sabbe te antarāyā sabbe te upaddavā sabbe te dunnimita tā sabbāte avamaṃgalā vinassantu āyuvaḍḍhako dhanavaḍḍhako sirivaḍḍhako yasavaḍḍhako vaṇṇa vaḍḍhako hotu sabbadā dukkharogabhayā verā sokā sattu cupaddavā anekā antarāyāpi vinassantu ca tejasā jayasiddhi dhanaṃ lābhaṃ sotthi bhāgyaṃ sukhaṃ balaṃ siri āyu ca vaṇṇo ca bhogaṃ vuḍḍhī ca yasavā satavassā ca āyu ca jīvasiddhī bhavantu te*). Then go home.

Moreover, when the offering is made to [one of] the spirits of the land, the name of the spirit and its parents must be mentioned. The father of the Phra Phuum [spirits of the land] is called Kaayathat and the mother is Santhaathibodeethewee. There are five spirits of the land. The spirit which protects the house is called Phra Chayamongkhon; the spirit of the land which protects the garden is called Phra Thamhoraa; the wat, Phra Waiyathat; the field and cowshed, Phra Yaochaphaeo; and the bridal chamber, Phra Sapphakhonthan. These are the names of the five spirits of the land.

When anyone makes an offering to one of the five spirits of the land, he should know about each one and know their names so that the correct name is used and the right spirit will receive the offering.

Apica Moreover, the *mae sue* of a baby born on a Sunday occupies a termite hill,[74] so it is advisable to bury the placenta in a termite hill; and the *mae sue* of a baby born on a Monday lives in a well, so it is best to bury the placenta in a well. Furthermore, the *mae sue* of a baby born on a Tuesday establishes itself in a shrine, so it is best to bury the placenta in a shrine; and the *mae sue* of a child born on a Wednesday lives in a bo tree, so it is advisable to bury the placenta where there is a bo tree.

The *mae sue* of an infant born on a Thursday occupies a pond or a big well, so it is best to bury the placenta in a pond or a big well. The *mae sue* of a baby born on a Friday lives in a big banyan tree, so it is best to bury the placenta near a big banyan tree; and the *mae sue* of a child born on a Saturday lives in a spirit shrine, so it is best to bury the placenta near a spirit shrine. Anyone who intends burying a placenta, should follow the text of *Khamphee prathom chindaa*, then the baby will be cool and contented in every way, as the masters have explained here.

Apica Moreover, if an infant aged from seven days to one month gets sick while it is by the fireplace, for instance, it twists and turns, its back is hot, it starts in its sleep, cries all the time or laughs and cries deleriously or while asleep, they say that it is the *mae sue* scaring the baby.

To treat it, offer a four cornered tray with fish and meat dishes, liquor and rice, reciting this *gāthā* three times: (*yatohaṃ bhagini ariyāya jātiyājāto nābhijānā misañciccapāṇaṃ jīvitāvorope tātenasaccena sotthiṭehotu sotthigabbhassa*). Then take the offering to the place where the placenta is buried and the baby will recover. If not, make this medicine to apply to the spine in the hope of preventing all kinds of *taan* and *saang*:

[106] Nutmeg seeds, rattan stems and sappan wood. Grind these 3 items together with grease from a python and apply; to treat all kinds of *taan* and *saang*.

Apica Moreover, if a baby at the fire has constant flatulence, is blue in the face, has cold hands and feet and convulsions, they say that the spirit of its own placenta has possessed the child.

To treat this, offer a round tray. Collect any amount you like of rice which has fallen from the mortar to the ground. Powder the rice, and mould it to the shape of an *ueng yaang* [type of bull frog] and a frog, and place seven water hyacinth flowers, meat, fish, liquor and rice on the tray and offer it at the base of the mortar, reciting this mantra three times: (*om pasasakako akāsarakāradathāpāya* [with] great joy three times *om* completely hidden [repeated] *savahā*). If the child is not better, then next have this medicine prepared to be taken or applied:

[107]

thian dam		
hing yaang pho		
khing	dried	
Mix one part of each of these with		
thian daeng		2 parts
krathiam		3 parts
kraphang hom	leaves	8 parts

Prepare pills from these 6 ingredients. To be taken mixed with hot water and applied to the abdomen, the spine, the crown of the head, the palms of the hands and soles of the feet, underarms and groin, base of the neck, the legs and the calves. This is powerful medicine. We are confident that it will work.

Apica Moreover, if a baby is born in the year of the rat [*chuat*], that is the [year under the sign of the] female *devatā*, and the auspicious tree is the coconut palm.

If a baby is born in the year of the ox [*shaluu*], that is the [year of the] male human being, and the auspicious tree is the palmyra palm.

If a baby is born in the year of the tiger [*khaan*], that is the [year of the] male ogre, and the auspicious tree is the *rang*.

If a baby is born in the year of the hare [*thoh*], that is the [year of the] female human being, and the auspicious tree is the silk-cotton tree.

If a baby is born in the year of the naga [*marong*], that is the [year of the] male *devatā*, and the auspicious tree is the pink cassia.

If a baby is born in the year of the snake [*maseng*], that is the [year of the] male human being, and the auspicious tree is the *pho baai* tree.

If a baby is born in the year of the horse [*mamia*], that is the [year of the] female *devatā*, and the auspicious tree is the banana (the banana tree) [sic].

If a baby is born in the year of the goat [*mamae*], that is the [year of the] female *devatā*, and the auspicious tree is the coral.

If a baby is born in the year of the monkey [*wok*], that is the [year of the] male ogre, and the auspicious tree is the jack fruit.

If a baby is born in the year of the cock [*rakaa*], that is the [year of the] male ogre, and the auspicious plant is the bamboo.

If a baby is born in the year of the dog [*cho*], that is the [year of the] female ogre, and the auspicious plant is the *bua bok*.

If a baby is born in the year of the swine [*kun*], that is the [year of the] male human being, and the auspicious plant is the lotus.

Here end the words of the great *thera* Tamyae, the author of *Khamphee prathom chindaa* and *Khamphee khanpharaksaa*, describing [events] from the seventh day of pregnancy until delivery and up to the time when the baby is by the fireplace.

The masters say that a doctor or mid-wife who is to take care of a pregnant woman until the birth of her infant should first pay homage and make an offering to the great *thera* Tamyae, then all will be well.

Phrakhamphee prathom chindaa, Book I, Part 4. Summary from [*Khamphee*] *sangyot* describing the good and bad characteristics of six types of women, their effects on the quality of their breast milk, and the resulting benefits and harm to their infants.

Ahameva karittiyāya tassa saṃyojanassa ṭhi tokho isiriddhiyādharo nāmalabhatilokiyajhānaṃ abhiññāyalakkhaṇaṃ itthiyāsuddusaṃ chabbaggiyāpi karissāmīti (*isi*) 'There was an ascetic' (*riddhiyādharo nāma*) 'called Ṛddhiyādharadābasa' (*labhati*) 'once,' (*lokiyajhānaṃ*) 'who was possessed of great knowledge of worldly matters.' (*Abhiññāya*) 'He was very perceptive and understanding,' (*ṭhitokho*) 'and he asserted that' (*lakkhaṇaṃ*) 'of the qualities of women' (*suddusaṃ*) 'both good and bad' (*chabbaggiyā*) 'there are six types.' (*Ahaṃ*) 'I,' (*komārabhaccoeva*) 'Komārabhacca', (*karissāmi*) 'will record' (*tassa saṃyojanassa*) 'this according to *Khamphee sangyot*' (*karittiyāya*) 'in detail' (*iti*) 'thus.'

As shown in *Khamphee sangyot*, there once was an ascetic of great wisdom, called Ṛddhiyādharadābasa, who knew about women and their ways, both good and bad. He was a teacher of Jīvaka Komārabhacca, so Jīvaka Komārabhacca saluted him and asked him about diseases of children.

'Sir, children born into this world get many different diseases. They are not the same. In *Phrakhamphee prathom chindaa*, on the origin of *saang*, they say that when infants born on the second,[75] fifth or sixth day of the week get sick, their illnesses should be mild; so why are they prey to severe sickness? On the other hand, it is supposed to be very bad for babies born on the first, third, fourth or seventh day. They should be difficult to rear and should have severe illnesses. So why do the sickly ones have mild illnesses and recover? Why do those born on good days turn bad and those born on bad days turn out to be good? Those born on bad days, for example, are easy to cure, those born on good days difficult? The bad ones, those born on the first, third, fourth or seventh day of the week cannot thrive. They say in *Phrakhamphee prathom chindaa* that *saang* is very severe in those babies and that they are very hard to rear. All the babies born on those days will not die, will they? And they say that it does not matter about the babies born on the second, fifth and sixth days because they are easy to rear. If that is so, may we conclude, Sir, that babies born on those days are immortal?'

The ascetic, Ṛddhiyādharadābasa, explained, 'Every creature born on earth in the cycle of existence, even if it is born on a good day and escapes severe *saang*, can, nevertheless, be difficult to rear because the mother's breast milk is itself bad for the baby. Also, an infant born on a bad day who should get a bad form of *saang* can be easy to rear. It all depends on the mother's milk; if it is good, the baby will thrive. This is all because a woman's milk can be good or bad. There are six kinds, as follows.' The ascetic then gave a brief description of two kinds of milk that is not good for infants.

(1) One kind of woman has a body odour like water after washing meat. She has red eyes, a creamy complexion, pendulous breasts and small nipples. She has a harsh voice like the caw of a crow; the palms of her hands are long, her feet are long, her trunk is long, her nose is long, her lower eyelids droop and her navel is deep. She is of medium size - neither fat nor thin - and eats a lot. This kind of woman is called *yakkhinee* [ogress]. She is a passionate woman. A baby fed on her milk will be sickly. Do not choose this type of woman for a wet-nurse.

(2) One kind of woman has the odour of a man, red eyes, white skin and each breast looks like the neck of a calabash. Her lips are round and her voice is as strong as a goat's. The sole of one foot is large; when she is speaking, her lips do not close, and when she is walking, she is clumsy and trips and kicks things. She is called *hatsadee* [elephant] and is a passionate woman. If a baby is fed with her milk, it is as if it were fed with poison. Do not select this type as a wet-nurse.

They say that these two kinds of women are extremely passionate. It oozes from every pore. A healthy baby allowed their milk will get sick because the milk is bad. As has been stated, this milk provides no resistance to disease.

Next, the characteristics of four desirable kinds of wet-nurses whose milk is not bad for babies.

(1) One kind of woman has a very delicate odour, like that of an orchid; erect shoulders, a slender waist and a straight back. She is small and dark, with bright cheeks, long tapering hands and feet, and her breasts are like lotuses that have just opened. She has a pink complexion and her voice is like the sound of a conch being blown. Her breast milk tastes sweet and creamy. She has the five attributes of a beautiful woman.[76] She is an excellent person to choose to suckle an infant.

(2) One kind of woman has the odour of a lotus, a voice like the sound of a horn, broad shoulders, firm hips, very round cheeks, beautiful slender hands and feet, breasts like full-blown lotuses and a yellow complexion. Her milk is sweet and thick. This woman has the five attributes of a beautiful woman and she is an excellent choice to suckle a baby.

(3) One kind of woman has an odour neither definitely fragrant nor offensive. Her waist is round and just right, her eyelashes curl up, her nose is high, her breasts rounded, with upturned nipples like lotuses just opened, and her milk is sweet and slightly creamy. She has the five attibutes of a beautiful woman and is an excellent choice to feed an infant.

(4) One kind of woman has a fragrant and hot-and-spicy odour, a voice like a cicada, a smiling mouth, eyes like a deer, hair coarse and straight, broad shoulders, broad hips, a beautiful forehead, abdomen like the leaf sheath of a banana tree, breasts erect and milk as white as a conch. Her milk tastes creamy and is rather thick. It is easy for her to rear children. This woman has the five attributes of a beautiful woman and is an excellent choice to suckle a baby.

These four kinds of women with the five beautiful features were chosen to nurse the Lord Buddha. Their milk is called the divine potion [*thip osot*]. It is like the nectar of the gods [*nam suraamrit*]. These four kinds of milk will enable a child to resist disease, even if it becomes ill, because the milk has medicinal properties and will not upset him - it is excellent.

There are four classes of women: the royal class, rich and noble class, merchant and farmer. A woman should be observed to see whether she has good or bad features as described above.

A doctor who is going to look after a child should first examine the milk of the wet-nurse and of the mother. If he finds it unwholesome, he should first have medicine prepared to cleanse the milk, then it will be free from impurities and safe from harmful effects.

If a doctor wants to know whether milk is good or bad, he should get the wet-nurse to express some of her milk into a basin of water. If the milk is as white as a conch and sinks down into the basin in the shape of a lotus seed, the milk is the best quality. If the milk disperses, then agglomerates and sinks, settling without becoming spherical, then it is the second best quality.

Apart from these two kinds of milk, even if a woman is of very high class or rank or very healthy, and has lots of merit from a previous existence, if her milk is sour, bitter, astringent, insipid or tasteless, and smells fishy, this milk is not good, as has been said.

There are still three other kinds of abnormal milk. These are [from]: the woman who suffers from dysmenorrhoea; the woman who is unable to stay by the fire and whose milk is not homogeneous; and the woman who lactates while pregnant, whose milk is watery and streaked with blood. Feeding a baby with bad milk from one of these women is like giving it poison, and it will be a sickly child.

The doctor who is to look after a baby should first investigate the state of health of the wet-nurse and what kind of woman she is. If she is found to have any abnormalities or harmful features, he should first have a preparation made to restore the blood and improve the flow of milk, and to act as a tonic for the elements, so that the condition of both the blood and the milk is perfect, then there will be no further danger. If the milk floats in water and does not agglomerate, it is because of a disorder of [the element] blood [toxaemia]. First have medicine prepared to restore the blood and rid it of toxins, then it will be in perfect condition, and the milk will be satisfactory.

Medicine to restore the blood:

[108] *thian thang* 5
kot so
kot khamao
samo Thai
samo phiphek
phak chee lom fruit
phak chee laa fruit
kluea sinthao
nam prasaan thong
sattabut flowers
bia tua phuu
sang
mahaa hing
phrik
khing
kaarabuun

Equal parts of each of these 20 ingredients to be ground together with purified croton [*salot*] fruit [see prescription no. 556] equivalent to half the total quantity of the rest of the ingredients. 2 *salueng* to be taken mixed with hot water. This will loosen the bowels, and expel bad, disordered blood, even in the baby.

Then prepare this tonic for the blood:

[109]	*thao wan priang*	root	1 *salueng*
	kamlang wua thaloeng		1 *salueng*
	khrang		1 *salueng*
	faang		1 *salueng*
	thian thang 5	of each	1 *salueng*
	chan	seeds	1 *salueng*
	tree katuk		1 *salueng*
	tree phalaa		1 *salueng*
	kot so		1 *salueng*
	kot hua bua		1 *salueng*
	chan thang 2		1 *salueng*
	phak chee thang 2	fruit	1 *salueng*
	yaa rang kaa		1 *salueng*
	muuk man	bark	1 *salueng*
	haeo muu	rhizome	1 *salueng*
	sakhaan		1 *salueng*
	chaa phluu	root	1 *salueng*
	chetta muun phloeng		1 *salueng*
	faang sen		1 *salueng*
	lueat daeng [raeng]		2 *baht*
	kham foi	flowers	10 *salueng*

boraphet		4 *baht*

These 33 items may be boiled together or powdered to be taken to improve the blood and the fire element, as well as purifying the breast milk. Then prepare this medicine to be taken to purify the milk.

Medicine to purify breast milk:

[110]	*kot thang* 5	
	thian thang 5	
	krung khamao	
	khing	dried
	kraphang hom	root
	chamot ton	

Mix with 1 *thanaan* of water,[77] then reduce to 1/3 its volume by boiling. Offer this to her, and all will be well. This is very effective medicine to purify breast milk.

If you put the milk in water and it looks green, like water used to boil mussels, taste it. If it tastes sour, it is because of a disorder of [the element] wind. First prepare medicine to treat the wind, then to purify the milk.

Application for the nipples:

[111] kot so

Pulverize, mix with ghee, and apply to the nipples to counteract disease in the infant. Very potent.

Decoction to purify the breast milk:

[112]	***Wirunlaha naaphee thi khun***		
	waan nam		1
	haeo muu		1
	samo Thai		2 [?1]
	phetsanukam	root	1
	khing		1
	utta phit		1

Equal parts of these 6 items to be mixed together and reduced to 1/3 volume by boiling. To be taken to purify the breast milk. An excellent remedy.

If the milk dissolves in the water, taste it. If it has an astringent taste, it is because of the element fire, and a disorder of *kamdao* [internal heat]. First prepare medicine to treat the element fire, then prepare medicine to purify the milk.

Decoction to purify the breast milk:

[113]	*kot thang* 5	
	thian thang 5	
	sai yoi	root
	phikun	bark
	haeo muu	
	chaang	tusk
	kwaang	young horn
	saniat	root

khok kra-om

Reduce equal parts of these 17 ingredients to 1/3 volume by boiling. To be taken to purify the breast milk.

If the milk tastes fishy, and smells musty and disagreeable, like a goat, it is because the elements earth and mucus are disordered. First, treat the elements earth and mucus, then prepare medicine to be taken to cleanse the milk.

Application for the nipples:

[114] *khok kra-om*
din ping

Mix with alcohol. First apply this for a full three days, then give the following decoction to be taken.

Decoction to cleanse breast milk:

[115]	*matuum*	under-ripe fruit
	haeo muu	
	khing	dried
	khat mon	root

Equal parts of these 4 items to be mixed together and reduced to 1/3 volume by boiling. To be taken to rid the breast milk of a fishy smell. Excellent.

Decoction to purify the breast milk:

[116]	*samo Thai*	
	khing	dried
	haeo muu	

Equal parts of these 3 items to be combined and reduced to 1/3 volume by boiling. To be taken to purify bad breast milk.

Decoction to improve the breast milk:

[117]	*song baadaan*	root
	khan sung	root
	waan keep raet	
	waan ron thong	
	waan lueang	
	nam nom raatchasee ton	
	nam nom raatchasee khruea	

Boil together equal parts of these 6 items and reduce to 1/3 volume. Add alcohol before it is taken. To purify bad breast milk.

Medicine to be taken when the milk will not flow:

[118]	*sadao*	bark
	mahaat	bark
	mai sak	bark
	takhop	root
	makok nam	root
	makok bok	root

Equal parts of these 6 items to be powdered. Prepare pills using coconut milk as excipient. To be taken. This will cause the milk to flow. A potent preparation.

Medicine to be taken when the milk will not flow:

[119]	*masaang*	bark
	phutsaa	under-ripe fruit
	makok	fruit
	makhaam pom	
	mawaeng khruea	fruit
	khanthatsakon	root

Equal parts, 6 items. Reduce to 1/3 volume by boiling. An excellent remedy to be taken when the milk will not flow.

When the milk is diluted, and it looks like water mixed with blood or like serum, the element water is disordered, because the woman has amenorrhoea and is in the early stages of pregnancy. The baby might get sick if it is fed this milk. First prepare this medicine to treat the element water, then to cleanse the milk.

Application to purify the breast milk:

[120]	*sang*	
	ubon	flowers
	kot so	

Mix these with milk and apply to the nipples first, then prepare the following medicine to be taken to purify the breast milk.

Decoction to purify bad breast milk:

[121] *ton thao yaai mom*
thep thaaro
lamphan
samo Thai
utta phit

Equal parts, 5 items. Reduce to 1/3 volume by boiling. Very effective when taken to cleanse bad breast milk.

In the case of amenorrhoea:

[122] Pure fresh cow's milk and coconut milk mixed together are very effective, taken or applied, to counteract any harmful effects in the infant.

Also:

[123]	*khaao tok kanyaa*	
	anchan khaao	root
	khanthatsakon	
	kot chadaa mangsee	
	chaang	molar tooth

Equal parts, 5 items. Powder and mix with honey. A potent mixture. To be taken to counteract 8 kinds of disorders in infants.

Here, three more kinds of harmful milk are described. These are [from] the mother who is unable to remain by the fire whose abdomen is as blue as that of a langur. When she leaves the fire and feeds her baby, it might make the baby sick, because her milk is one of these three harmful kinds.

That is: the milk is green and watery, like water after boiling mussels; the milk is thin and sour tasting; or it is frothy. These three kinds of milk give babies symptoms such as diarrhoea, flatulence, a high temperature and colic, because of imperfections in the milk.

When a doctor is going to treat an infant, he should first examine the wet-nurse. If he knows that her milk is imperfect, he should first have medicine made to correct this, then the milk can be given to the baby, and this will counteract and rid the child of its diseases.

Application [for the nipples] if the milk has imperfections:

[124]	*tree katuk*	
	chuk rohinee	
	nom sawan	root

Equal parts, 3 items. Mix with cow's milk, and boil over a fire. Allow to cool, then apply to the nipples. Before feeding the infant, wash the nipples with coconut milk. Excellent to counteract the three harmful effects of imperfect breast milk and the ten harmful effects in infants.

Medicine to be taken to treat imperfect milk:

[125]	*dee plee*	
	thap thim	flowers
	matuum	under-ripe fruit
	faek hom	root

Equal parts, 4 items. To be taken mixed with honey. Very effective.

Also:

[126]	*thian thang* 5	
	lot	bark

Equal parts, 6 items. To be taken mixed with honey, or to be applied to the nipples. A very good remedy for unwholesome milk.

Also:

[127]	*khamin khruea*	
	muuk luang	fruit
	khamin oi	
	makhuea khuen	fruit and root
	cha-em	root
	masaang	bark

Equal parts, 7 items. Reduce to 1/3 volume by boiling. To be taken to counteract sickness caused by imperfect milk. Very potent.

Medicine for the elements, to prevent defects:

[128]	*yaa peen to*		2 *salueng*
	kaphrao	leaves	6 *baht*
	taan mon	leaves	1 *baht*
	sawaat	leaves	6 *salueng*

4 items. Prepare pills using alcohol as excipient. Give only one pill to a one month old infant. Keep increasing the dose according to the age of the child. This should be able to counteract [disorders] from morning to midday. It is very good.

Medicine for the elements, to prevent defects:

[129]	*chan*	seeds	
	chan	arils	
	krawaan		
	kaan phluu		
	dee plee		
	khamin oi		
	1 *fueang* of each		
	krachaai		1 *salueng*
	kaphrao	leaves	
	taan mon	leaves	
	khon thee so	leaves	
	1 *baht* of each		

10 items. Prepare pills using alcohol as excipient. To be taken mixed with alcohol. If the infant has reached one month of age, one pill should be given. The dose to be increased depending on the age of the child. This medicine should counteract [disorders] from midday to nightfall and from nightfall to 5 a.m.

To treat an infant who has been fed bad milk:

[130]	***Bencha kot***		
	kot so		
	kot khamao		
	kot phung plaa		
	kot chulaa lamphaa		
	kot hua bua		
	kaan phluu		
	chan thet		
	cha-em		
	1 *salueng* of each		
	nam taan	granulated	1 *fueang*

9 items. Prepare pills using aromatic water as excipient. To be given mixed with honey or lime juice. To treat babies, to counteract impurities in breast milk and to treat the poison of *saang* in the throat and chest. It is also very effective against coughs and hiccoughs.

A doctor who intends treating children, should [always] look for impure milk in wet nurses, as explained above. If he finds it is harmful, he should first have medicine prepared to restore the blood, then a tonic for the elements, medicine to increase the flow of milk, and then a lotion to be applied to the breasts, so that the milk will be free from impurities.

All medicines to nourish and restore the blood are given in *Phrakhamphee mahaachotarat* and *Khamphee sangyot.* They have been included here as a guide to the poor people who have to look after themselves. Royalty and high class people who have much merit are excepted, because they will have chosen wet-nurses who are free from defects, whose milk is pure and safe, so they will not need to be treated every day like us.

Medicine to rid breast milk of blood:

[131]	*Intthachon* [see no. 283]		1 *tamlueng*
	yaa dam		1 *baht*
	maaraa	nest	2 *baht*
	dee kluea		2 *baht*

These 4 items to be ground together and taken. Very effective.

Medicine to rid breast milk of blood:

[132]	*thian thang* 5		1 *fueang* of each
	chetta muun phloeng		
	dong dueng		1 *salueng* of each
	yaa dam		
	krathiam		
	kaarabuun		1 *baht* of each
	salot	purified fruit, [see no. 556]	an amount equal to the whole

These 11 items to be powdered together and taken mixed with hot water. If the elements are heavy, take only 1 *fueang*. If the elements are light, take 2 *phai*.[78] To be taken to expel *lom* and to get rid of poisons.

If severe diarrhoea follows, then it will cease if a decoction is made of:

[133]	*fak khieo*
	nam taan mo

This medicine should counteract blood poisoning and bad breast milk still existing after one, two, three or four years. This might change to tuberculosis or spread as abscesses in the abdomen. This will clear it up completely. It is extremely good.

Medicine to cleanse the breast milk of blood:

[134]	*sahatsakhun thang* 2	
	chan	seeds
	chan	arils
	thian thang 5	
	waan haang chaang	
	haang chang	root
	tong taek	root
	tree katuk	
	krathiam	
	yaa dam	
	2 *baht* of each	
	khaa	dried

phlai dried
kaan phluu
1 *baht* of each
hom daeng 3 *baht*
saan som
din prasiu khaao
1 *salueng* of each

Powder these 23 items together and mix with a triturate of tamarind fruit pulp in water. 1 *salueng* to be taken each day. This is a cleansing medicine which should completely counteract the harmful effects of bad breast milk.

The masters say that doctors who do not follow *Khamphee shanthasaat* because of blind avarice and self-righteousness should be called blind and wicked.

It has been shown that a doctor who has not studied *Khamphee shanthasaat* does not know the origin of *saang* and the properties and therapeutic value of drugs, but takes only from the texts that others have written and uses these to treat people. There are four reasons for this: he is greedy for other people's money; he is under the misconception that he knows better than others; he does the wrong thing without realising it; and he is bad tempered with his patients. These are not genuine doctors. Many people like these have been executed in the city of Solasa. You should all know about this.

Also, the action of a doctor who does not know the origin of disease and gives the wrong treatment is, according to the Pāli texts, (*paṭhamaṃ sattiyathā*) 'the first time equal to killing with a spear;' (*dutiyaṃ aggiyathā*) 'the second time like burning the patient with fire;' (*tatiyaṃ assanīyāthā*) 'the third time like striking him with a thunderbolt.' (*Javaraṃ*) 'Then the disease' (*kuppitā*) 'becomes stronger' (*satasahassaṃ*) 'by 100 to 1000 times.' (*So vejjo*) 'Such a doctor' (*kālakiriyaṃ* 'when he dies', (*nirayagato*) 'will be reborn in hell,' (*nirayapālo*) 'and all the guardians of hell' (*parivārito*) 'will have him in their power.' (*Tayā*) 'You' (*veditabbo*) 'should know' (*iti*) 'this.'

NOTES

1 *tamraa, khamphee* and *phrakhamphee* all mean 'book' or 'text'.

2 *Jīvaka Komārabhacca:* the father of Thai medicine.

3 *brahmacārī* (Pāli): usually refers to persons observing chastity. In this case, messengers from Brahmā. Cf. T.W. and C.A.F. Rhys Davids, trans., *Dialogues of the Buddha,* translated from the Pali of the *Dīgha Nikāya,* Part III, Sacred Books of the Buddhists, Vol. IV (London: 1957), pp 82 ff.

4 Jambū Dvīpa: ancient name for India. Parts of this creation story may be found in Frank E. Reynolds and Mani B. Reynolds, trans., *Three Worlds According to King Ruang: A Thai Buddhist cosmology* (Berkeley, California: 1982). See also Maneepin Phromsuthirak, 'Hindu Brahmā in Thai Literature,' *JSS,* Vol. 69, January-July 1981, pp 43-57.

5 *vidyādhara* (Skt): neither man nor god, yet possessing great knowledge and supernatural power.

6 *lohit bangkoet maa tae hatthaya:* could be interpreted to mean 'the blood which comes from the heart'. According to DT, it means 'blood which affects the heart'. This interpretation has been used throughout this section.

7 *khwan kin thuean:* her spirit has left her; she has lost her vitality. See note 61.

8 *tamlueng* : a fruit; also a measure of weight. See note 67. The scientific names and other details of many of the plants, animals and minerals mentioned in the text are included in Appendix I, which lists the prescription ingredients.

9 *yaa thaat:* medicine to aid digestion; (lit.) medicine for the elements. These are the elements of the body, of which it is composed. There are four main categories: earth, referring to parts which are solid; water, liquid; wind, which have the quality of movement; and fire, heat. This theory of medicine, including the humoral theory of the *tridoṣa,* wind, bile and mucus, has been adopted in part and superimposed on indigenous Thai medical theory. Its origin is Indian *āyurvedic* medicine.

10 *ritseeduang* : a class of diseases in which lumps occur.

11 *ritseeduang haeng* (lit.) dry *ritseeduang:* tuberculosis.

12 The relationships of left and female, and right and male recur often in this text. This dualism has been discussed at length by various scholars in Rodney Needham, ed., *Right and Left: Essays on dual symbolic classifications* (Chicago: 1973).

13 *bencha khan* *(pañca khandha,* Pāli): the five senses: material qualities, feeling, perception, coefficients of consciousness and consciousness. T.W. Rhys Davids and William Stede, *Pali-English Dictionary* (London: 1966), p.233. Cf. Book II, note 2.

14 Cf. Reynolds and Reynolds, *Three Worlds ...,* Chapter 5.

15 Bodhisattva: a being of (or destined for) enlightenment. Edward J. Thomas, *Life of Buddha as Legend and History,* 3rd edn. (revised) (London: 1975), p.1.

16 *thera* (Pāli): a venerable Buddhist monk. The traditional Thai midwife is called *mo tamyae*; '*mo*' meaning 'doctor' or a person especially skilled in a particular art. The use of the word '*tamyae*' might have originated in the name of this *thera* or his name could have been given to him because of his skill in obstetrics.

17 Phra Khodom (Gotama, Pāli): The previous six Buddhas were Vipassin or Vipaścit, Sikhin, Vessabhū or Viśvabhū, Kakucchanda or Krakucchanda (Kakkusantha, Thai), Koṇāgamana or Kanakamuni and Kassapa or Kaśyapa. Thomas, *The Life of Buddha ...*, p.27.

18 *puna ca paraṃ* (Pāli): and again; something else.

19 Many Thais believe that they will die on the same weekday as they were born. (VJ) Consequently, the day of conception, the day of birth and the day of death might all be expected to be the same if the statement on conception and birth is also believed.

20 *saang:* a generic name for children's diseases which usually start in the buccal mucosa and the throat. Possibly varieties of *Candida.* (VJ)
saang phloeng, also called *saang fai:* fiery *saang.*
Names of diseases are not translated in the text unless they have meaning in Western medical terminology, since translation does not usually convey the meaning in Thai terms.

21 *saang nam:* watery *saang.*

22 *saang daeng:* red *saang.*

23 *saang sako:* vigorous *saang.*

24 *saang wan:* misprint for *saang wua.* Also called *saang kho:* cow *saang.*

25 *khat bao:* could also mean an obstruction to the flow of urine or inability to urinate.

26 Months are lunar months and the duration of pregnancy is estimated to be ten lunar months.

27 *saang chaang:* elephant *saang.*

28 Strong salads consist of unheated, freshly marinated fish, sour and hot flavours, sugar and salt. The fish is pickled or soused by the action of the vinegar and other substances used as marinade. (VJ)

29 *saang khamooi:* robber *saang.* Synonym, *saang chon.*

30 *khai ram phe ram phat:* '*khai*' can mean fever or disease. This is a type of illness.

31 *sannibaat:* a disease category. In each of its several forms, the overall signs are muscular tremor, mild tetanus and Parkinson-like movement. (VJ) According to the theory of the elements, *sannibaat* results when each of the *tridoṣa* (three humours), wind, bile and mucus, is abnormal. See Mulholland, 'Thai Traditional Medicine: The treatment of diseases caused by the *tridoṣa*,' *South East Asian Review*, Vol. III, No.2 (February, 1979), pp 29-38.

32 *bat:* a tray, two or three inches deep, usually made from the petiole or lamina of a banana leaf. (VJ)

33 mantra: a spell to protect against danger or to promote health and wealth.

34 The scientific names and other details of most of the prescription ingredients are given in Appendix I.

35 *bot tham thaeng wai:* grind together and prepare a mass and roll it into a pencil-shaped stick. This is then either made into pills, later to be mixed with a liquid before being taken, or powder is obtained by rubbing the stick on a stone slab. The powder is then mixed with a liquid and either taken or applied to the body. Since it is not always clear whether the ingredients are obtained in dried or powdered form, the term 'mix' has been used frequently to indicate grinding, powdering and similar methods used in dispensing. Also, the term 'to be taken' is used in preference to 'to be given' to make it clear which medicines are for internal use.

36 The experienced doctor knows the quantity of any particular drug to be given. (DT) According to Dr Chalerm Phongsanit, a lecturer at Wat Pho Traditional Medical College, the quantity varies depending on the preparation. For example, one part used in a mixture with an aqueous vehicle is normally 1 *baht* (approximately 15 grams).

37 The method used to prepare a decoction, a common method of administering medicaments.

38 *sia krabaan:* a special ritual for the expulsion of evil spirits when someone is seriously ill. This is described by Phya Anuman Rajadhon in *Five Papers on Thai Custom*, Data Paper: Number 28, Southeast Asia Program (Ithaca, New York: 1958), pp 5-8.

39 *gāthā* (Skt): a verse or song; in Thai, also a spell.

40 *salueng*:: a measure of weight. 4 *salueng* = 1 *baht* (approximately 15 grams).

41 *devatā* (Pāli): an order of beings, according to an ancient Brahmanical system, occupying six seats or abodes of happiness, placed in rising succession above the abode of man. Benign spirits. *Mc*, p.423. A god, a spirit.

42 *bat phraket:* an offering to ward off some cosmological misfortunes. Dr B.J. Terwiel, personal communication. Ketu is considered in astronomy as the ninth planet and in mythology as the body of a demon which was severed from the head of Rāhu by Vishnu at the churning of the ocean, but rendered immortal by having tasted the elixir of life. *Mc*, p.119.

43 Because beings or lives which have come to be reborn are still naturally *anulomapatiloma* - in regular order and reversed or contrary - and cannot yet be properly begun. This is part of Buddhist cosmology and it is not Buddhist practice to go into it. Personal communication SN Ian Govinda, Wat Bovornivet, Bangkok, 1981.

44 The number of items can be seen to be calculated, not from the number of drugs, but from the number of parts, including, for example, 5 items counted in the 5 *thiang*.

45 *atisaan:* dysentery; the last stages of a disease where blood is mixed with the excrement; a moribund condition. *Mc*, p.957.

46 *baht:* a measure of weight = approximately 15 grams.

47 *kam mue, yom mue kam mue:* (lit.) a handful. A measure of weight. 150 grains of paddy = 1 *yip mue* (a pinch). 4 *yip mue* = 1 *kam mue*.

48 *yaa sadao luuk:* medicine to induce labour; an oxytocic remedy.

49 *lohit tee khuen:* (lit.) blood increasingly agitated. The symptoms include sweating and difficulty in breathing, which occur when the uterus does not contract, for example, and the mother cannot expel the placenta. A very serious condition. If the placenta is not expelled, she will die in four or five hours. In modern terms, septicaemia caused by bacterial infection. (PT)

50 *peesaat (pisāca,* Pāli): an evil spirit.

51 *thanuu kaaka: thanuu* arrow; *kaakaa* crow.

52 *lom lohit:* blood disease. The term ' *lom*' is used in several different contexts. Here it means 'disease'. Commonly, it means 'wind' or 'gas'; and it is also the name of one of the body elements, in which case it is called 'wind', equivalent to the *āyurvedic 'vāyo'* or *'vāta'*, implying movement. This has been discussed by Scott Bamber in *Lom*: *An examination of a term used in association with illness in traditional Thai medicine.* BA (Asian Studies) Honours sub-thesis, Australian National University, 1982.

53 Cf. Reynolds and Reynolds, *Three Worlds* ..., pp.120 ff. Also V. Fausböll, ed., trans. T.W. Rhys Davids, *Buddhist Birth Stories* (London: 1880), p.66.

54 *taan:* a generic name for children's diseases caused by parasites, usually worms.

55 *khamao* (lit.) soot. It is black and occurs on the upper lip under the nose and in the mouth. (DT) It is possible for it to occur anywhere on the upper part of the body and on the head as well as in the mouth. Sek Soralamp. (Personal communications).

56 *fee:* an abscess, boil or pustule. Types of boils.

57 *tua ron:* (lit.) a hot body. A high temperature.

58 *saphan* or *taphan:* a type of disease, particularly of infants, caused by the change in temperature experienced by the new-born child on leaving the womb and coming into contact with the open air. *PPPT*, p.328.
saphan fai: fiery *saphan*.

59 *sen en* or *en:* frequently translated as 'tendons', covers a wide range of meanings, but usually refers to long, hollow, tubular organs of the body such as tendons, cartilages, ligaments, muscles and the penis. It may refer to blood vessels and finer structures.

60 This statement appears to have been omitted in error in this and the 1914 edition. This information is supplied by (DT).

61 Cotton is tied around the wrists to prevent the *khwan* (spirit or vitality) escaping. See note 7.

62 The time of day when medicinal plants are collected is believed to be important.

63 *luuk prakham:* (dried) seeds of *prakham kai* (see Appendix I) made into a necklace to be worn by a child as a protective charm.

64 Names of illnesses.

65 *Bencha taan:* also the name of a slightly different recipe, no. 253, and mentioned after nos. 527 and 608.

66 *fueang:* a measure of weight = 1/2 *salueng* (approximately 2 grams).

67 *tamlueng:* a measure of weight = 4 baht (approximately 60 grams). Also the name of a fruit. See note 8.

68 *la:* a mouth disease; pustules or small, inflamed elevations of the skin, either convex or flat, of which there are various kinds, of different colours.

69 Liver hangs down: the liver is enlarged.

70 Lying (or baking) by the fire: traditionally, a Thai mother remains by a fire in a closed room, with her baby, from the time of birth, for one or more weeks.

71 *phraai* and *kumphan:* water spirits (usually malicious) and demons. *So*, pp 91, 648.

72 The direction is fixed to ensure that the prevailing wind does not carry the bad odour back to the house.

73 Knowledgeable in the three *vedas:* in Buddhism, means one who has realised three kinds of knowledge: remembrance of former rebirths, the divine eye and extinction of all cankers. Nyānatiloka, *Buddhist Dictionary: Manual of Buddhist terms and doctrines*, 4th revised edn., ed. Nyanaponika (Kandy: 1980), pp 220, 221.

74 *mae sue:* spirits, sometimes called guardian spirits, but clearly capable of harm, from whom children are bought to redeem them from the spirits after three days, to become human on the fourth day.

75 The first day is Sunday.

76 *bencha kalayaanee* (*pañca kalyāṇī*, Pāli): the five attributes of a beautiful woman: beautiful hair, beautiful lips, beautiful teeth, beautiful complexion, lasting beauty. *So*, p.535.

77 *thanaan:* a measure of volume, equivalent to the capacity of a coconut shell; now superseded by *thanaan luang*, one litre.

78 *phai:* a measure of weight = 1/4 *fueang* (approximately 0.5 gram).

[Book II]

Prathom chindaa, Book II, Part 3 [sic]. A brief description of women, babies, *paksee*[1] and harmful *peesaat*, three kinds of harmful milk and the origin of *saang chon*, *saang daeng*, *saang lueang*, *saang ninlapat*, [*saang*] *nin* and *la*.

Puna ca paraṃ A summary of the origin of the first diseases of infancy follows. Doctors should understand this.

Nonthapaksee give infants flatulence and make the abdomen and back hot. *Kaanlapaksee* make children vomit through the mouth and nose. *Asunnonthapaksee* make a baby cry and start in its sleep, frightened and convulsed with fear. *Theppheepaksee* cause flatulence, cold and numb hands and feet, and a hot head. Any baby affected by all these four diseases between the ages of eleven months and one year and six months will die within one year.

Saang is caused by the weather. There are eight kinds of *saang*. Any baby which develops this is called *amanutsaruup* [not human] and doctors will find it very difficult to cure. The dangers it faces are:

- When the infant leaves the fire, *khamao* develops.
- When it knows how to hold up its head, the body elements cause diarrhoea and vomiting, *taan*, *saang*, rubella and rubeola [*hueat hat*].
- When the baby can stand supporting itself, the crown of the head makes a clicking noise and the tendons move.
- When the child starts to eat food to which it is unaccustomed, *taan* and *saang* occur.
- When it learns to walk, the liver, lungs, intestines and abdomen move, and the child suffers from the ill effects of abnormalities of the elements of mucus and blood, and from *taan* and *saang*. When these changes occur, the child has *sunthonwaat saang*. This *saang* has many pustules covered with mucus, making the child ill and ten kinds of *saang* occur.[2]

These are *saang daeng*, *saang khaao*, *saang khamao*, *saang khum*, *saang chaang*, *saang sian*, *saang khwak*, *saang fai*, *saang chon* and *saang tamoi* [a painful pustule under the skin of the toes]. If it is *saang chaang*, the neck is bruised; if it is *saang sian*, the baby has an itchy rash like heat rash; with *saang khwak*, the neck is itchy; and *saang chon* produces sores which form a pattern like that of a spiny eel [yellow and brown patches and marks]. This induces general pain all over the body. The mother is forbidden to eat ten kinds of flesh, as these diseases are very difficult to cure.

[The type of infant] called *athitsaruup*[3] has a large or deep crown. When by the fire, *khamao* comes and then goes, but at the fire, the dominant elements causing disease are mucus and blood.

[Concerning the effects of] *nonthapaksee*; if the mother became pregnant in the fifth, sixth or seventh month of the year, gave birth on the first, third, fifth or seventh day [on a Sunday, Tuesday, Wednesday or Saturday] and the baby was born in the afternoon, then it will be difficult to rear, because it will have *saang daeng*, *saang chon*, *saang fai*, *saang sako*, *saang ninlapat*, [*saang*] *nin* and *la*.

Puna ca paraṃ In *Phrakhamphee prathom chindaa*, Book II, Part 1, the masters next refer to the eight features of woman. For example, the woman who has the eight attributes of womanhood has a perfect figure, and is called *noralak benchakalayaanee.* Her blood is darkened and bitter, whether the 32 parts of her body are [her skin is] black, brown, white or yellow, or a mixture of white and yellow.

Manutsaruup [human form], with a medium figure, has five features, whether she is white or dark. If a woman has none of these five, she is *aatukaruup* and *phaanonruup*, whether she is white or dark. *Chayaruup* has four features, whether she is black, brown, white or yellow. The appearance of women should be considered in this way.

Furthermore, a woman who is white and round shouldered will not be able to rear a baby; a woman who has pop-eyes, with the whites of her eyes greater than the dark part, will not be able to rear her baby; a woman whose breasts are separated and on the sides is prone to miscarriage; and a woman whose breasts are pendulous and turned out to the sides, has a rounded waist, erect shoulders, a straight back, tapering arms, creamy yellow complexion like the *kaaraket* flower, eyes like the hog deer, and smells as fragrant as the *kaaraket* flower is *noralak* and has the eight features of womanhood.

Moreover, there are four kinds of birth place. It is said of a place that has muddy water, salt and sweet water, and sweet water, that when those born there become ill, it is because of mucus. *Kamdao* [internal heat] is the primary cause of illness in people born on a plateau. Wind is the primary cause of illness in people born in a place which has both muddy water and rainwater. Leprosy is the prevalent illness in people born in scrubby country with pebbles and sand. Here is explained the place of birth as the predisposing factor of disease.

Puna ca paraṃ Next, the four types of infant are discussed, that is, *athitsaruup*, *haritaruup* [green], *manutsaruup* and *mahatsaruup.* All infants, male and female, born into this world will assume one of these forms.

Mahatsaruup: The crown is open, the penis is swollen and the testes hang down. While by the fire, this child never has *taan*, *saang* or *khamao* because the mother's milk is warm. After leaving the fire it has *khamao* and *saang* , and the intestines are enlarged and coiled up. When the baby cries, it sounds like a cat's miaow. It has flatulence and vomits through the nose; *haritathaat*[4] makes the baby tremble and the first severe illness occurs.

Athitsaruup: While at the fire, this baby has *khamao* but not very much. *Saang* develops on the tongue and up to the tip of the tongue. After the *saang* has gone, but while still at the fire, the infant has diarrhoea and vomiting. Mucus is the element which brings on two kinds of *saang.*

Haritaruup: While at the fire, *khamao* occurs in the chest and up to the tip of the tongue. In five days it descends and upsets the stomach causing diarrhoea, vomiting and cough. Blood is the element which causes two kinds of *saang* to occur.

Manutsaruup: There is no *khamao, taan* or *saang* while the infant is by the fire, but after leaving it, eight kinds of *saang* develop and [the element] internal heat is the cause. One pustule of *saang* comes from the abdomen to the chest; one ascends from the chest to the throat; another pustule moves up from the throat and appears on the chin and on the palate; and arising from the palate, three pustules develop in the crown of the head and three in the middle of the spine.

Furthermore, when the child of the *mahatsaruup* type has left the fire for three to six months, if it is the year of the dog, then *theppheepaksee* and *asunonthapaksee* arise.[5] The year of the swine is the time for *kaanlapaksee* and *asunonpaksee* to come; *nonthapaksee* and *saang chon* are severe; *kaanlapaksee, saang daeng*, and [*saang*] *ninlapat* develop; and *theppheepaksee, saang fai pathommakan* and *asunonthapaksee* are severe and spread. They say that the infant called *mahatsaruup*, with the large crown, swollen penis and testes hanging down, has no *khamao, taan* or *saang* while by the fire. *Haritaruup*, with the line on the crown of the head, develops slight *khamao* at the tip of the tongue after leaving the fire. This is called male *saang daeng. Athitsaruup* has a sunken fontanelle. *Saang* develops while by the fire, then is hidden. It is very difficult to cure. The *manutsaruup* baby gets *saang chon*. While the mother is pregnant, she craves for fishy and meaty food, and this makes the infant thin and dehydrated when it is from three to six months old. This is very hard to cure. The *saang* of *mahatsaruup* is *saang nin*; of *athitsaruup*, male *saang daeng*; and of *amanutsaruup*, it is *saang chon*. All infants are affected by [one of] these eight types of *saang*.

Puna ca paraṃ Next are mouth paints for *la*, *saang* and *khamao*:

Mouth paint for *la*:

[135]	*chaat horakhun*	
	phimsen	
	nom phichit	leaves
	mara	leaves
	khee malaeng saap	
	nguu lueam	bile

Equal parts of these 6 items to be mixed together and powdered. Add a little salt and prepare a stick. Apply to *la* and pustules of *saang* on the tongue and they will go. An excellent remedy.

Another:

[136]	*chaat horakhun Thai*	
	chaat horakhun cheen	
	chaat kon	
	chamot	
	phimsen	
	nam prasaan thong	
	see siat	
	chunsee	
	khee malaeng saap	
	makok	roasted seeds
	raak din	roasted

Equal parts, 11 items. Prepare a stick, mix with salt water and apply to *la* and *saang* and it will go.

Another:

[137]	*thong laang bai mon*	leaves

nam prasaan thong
nam taan tanot
Equal parts, 3 items. Prepare a stick. Use for application to *la* and it will go.

This is an oily paint for *khamao*:

[138] *waa* bark sap 1 cupful
nam phrik Thai 1 cupful
nam kraam chaang 1 cupful
nam see siat thet 1 cupful
ngaa oil half a cupful
Boil down these 5 items until only oil remains. Apply to the *khamaao* and it will go. Excellent.

Another:

[139] *thian thet*
ching chaa chaalee leaves
Mix with honey and apply to the *khamao* and it will go. Very effective.[6]

Another:

[140] *yaa dam*
krathiam
nam prasaan thong
Grind together and apply to *khamao* and *saang*.

To counteract the poison of *saang*:

[141] *sawaat* fruit
krathiam
nam prasaan thong
kaarabuun
nam puun sai
ngaa fresh oil
Equal parts, 6 items. Mix and apply to relieve the pain and to counteract the poison of *saang*.

To treat *saang* which has gone down to the stomach and upset it:

[142] *maeng lak* leaves
phak sian phee leaves
boraphet leaves
kwaang horn
chaang tooth
waai takhaa
chan daeng
neraphuusee
Equal parts, 8 items. Prepare pills. To be taken mixed with river water.

[143] ***Yaa lueang noi*** to treat the poison of *saang:*
saan som

nam prasaan thong	
makruut	seeds
manao	seeds
som saa	seeds
mangua	seeds
marum	bark
thong laang bai mon	bark
hom daeng	
dee plee	
kammathan daeng	

Equal parts, 11 items. Prepare pills. To be taken mixed with *nam makruut*, *nam mangua* or bark sap of *thong laang* as required, depending on the disease.

[144] ***Yaa lueang yai***

phrik Thai	
khing	dried
krachaai	dried
kathue	dried
phlai	dried
khamin oi	dried
krathiam	dried
hom daeng	
saaraphat phit	fruit
sang karanee	aerial parts
waan keep raet	
waan ron thong	
prakham dee khwaai	fruit
phak kaat	seeds
saan som	
din prasiu khaao	
kammatham daeng	
chan	seeds
chan	arils
manaao	seeds
dee plee	

Equal parts, 21 items. Pills. To be taken mixed with alcohol to counteract the poison of *taan* and *saang*.

[145] ***Mahaa nin***

chan	seeds
chan	arils
nam prasaan thong	
thian thang 5	
khamin oi	
khing	dried

krathiam fresh

Equal parts, 11 items. Add an equivalent amount of earthworms, roasted until almost burnt. Prepare pills to be taken with river water to treat the poison of *taan* and *saang*.

A purgative for infants:

[146] *phlap phlueng* leaves
phlai
phak kaat seeds
waan nam
nguu lueam grease

Equal parts, 5 items. Make a mass, heat over a fire, wrap in a cloth and apply [as a poultice] to the ribs. To dislodge mucus within the rib-cage, so that it will slip down into the stomach. A potent treatment to counteract the poison of *taan* and *saang*.

[147] ***Ketsaraa ru semha***
bua luang pollen
bunnaak pollen
khrai hom
chan khaao
cha-em
khing
raatcha phrik seeds
khee kaa thang 2 root
nam prasaan thong
yaa teen nok

Equal parts, 11 items. Reduce to 1/3 volume by boiling. Before it is to be taken, add some syrup. To be taken according to the strength of the infant to treat a raised temperature caused by mucus and internal heat, to treat the poison of *taan* and *saang*, and to improve the appetite and the digestion.

To dislodge putrid mucus:

[148] *yaa dam*
mahaa hing
kaphrao leaves
phak sian phee
kradom fruit
boraphet
nam prasaan thong
khamin oi

Equal parts, 8 items. Pills. To be taken according to the strength of the child, mixed with water, to dislodge putrid mucus.

Purgative for infants:

[149] *salot* 9 seeds

Place 3 seeds in each of 3 balls of cooked rice. Bake over the fire until almost burnt [well done]. Add

kaan phluu	8 flowers	
phlai		
phimsen		

Prepare pills the size of peppercorns. To be taken according to the strength of the child.

Purgative for infants:

[150]	*kaarabuun*		1 part
	rong thong		1 part
	phrik Thai		1 part
	khing		1 part
	yaa dam		2 parts
	salot	fruit	8 parts

6 items. Prepare pills the size of peppercorns, using *makhaam* fruit juice as excipient. Dose for a one year old child, 3 pills. If the elements are heavy, 5 pills to be taken mixed with alcohol.

[151] ***Thep samrit*** to improve the body elements:

saan som	
din prasiu khaao	
nam prasaan thong	
som poi	pods
prakham dee khwaii	fruit

Equal parts, 5 items. Prepare pills the size of a *phutsaa* seed,[7] using lime juice as excipient. One pill to be taken mixed with alcohol or lime juice as required. If this is not effective, increase the dose to 3 pills.

To treat constipation:

[152]	*mai sak*	charcoal
	chan	roasted seeds
	rong thong	

Wrap in a lotus leaf which has dried in the pond. Roast in a fire until scorched and shrivelled then mix together. Combine with lime water and give the resulting sediment to the baby to eat.

Medicine to relieve retention of urine:

[153]	*khok krasun*		1
	khee lek	the leafy tops of new shoots	1
	khamin oi		7 pieces

Boil together until reduced to 1/3 volume. To be given to the baby to take, then it will urinate.

Another:

[154]	*bua luang*	the [alkaline] ash of the leaves

To be taken mixed with honey, then the urine will flow.

Medicine to treat severe diarrhoea in young babies:

[155] *matuum* — under-ripe fruit
thap thim — fruit
dee plee
naat — root
khing — fresh
Equal parts, 5 items. To be taken mixed with honey.

Another:

[156] *khon thee so* — leaves
phak sian phee — leaves
phlai
khamin oi
yaa dam
mahaa hing
Equal parts, 6 items. To be taken mixed with proof spirit [*nam yat lao*] to treat *taan* and *saang.*

Another:

[157] *mahaa hing*
nam prasaan thong
chan — seeds
samo thet
kaarabuun
Equal parts, 5 items. Add an amount of *chetta muun phloeng* equivalent to the whole. Prepare pills. To be taken mixed [with a liquid].

Puna ca paraṃ Whether a baby is fifteen days old or one, two, three or four months, *khamao, taan, saang,* blood disorders, *krasaai* [*krasai*], and diseases of the 37 tendons develop from the first month and nine kinds of *saang* arise. One kind occurs internally. It affects the intestines, stomach, liver, lungs and heart - these are called *bencha khan.*[8] Those who understand can distinguish [between the various types of *saang*]. Namely:

Saang faai is like this:

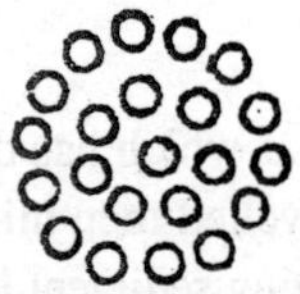

It does not matter whether it comes up on the tongue or in the mouth.

Saang khum is like this:

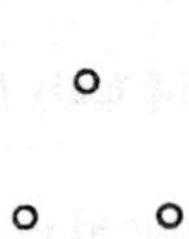

If the centres are a dull white, the *taan* will be gone in two days.

Saang khaao plueak occurs on the tongue and mouth and looks like a cow's tongue. In two days it will descend to the abdomen. *Saang khaao* [*plueak*] is like this:

o o o
o o o

Saang khwaai is like this:

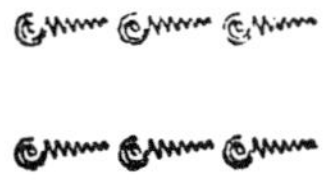

If it turns black, the baby will die in twelve days.

Saang maa looks like this:

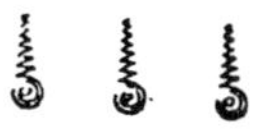

After two days it merges together and turns black and blue. This is very severe.

Saang chaang looks like this:

o o o
o o o
o o o

If it is concave, with red centres, it will cause diarrhoea.

Saang chon looks like this:

o o o o
o o o o
o o o o
o o o o

It develops in the intestines and liver and in the spine. When it is ripe, it comes up like a large flower of elephant yam, thus:

and the *saang* looks like this:

o

o o o

o

and if it is red, it becomes pitted.

Saang fai looks like this:

o o o
o o o
o o o

It is very bad if it is black in the middle of the tongue and red at the edges. The baby will die if ever it bleeds.

Before treating *saang*, the doctor should first consider the symptoms and make a diagnosis. If it affects the intestines and stomach, it causes diarrhoea; if it affects the heart, the child passes blood and fresh mucus; if the liver is attacked, a little blood is passed; and if the larynx is affected the mouth and throat become dry. *Saang* outside the intestines and in the chest causes thirst.

Furthermore, if a baby wakes up with a red mouth and is dribbling, *saang* has started at the tongue and has entered the throat. When fed, the infant will cough and vomit, then the *saang* will go down and upset the stomach. Later, the child will be thirsty, then the spine will stiffen. This is influenza [*khai wat*] caused by *saang chon*, and the baby gets thin and yellow and looks as if it has birth marks on its body. *Saang faai* is white and causes dribbling when it affects the lips. If it turns yellow, the doctor should treat it with medicine called *la-ong phrabaat*. *Saang ritseeduang* causes very bad sores in the mouth. When it is ripe, it will cause abdominal cramps. Treat it with this medicine:

[158]	*yaa sai*	
	taan mon	leaves
	kaphrao	leaves
	sawaat	leaves
	maklam khruea	leaves
	phak khraat	
	mayom tua phuu	leaves
	makruut	
	chamot	

Equal parts, 9 items. Pills to be taken mixed with alcohol and a little opium to treat abdominal cramps.

To counteract *la-ong phrabaat*[9], which at first is white [in the mouth], then yellow and produces excessive salivation, recite these powerful words seven times (*Ummāgarūpamukkhā vā gantvā svāha ummāgarūpamukkhā vā gantvā svāha*) at the same time blowing on some

[159] *maak* and *phlai* [to transfer the power of the words to the medicine]. Chew these, then put the chewed mass in the child's mouth to treat *la-ong phrabaat*.

Medicine to treat *la-ong phrabaat*:

[160]	*kaphrao*	leaves	1
	phrik		7
	khing		7
	krathiam		7
	kluea		7

Make a decoction to be taken.

Another:

[161] *nam prasan thong*
fin
benyakaanee
nam taan
krathiam

Add a little salt, grind finely, dip some cotton in the mixture and place this in the child's mouth to be sucked. For *la-ong phrabaat* on the tongue and in the mouth.

To treat *la-ong phrabaat* which has gone down to the stomach and upset it:

[162]	*benyakaanee*	galls
	neraphuusee	
	chan daeng	
	nguu lueam	bile

Equal parts, 4 items. Pills to be taken mixed with alcohol.

Medicine to treat *la-ong phrakrit*:

[163]	*thao yaa naang*	root
	nguu lueam	bile

To be taken mixed with alcohol.

Medicine for *saang daeng*:

[164]	*raet*	molar tooth
	chaang	molar tooth
	kwaang	horn
	samun waeng	
	neraphuusee	
	chan daeng	
	nguu lueam	bile

Equal parts, 7 items. Prepare pills using alcohol as excipient. To be taken and applied.

Another:

[165]	*nam prasaan thong*	
	khing	
	krathiam	
	khamin oi	
	phlai	
	phimsen	
	nguu thap thaang	bones
	raet	horn
	chaang	tusk
	raet	molar tooth
	chaang	molar tooth
	suea	eye tooth
	chorakhe	eye tooth
	muu	tusk

Equal parts, 14 items. Prepare a stick. To be applied to *saang daeng, dam, khaao* and *lueang*.

Another:

[166]	*raet*	molar tooth
	chaang	molar tooth
	chaang	tusk
	raet	horn
	suea	eye tooth

chorakhe	eye tooth	
muu	tusk	
nguu thap thaang	bones	
kot thang 5		
khamin oi		
phlai		
taphaap nam	bile	
nguu lueam	bile	
phimsen		

Equal parts, 18 items. Pills to be taken mixed with alcohol to treat all kinds of *saang.*

Another:

[167]

hoi eerom	calcined	
muek hom		
khan sung	root	
chaat horakhun		
nam prasaan thong		

Equal parts, 5 items. Reduce to a powder, then mix with fresh sesame oil. To be applied to *saang.*

Medicine to treat *saang chon*:

[168]

boraphet		
khon thee so	leaves	
kaphrao	leaves	
angkaap	leaves	
phluu kae	leaves	
phlai		
khamin oi		

Equal parts, 7 items. Pills. To be taken mixed with alcohol.

Another:

[169]

chetta muun phloeng		1
din kin		2
utta phit	rhizome	2
tree katuk		3

Equal parts [sic], 4 items. Pills to be taken mixed with alcohol to treat *saang chon.*

Another:

[170]

khamin oi		
phrik		
khing		
krathiam		
kraphrao	leaves	

Equal parts, 5 items. Pills. To be taken mixed with alcohol to treat *saang chon.*

[171] ***Bencha naaraai***

raatchadat	fruit	
yaa dam		
prakham dee khwaai	fruit	
khamin oi		
nguu lueam	bile	

Equal parts, 5 items. To be taken mixed with alcohol to treat *saang chon* [causing] the passage of mucus and blood.

Another:

[172]

khaa		1 part
phlai		2 parts
yaa dam		3 parts
khamin oi		4 parts
kaphrao	leaves	5 parts

5 items. Pills. To be taken mixed with alcohol to counteract the effects of *saang chon* in the upper chest.

Another:

[173] *phak khraat*
taan mon
khop chanaang thang 2
Equal parts, 4 items. Mix with water and add

phrik	7
khing	7
krathiam	

To be taken to kill [intestinal] parasites and get rid of offensive faecal smell.

Another:

[174]

taan dam	
taan khamooi	
phrik Thai	
phak sian phee	
kum thang 2	
kluea	
suea	bones
nguu lueam	bones
kaarabuun	

Boil with fresh sesame oil. To be taken or applied. If applied for stiffness to the back caused by *saang chon* it will cure it.

Another:

[175] *phlai*
khing
khaa
khamin oi

Equal parts, 4 items. Mix with lime juice and warm over a fire. To be taken or applied.

Medicine to expel *saang*:

[176]	*salot*	fruit	
	makaa	leaves	
	raatcha phrik	leaves	
	yaa tai bai		
	khamin oi		
	kaphrao	leaves	

6 items. Use 1 part of *salot* and 2 parts of each of these 5 kinds of leaves. Make pills the size of kapok seeds. To be taken according to the strength of the child.

Another:

[177]	*phak kaat*	seeds	1 part
	thian dam		2 parts
	salot		3 parts

3 items. Prepare pills the size of peppercorns, using lime juice as excipient. To be taken according to the strength of the child to dislodge mucus and purulent serum.

Eye drops:

[178]	*kathok rok*	root	
	khamin oi		
	hoi khong	shell	

Soak these three ingredients in water. [The resulting supernatant liquid] to be used as eye drops to treat indistinct vision.

Another:

[179]	*phak khraat*	root	1
	khamin oi		1
	phan nguu daeng	root	1
	kluea		7 crystals

Soak in water. To be used as eye drops to prevent *saang* from affecting the eyes.

Medicine to treat all forms of *to* that make the eyes white:[10]

[180]	*phlai*		
	angkaap	root	
	anchan khaao	root	

Equal parts, 3 items. Prepare a stick using lime juice as excipient. Use to prepare eye drops to get rid of *saang chon*.

Medicine to treat the tendons:

[181]	*mara*	leaves	
	haang chorakhe	leaves	
	tamlueng shaek (tamlueng tua phuu)	leaves	
	khamin oi		

din prasiu khaao

Make a poultice from equal parts of these 5 ingredients.

Medicine for the tongue:

[182] *nam prasaan thong*
kaan phluu
bai naat
khrai hom
khamin oi
kaphrao leaves

Equal parts, 6 items. Mix with lime juice, then prepare pills. Before it is taken, add Borneo camphor and honey. Give when the baby is unable to suck.

Medicine for babies who cannot eat:

[183] *boraphet*
kaphrao leaves
khrai hom
khamin oi
nam prasaan thong

Equal parts, 5 items. To be taken mixed with honey, then the baby will be able to eat.

Siddhikāriyaḥ[11] We will discuss serious diseases of infants: *taan* and *saang*, mother's milk and *mae sue*, *nonthapaksee* and *putsakapaksee*. If a baby has a fever which makes it tremble all over, a high temperature, restlessness, and a great thirst, it should be understood that it is because of *nonthapaksee*.

If *putsakapaksee* cause disorders and make the baby ill, have this medicine made:

[184] *thua paep* root[12]

Mix with fresh oil. To counteract all ill effects, such as those of *putsakapaksee*.

Another:

[185] *kaphrao* leaves
phak waen root

Prepare from these 2 ingredients pills the size of *sadao* fruit. Tie the wrists and ankles of the child [with thread] to protect him against all the *paksee*. If the wrists and ankles are not tied, it will be just the same if the medicine is heated and applied to the hands and feet.

Another:

[186] *sadao* flowers
krameng
phrommi
thua rae leaves
rak khaao leaves

Mix with water, then with fresh oil. To be applied to the child's body to counteract the harmful effects of all *putsakapaksee*.

Another:

[187]	*taen*	nest
	phak waen	
	angkaap	leaves
	makham kai	leaves
	samun waeng	
	ulok	leaves
	anchan khaao	leaves

To be applied to the child's body, mixed with fresh oil, to counteract all harm.

[188]	***Bencha phangkhee***	
	makhwit	the leafy tips of new shoots
	pho baai	the leafy tips of new shoots
	thong	the leafy tips of new shoots
	matuum	the leafy tips of new shoots
	maduea	the leafy tips of new shoots

Mix together and apply to the child's body, then bathe the child, to counteract bad luck and [the element] blood.

Also, prepare an offering of:

[189] sweet biscuits, honey, beans, sesame and liquor, decorated with fragrant flowers. Make the offering, then take it to a three-way intersection at night, to counteract any harm which might befall the child.

Another:

[190]	*mai phai*	skin
	chan takhian	
	noei	

Burn these 3 ingredients and fumigate.

Siddhikāriyaḥ Here we will describe the four kinds of *peesaat* that harm babies: *nonthapaksee, kaanlapaksee, asunnonthapaksee* and *theppheepaksee.*

(1) *Nonthapaksee* affect infants while they are at the fire, entering the intestines. They cause disorders of [the element] mucus, pain all over the body and vomiting through the nose.

(2) *Kaanlapaksee* Five months after the mother has left the fire, the *peesaat* come out of the baby's intestines and cause the intestines to coil up tight and make loud noises, and the baby cries for a short time, then sighs heavily and cries in its sleep.

(3) *Asunnonthapaksee* make infants thirsty, unable to sleep or eat and hot. The *peesaat* are in the liver.

(4) *Theppheepaksee* make the baby wave its hands and feet about. Three or four months after leaving the fire, the child's eyes roll from side to side and upwards, and the crown of its head is sunken.

It is said that *nonthapaksee* enter through the intestines and leave by the anus; *kaanlapaksee* leave by the urethral passage; *asunnonthapaksee* enter by the nose and leave through the eyes; and *thepheepaksee* enter by the breast and leave through the feet.

For relief from *nonthapaksee:*

[191] *bai naat*
mahaa hing
Mix, and apply to the child's body to frighten off *nonthapaksee.*

For relief from *kaanlapaksee:*

[192] *saap raeng*
saap kaa[13]
khwaai horn
Mix together, burn and fumigate to frighten *kaanlapaksee.*

For relief from *asunnonthapaksee*:

[193] Mix together and burn birds' feathers and crows' feathers to frighten *asunnonthapaksee.*

For relief from *theppheepaksee*:

[194] Mix together crinum lily [leaves] and arsenic and burn to frighten *theppheepaksee.*

Nonthapaksee enter at the break of day and go at sunset; *kaanlapaksee* enter when the baby goes to bed and leave at sunrise; *asunnonthapaksee* come at noon and go at midnight; and *theppheepaksee* enter in the evening and go before dawn.

Moreover, during the fifth, sixth, seventh and eighth months, Phra Seephromyak is in possession of greater power than all the other *peesaat,* and [this demon] enters infants and harms them. During the ninth, tenth, eleventh and twelfth months, Phra Seehatsabodee is in possession of greater power than all the other *peesaat,* and enters infants and harms them; and during the first, second, third and fourth months, it is Phra Seekumaarayak who is the demon in possession of greater power than all the other *peesaat* and harms babies.

Nonthapaksee enter when a baby is frightened by the cry of a dumb animal, and go away when animals fight. *Kaanlapaksee* enter when a tree falls and animals fight, and go when animals fight. *Asunnonthapaksee* enter when someone comes from afar, bringing two or four legged animals. They go when people quarrel. *Theppheepaksee* come with the sound of wind blowing and thunder and the music of gongs and drums. They go with the sound of a human weeping.

They used to have two *krabaan* made if a baby was sick and vomited after its feed, and had diarrhoea and could not sleep. On one, they put models moulded from earth, of all the animals; and on the other, models of all the spirits. They also took a new pot and moulded from dough a mother with two children holding each other, and put them in the pot. Then they put the milk of a coconut and a lighted candle in the mouth of the pot and set it afloat, together with the *krabaan.*[14]

And in *Khamphee prathom chindaa,* Book I, Part 4, on *sangyot,*[15] the masters speak of three kinds of women who have unwholesome milk: one who eats food that is incompatible with her elements, one who eats things not normally eaten as food, and the passionate woman who always has her mind on her femininity. A baby fed with milk from a woman of one of these three types will be made sick. This is explained in *Khamphee sangyot.*

Medicine to purify unwholesome breast milk:

[195] *krung khamao*
khing
kraphang hom
kot thang 5
chamot
Equal parts, 9 items. Boil with 5 *thanaan* of water. Reduce to 3 *thanaan*. Give to the mother of a young infant to take to purify her milk.

The masters say that the person who is to take care of such a baby should do so with a firm but soft voice, forbid the wrong food, and feed the child with milk. If it has a fever:

[196] Combine 3 parts of fresh buttermilk with one part of water and mix with coconut milk. To be given to infants to counteract the effects of unwholesome breast milk.

Another:

[197] *tree katuk*
chuk rohinee
Powder together, add cow's milk and boil. Give it to the child as a remedy for fever caused by [the element] internal heat.

[198] ***Phalaathikhun***
lamphan
khing dried
haeo muu
utta phit
Boil and give to the mother of a young infant to take to purify her milk.

Another:

[199] *khok kra-om*
Mix with water and apply to the child's body and to the mother's nipples to dry them, then wash off. Then give some of the medicine to the child to take to counteract the *tridoṣa*.[16]

Also, look at the milk and taste it. If it is astringent, drop some into a basin of clear water. If the milk disappears, it is still affected by internal heat. If it is thick and white and sinks, it is quite pure and harmless.

Another:

[200] *mai thao yaai mom*
thep thaaro
lamphan
utta phit
Boil together until reduced to 1/3 volume. To be taken by the mother to purify her milk.

Siddhikāriyaḥ Here we will describe *saang chon*. It looks like this:

o o o
o o o
o o o

The *saang* first appears when the infant is three days old, with four pustules in the spine and four in the crown of the head.[17] When the baby is three months old it might occur in the mouth as one pustule at each of the angles of the jaw. The heads of the pustules are black and their bases are red. As a result, the baby has diarrhoea during the period of time from the age of three months to ten years (or ten months) [sic].[18] The diarrhoea produces faeces like liquor ferment. After three months, the body is covered [in yellow and brown patches and marks] like the pattern of the spiny eel and the major pustules make the whole body sting. After six months, the *saang* withdraws into the spine and intestines and the edge of the liver. If it enters the liver, the faeces are black; if it enters the ileum, the faeces are as green as a leaf; and if it enters the heart, the child vomits fresh blood. [The throat gets dry if the *saang* enters the throat.][19] If the *saang* enters the stomach, it causes hunger and thirst; if it enters the abdomen, the back becomes humped, the child has difficulty in urinating, has urinary calculi and the urine is white like lime water. When the *saang* moves inside the body, one major pustule comes up in the supra-pubic area and there are 30 followers.[20] There is one major pustule in the liver, with 60 smaller ones; one in the abdomen, with 40 followers; one in the upper chest, with 50 lesser pustules; one in the heart, with 70; one in the throat, with 80; one in each eye, with 20 followers to each eye; a total of 350 [370] followers of *saang chon.*

If the doctor wants to be sure, he should inspect the *saang* in the crown of the head, or that in the eyes. When death is near, the throat is obstructed, so that the baby can neither eat nor take milk.

The followers from the crown come up in the gums on both sides of the mouth, in the lower jaw and they are coloured red, black, white or yellow. If ever they break, the baby will die instantly. When they have erupted in the gums, the throat and at the roots of the teeth, then the two pustules in the eyes descend to the spine, where they combine and produce six heads.

The *saang* appears once at three months of age, [again at six months][21] and once more at nine to eleven months. When this happens, the child has foul-smelling, liquid diarrhoea. Drastic purgatives and medicine to expel flatus should not be given if the baby passes blood or pus, as it is very difficult to cure this and strong purgatives will kill the child. When the major pustules of *saang chon* erupt in the cheeks, if there are any followers, there are five, six or seven in the spleen, causing it to hang down to the lower edge of the ribs, and the baby has a high temperature, yellow eyes, gastric pain, goose flesh, a hollow chest,and is thin and yellow. If the followers occur at the edge of the liver, they form a pattern like the iris of the eye, then spread out and merge together; if they develop in the intestines, the intestines swell up, the abdomen turns yellow and the child has continual diarrhoea; if they erupt between the spinal vertebrae and get into the bones, this is very hard to cure and the patient usually dies. If *saang chon* breaks out in the foot at birth, then a day after birth there are five pustules like this:

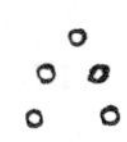

one on the sole of each foot, one in the middle and three on top. In boys, there are five pustules on the right foot. If three pustules erupt on the left foot, the baby will die.

Khamao comes after the time of lying by the fire because the *saang lom* originates in the feet. After three months the *saang* in the feet subsides then emerges at the knee-caps. The doctor should make a careful examination, because the *saang* that comes up from the feet to the knees and thighs looks like this:

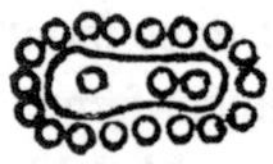

and it comes out on both shins like the rough skin of a young stingray. This *saang* then develops close to the spine and in all the bones and tendons. When it reaches the supra-pubic area, one pustule erupts in the intestines, one in the abdomen, one at the edge of the liver, one at the heart, one in the throat and one on each side of the palate. In addition, one pustule comes up on the right side of the body, from the abdomen, and one on the left, from the waist and neck; and one comes from the intestines and emerges at the middle of the back between the shoulders.

The following summary is included to make it clear to doctors. The followers of *saang chon* which can be fatal and can occur in all infants, affect the whole body in many ways. Whenever the major pustules of *saang* arise in all the important organs, then the small pustules which accompany them follow from the supra-pubic area to the navel. First, one pustule comes up with eight followers, which then erupt as sores with raised heads like tubers of the elephant yam, but there is something resembling daphnia [*rai nam*] to be seen and they all merge, then spread up to the stomach and the edge of the liver. If the major pustule comes from the intestines, it causes diarrhoea; if it reaches the stomach, it causes great thirst; if it reaches the edge of the liver, it causes the child to pass blood; if it enters the spleen, it produces heat in the body, the abdomen and the back, and makes the baby agitated and distressed so that it becomes fatigued and collapses. After one day this subsides, then one pustule erupts in the right eye first, [and on the seventh day, this pustule crosses over to the left eye].[22] On the eighth day, it disappears. Then the *saang* in the liver and spleen affects the heart, after which three pustules obstruct the throat. On the ninth day the baby will die and when it is dead the pustules will appear in the spine - some red, some black and some blue. If any doctor wishes to know the origin of *saang chon*, he should investigate these things. *Saang nin* looks like this:

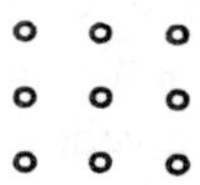

One day after birth, there are three pustules in the crown of the head which descend to erupt as five pustules in the spine. While the baby is by the fire you cannot tell whether there is *khamao* because of the three pustules on the crown of the head. After leaving the fire, there will be *khamao*, *taan* and *saang*. To be certain of his diagnosis, the doctor should examine the pustules on the baby very carefully. The *saang* in the crown will move to the palate, where it will erupt with one, three or four heads; and when this happens, there is no *khamao* while by the fire or afterwards. Two or three months later the *saang* spreads to the gums and jaws, causing general aches and pains, vomiting, diarrhoea, thirst, flatulence and inability to eat. In three months it appears on the neck in a red pattern that looks like popped rice, and the anus and urethra are red. After another three months the *saang nin* subsides, and is replaced by *saang daeng*, which appears at the throat and the body orifices. If the *saang nin* was in the cheeks, then *saang daeng* erupts in the gums, in front of the teeth and in the upper jaw, at the angles of the jaw. If the doctor notices that the pustules in the gums and angles of the jaw have black heads and yellow bases, he must not treat this. If despite this warning he treats the baby, the doctor is forbidden to give drastic purgatives because, if he does, the child is sure to die. If the *saang* in the throat is red and goes away by itself, then it will certainly develop internally. Then, in three months time, the *saang* in the crown moves to the right side of the spine. If the baby is a girl, it comes up on the left side close to the backbone. It has six heads. Six months later, they all withdraw together and recur internally like this:

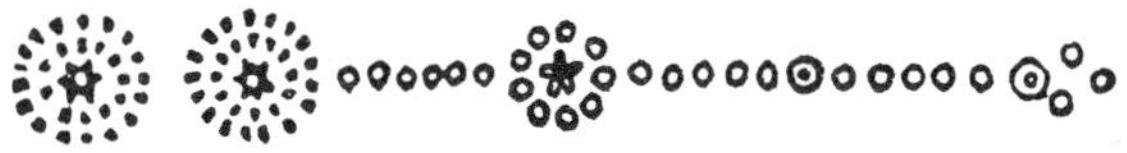

If the doctor is certain that this is the case, he should be very careful about the medicine he gives, as the disease will cause diarrhoea, vomiting, thirst, a high temperature and cold hands and feet, and the diarrhoea will last for seven days. Then the baby will have dysentery for nine days, then pass foul blood for seven days. *La-ong saang* follows, appearing in the mouth and throat, at first causing coughing. Then it breaks and cracks and comes up at both the underarms like the rough tubercles of red *boraphet,* like this:

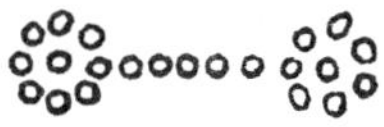

When it erupts in the throat it is like this:

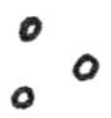

then, indeed, symptoms of *saang* will appear in the feet, and this is the sign of death.

The doctor should be able to distinguish between the symptoms of the various types of *saang* which afflict all infants. He should examine the baby's legs very carefully, from the ankles up, to see if the flesh is as rough as the skin of the feet. Whenever this occurs in a child, it has diarrhoea at first, then pants and gets breathless. The 70 followers of *saang daeng* then erupt on every bone, in the flesh, in the intestines, inside the long muscles of the back [beside the spine] and spread all over the body. And the major pustules of *saang* develop in the important parts - one in the supra-pubic area, one in the abdomen, one in the upper chest, one in the crown, one in the throat and one in the eye. And the sign of death will show in the eyes. The whites will be blood red. Once all these symptoms of *saang daeng* have ocurred at the same time, the baby will die in nine days.

Students of medicine should make a thorough investigation in order to decide whether the baby will live or die. This condition is very difficult to cure. If the wrong medicine is given, the baby will die in one or two days; if the right medicine is given, it will only prolong life for eleven, thirteen or fifteen days, but children are known to die from *saang daeng* in seven days.

They say if a boy gets *saang daeng*, it comes up on the right side, like this:

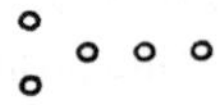

If it is a girl, it will appear on the left side, like this:

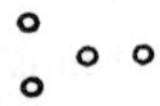

Seven days after birth, the umbilical cord drops off and the next day, *saang* begins in both feet. Then one major pustule of *saang* develops in the supra-pubic area and *la-ong* comes from the abdominal flesh and from inside the intestines to the throat. It looks like rice bran. Then it moves up from the throat to the tongue and lips, and the pustules in the mouth are called *khamao.* It withdraws from these three places to the supra-pubic area. Three months later, the *saang* in the feet moves up to the middle of the right shin if the baby is a boy, to the left shin if it is a girl. It looks like this:

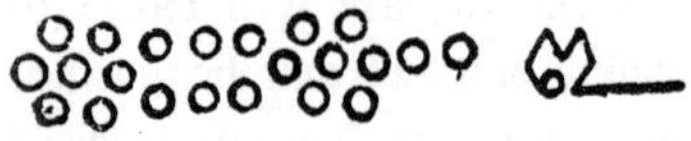

After six months, it reaches the knee-cap, and the *saang* in the supra-pubic area subsides. The symptoms are vomiting and various aches and pains. Provided that the doctor recognizes this and gives the right medicine, the child will survive; otherwise, it will die in seven, nine or eleven days. When *saang daeng* develops in the abdomen, it first appears in the mouth like this:

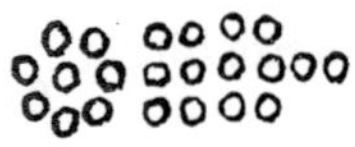

It moves up from the base of the tongue to the mouth, making the mouth and gums red and it spreads from the angles of the jaw, meeting and forming three pustules like this:

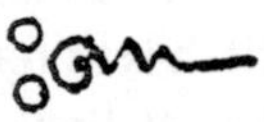

in front of the teeth. At nine to eleven months of age, the *saang* from the supra-pubic area comes up in the long muscles beside the spine, like this:

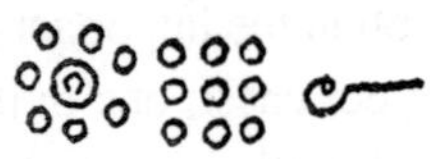

then the followers erupt in the intestines and in the flesh all over the body. In the intestines and stomach they look like this:

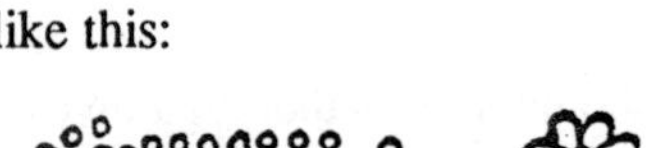

If they occur in the long muscles of the back, on the ribs and at the edge of the liver, they might cause diarrhoea, vomiting or thirst, and the baby might pass blood in the stools. At the age of one year and three months or one year and six months, the *saang* spreads out and attacks the throat, ears, eyes and the crown of the head; the child's condition gradually deteriorates and it becomes very thin and lethargic. It is unable to drink water or milk, cries in a husky voice, has sticky eyes and thin teeth, and when it sits down its knees come up to its ears. When this happens, the baby's vision is blurred and the corners of its eyes are yellow. At one or two years of age and when the child is near death, the *saang* appears at the hips, the legs, the middle of the back, the chest and all over the body. At first there are vermilion coloured spots, then these break and spread out like burns, with a distinct margin. In that case, *saang kaan*, which is called *ninlapat*, erupts in the throat with three pustules like this:

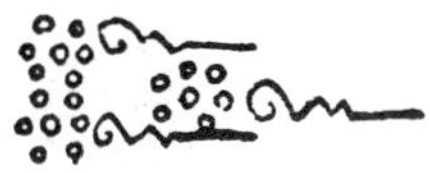

then *la-ong saang* appears in the mouth and comes up on the tongue like eggs, thus:

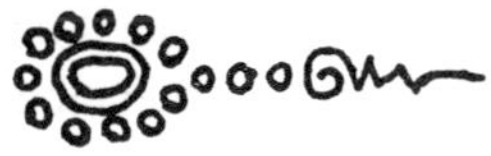

then spreads out and fills the mouth. When the doctor sees this, he will know that the child will die within two to three days. It is also said that if any baby gets the thirteen major pustules of this *saang*, that is its karma [fate].They say that *saang fai* looks like this:

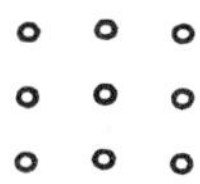

Khamao appears while the mother and child are by the fire immediately after birth, but it goes once they have left the fire. Three months after leaving the fire, the *saang* appears. There are five pustules at the right hip; if the baby is a girl, there are three pustules at the left hip and two in the middle of the sole of each foot, like this:

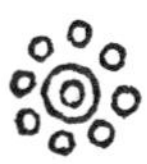

Three and a half months later, the *saang* in the middle of the soles of the feet subsides and moves up to the shins and it looks like this:

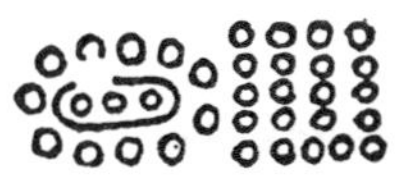

There are 50 followers. When the major pustules spread to the thighs, the followers disperse, and fifteen of them erupt on the left foot, with others at each joint. These cause generalized muscular pain and fatigue and a high temperature, so that the baby cries from afternoon to late at night and gets very little sleep. After another three months, the baby's feet are cold and an itchy rash develops on the body giving the appearance of sand having been thrown on the body; then the rash goes away. In three more months, spots erupt on the arms, legs or shins making the skin dry and black as if burnt. If this covers the whole area from the feet up to the waist, the baby will die when it reaches the waist and as death approaches the *saang* will appear on the legs, like this:

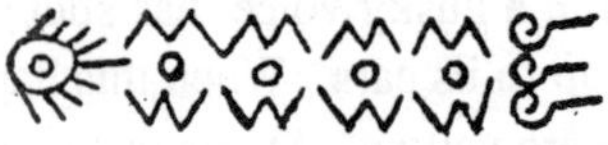

in the supra-pubic area, like this:

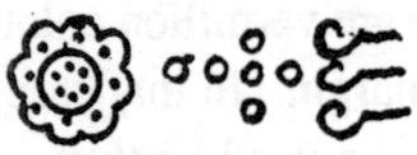

and on the abdomen, like this:

The doctor should be very careful if he recognizes these symptoms and treats them, as this is very difficult to cure and the baby will die if the treatment is unsuccessful.

There are nine kinds of *la* that occur in association with birth *saang*. If a doctor is to treat birth *saang*, he should examine the mouth and tongue in order to diagnose which kind of *la* the baby has. The pustules of *la* may be yellow, red, as black as ink, leaf-green with visible blood vessels, as dark as sapphires, the [reddish-purple] colour of the almost ripe jambolan, indigo coloured or white. In treating *la*, the type of *saang* affecting the child should be taken into consideration. *La* is very bad if it makes the inside of the mouth red and medicine should be administered with care. If the *la* gives a yellow coating to the tongue, **it is called *la-ong phrabaat*.** If the *la* is maize coloured, **it is called *saeng phrachan*** and with this the baby has diarrhoea and cannot sleep.

Medicine to treat *saang saeng phrachan*:

[201] *thian dam*
saan som
dee plee
Equal parts, 3 items. Prepare a stick using *mawaeng* fruit juice as excipient. To be mixed with *mawaeng* juice and applied to *saang saeng phrachan*.

If the pustules are red, **this *saang* is called *utthayakaan*.** At first, the eyes are yellow, the baby has spasms of the hands and feet, kicks in its sleep and neither the bowels nor bladder function.

Medicine to treat *saang utthayakaan*:

[202] *phimsen*
kluea sinthao
sakhaan
krathiam

Equal parts, 4 items. Prepare a stick. To be applied mixed with cow's milk.

If the pustules come first, **it is called *foi fai*.** After three days the back and the whole body hurt and breathing becomes difficult.

Medicine to treat *saang foi fai*:

[203]	*din prasiu khaao*	
	thong laang bai mon	bark
	rangap phit	leaves
	thian dam	
	haang chorakhe	

Equal parts, 5 items. Prepare a stick, using coconut milk as excipient. To be used, mixed with river water, as an application or lotion.

If ineffective:

[204]	*bai naat*	
	chan	arils
	phimsen	
	nam prasaan thong	

Equal parts, 4 items. Prepare a stick, mix with salt water or alcohol and paint the child's mouth.

If the pustules are leaf green with tiny blood vessels in them, by the fifth day they cause flatulence, diarrhoea and dry lips and the baby cries in a dry [husky] voice. To treat this:

[205]	*nam tao*	leaves
	phak hai	leaves
	praduu	leaves
	fak khaao	leaves
	prakham dee khwaai	fruit
	chan hom	

Equal parts, 6 items. Prepare a stick, mix with alcohol and apply. Then prepare the following mouth paint.

Mouth paint:

[206]	*thian dam*
	bai naat
	din prasiu khaao
	phrik Thai

Equal parts, 4 items. Mix with alcohol and use as a mouth paint.

If it affects the throat:

[207]	*maklam khruea*	leaves
	cha-em	

Powder and mix with honey. To be taken.

If the pustules are as dark as sapphires, it is called *ninlakaan* [black sapphire]. After one day it changes to *ninlafai* [fire sapphire], then after two days, to *ninlaphet* [diamond sapphire]. It is the same on both sides of the mouth. If *saang ninlakaan* lasts three days, half the body is paralysed and the baby cannot cry.

Medicine to treat *saang ninlakaan*:

[208]	*saaraphat phit*	fruit
	naat	root
	makruut	bark
	khon thee so	leaves
	phak hom hin	root
	thap thim	bark
	kaarabuun	
	phimsen	

Equal parts, 8 items. Prepare a stick. Mix with cow's milk and use as a mouth paint.

If this is ineffective, prepare the following:

[209]	*thua rae*	leaves
	kaan phluu	
	nam prasaan thong	
	kluai teep	root

Equal parts, 4 items. Prepare a stick using leaf juice of *tamlueng tua phuu* as excipient. Mix with river water, add some buttermilk mixed with 1/3 part of water and paint the mouth.

Lotion to counteract poisons:

[210]	*rangap thang 2*	leaves
	tamlueng tua phuu	leaves
	khok kra-om	
	yaa dap fai	
	chan hom	
	chabaa	leaves
	fak khaao	leaves
	khaa	

Equal parts, 9 items. Prepare a stick to make a lotion to treat the poison of *saang*.

[211] ***Kanlayaa thi khun***

krisanaa	
kralamphak	
khondok	
kot so	
kot khamao	
kot kaan phraao	
kot chulaa lamphaa	
kot chiang	
kot hua bua	
chan	seeds
chan	arils
kaan phluu	
krawaan	

neraphuusee
cha-em thet
phimsen
amphan thong

Equal parts, 18 items. Prepare pills, using aromatic water as excipient. To be taken mixed with rose water or aromatic water. A very spcial remedy for listlessness, loss of appetite, drowsiness and semi-consciousness caused by *taan chon.*

[212] ***Khieo noi***

rangap phit	leaves
nam tao	leaves
bai naat	
krameng	leaves
saniat	leaves
angkaap	leaves
tree katuk	
khamin oi	

Equal parts, 10 items. Pills to be taken mixed with alcohol, in doses depending on the strength of the child. To improve the appetite and to prevent the abdominal pain and diarrhoea caused by *taan chon.*

[213] ***Mahaa rot***

horaphaa	fruit
makhaam pom	fruit
phak chee	fruit
kot phung plaa	
kot hua bua	
kot so	
nam prasaan thong	
saan som	

Equal parts of each.

cha-em thet 2 parts

9 items. Make a stick. To treat the effects of *saang* on the tongue and blood and mucus in the faeces, this is to be mixed with alcohol to paint the mouth. To treat colicky pain, it is to be taken mixed with *nam kathue mok fai.* To treat diarrhoea, it is to be taken mixed with *maduea* bark sap. To alleviate all forms of *taan* and *saang,* to be taken mixed with *kaphrao* leaf juice.

[214] ***Sangkha samutthai***

malaeng mum	carcass
nam prasaan thong	
kaphrao	leaves
krawaan	fruit

Equal parts, 4 items. Prepare a stick, using alcohol as excipient. Mix with river water and use as a mouth paint.

Oily medicine:

[215] *khee wua* fresh
phluu kae leaves
krathiam
yaa dam
fin
nguu lueam bile
nam man ngaa

Mix together equal parts of these 7 ingredients. Boil until only oil remains. To be taken or applied as a mouth paint to treat *saang* in the mouth and on the tongue.

Oily medicine:

[216] *samo thet*
samo Thai
samo phiphek
mara leaves
nom phichit leaves

Equal parts, 5 items. Add sesame oil as required. Boil until only oil remains. A very special remedy to be taken or applied to treat any kind of foul smelling, putrid inflamation.

[217] ***Lueang noi***
phrik
khing
krathiam
hom daeng
phlai
khamin oi
din prasiu khaao
suphannathan daeng

Equal parts, 8 items. Prepare pills, using lime juice as excipient. To be taken mixed with alcohol to treat *taan* and *saang.*

[218] ***Lueang yai***
phrik
khing
khaa
krachaai
hom
krathiam
kathue
phlai
khamin oi
phak kaat seeds
neraphuusee
sang karanee

waan keep raet
waan ron thong
Equal parts, 14 items. Prepare pills using alcohol as excipient. To be taken mixed with alcohol to treat the poison of smallpox, boils, *taan* and *saang*, *taan chon* and very severe forms of *la-ong* and *khamao.*

Medicine for *saang* and *taan khamooi*:

[219]	*boraphet*	
	khon thee so	leaves
	kaphrao	leaves
	angkaap	leaves
	phluu kae	leaves
	phlai	
	khamin oi	

Equal parts, 7 items. Pills to be taken mixed with alcohol to treat *taan*, *saang* and *taan khamooi.*

Medicine to treat *saang daeng*:

[220]	*kammathan daeng*	
	yaa dam	
	din prasiu khaao	
	khamin oi	
	phlai	
	khat mon	leaves
	taan mon	leaves

Equal parts, 6 items. Pills to be taken mixed with alcohol to treat *saang daeng.* The masters highly recommend this prescription.

[221] ***Bencha pat***

chunsee		1
nam prasaan thong sat		2
kapi	partially burnt paste	3
kluea	roasted	4

Mix together these 4 ingredients. Powder, then add *phimsen.* Prepare a stick. Swab the throat[23] with the medicine if *saang daeng* or any other form of *saang* is severe. If it is applied in this way, the child will not vomit, not a drop. The medicine will only purge. If the child does vomit up the medicine immediately, it will not die. The treatment should be altered in accordance with the progress of the disease.

In Book II of *Khamphee prathom chindaa*, the masters have summarised the appearance and attributes of women, the kinds of *paksee*, all types of *saang*, the invasion of *paksee* and three kinds of evil *peesaat* and described the origin of *saang daeng*, *saang chon*, *saang fai*, *saang ninlapat* and all types of *saang.* It ends here.

Siddhikāriyaḥ A summary of the aetiology of all kinds of *saang* occurring in infants, so that doctors will be able to recognize them.

The origin of *saang fai*. *Saang fai* is the main illness of a child born on Sunday. When the mother is three months pregnant, she is constipated, has difficulty in urinating, blood in the urine, gastric pain, muscular tremor of the hands, feverishness, is thin and yellow, unable to walk far, has a feeling of obstruction in the supra-pubic area and lower abdomen, pain in the lumbar region, severe pain at the hips and craves for sweet things.

Description of *saang fai*. It has four major pustules. *Khamao* develops when the baby is born and it remains for seven days while the mother and child are by the fire, before it disappears. Then, if the baby is a boy, three major pustules of *saang fai* appear on the sole of the right foot and one on the left foot. If it is a girl, there will be three on the left foot. Two [sic] of the 40 minor pustules erupt on the legs and 20 on the arms.

Three months after leaving the fire, there is one major pustule in the centre of the sole of the foot. A month later, the feet are bruised and the child cannot eat or drink and tends to sleep longer. Six months after leaving the fire, another pustule comes up forming two heads together and these grow out of the flesh looking like slightly under-ripe jambolan fruit. After six to ten days they go away. After eight months, another pustule erupts, with three heads, at the ankle. After nine months, another major pustule of birth *saang* develops, with four heads and 40 followers which spread over the middle areas of both the upper and lower legs and on the knees. These minor pustules on the legs have heads the red colour of *mafai* fruit,[24] and are red and hard around the margins. They spread out like burns, and later, blisters form, then merge together. When they are ripe, they break, causing pain on the tops of the feet and up the legs as far as the hips or the waist.

The doctor is advised not to treat this condition, as those four major pustules in the abdomen will form a sore or abscess as big as a tuber of elephant yam [slightly round and about five inches in diameter]. This will become inflamed and spread to the supra-pubic area, anus, rectum and around the navel.[25] The baby will then pass blood, mucus, pus and offensive smelling liquid faeces,[26] because the major *saang* has passed through the ileum and colon and affected the liver and lungs, then emerged at the anus. The followers are painful, sting and make the baby feel hot as if burnt. When the child is going to die, the palms of the hands and soles of the feet are as red as a baby bird. Whenever the symptoms of *saang fai* occur together like this, the baby is sure to die within eight to eleven days.

A baby born on Sunday has *khamao* in the mouth because the mucus and internal heat [two of the body elements], being strong, make the child hot internally. This produces internal *khamao,* and internal *saang* and *khamao* develop as a result of the combination of [the elements] blood and mucus. Then the baby is unable to eat or drink because of the strength of the blood and mucus. Sometimes the mucus is putrid, then the infant passes mucus and blood; sometimes there are parasites. To treat it, first have this medicine prepared:

(1) **Medicine to treat *saang fai*:**

[222] *waan keep raet*
waan ron tong
neraphuusee

thian dam
thian daeng
cha-em thang 2
maklam khruea leaves

Boil until the volume has been reduced to 1/3. To be taken to lower the body temperature and to treat *taan* and *saang*. This can be made into pills and taken mixed with alcohol to treat blood and mucus in the stools.

(2) Medicine to treat *saang fai*:

[223] *yaa klet hoi*
san phraa hom leaves
phung do leaves
chueak khao fai

4 items. Prepare pills, using *nam prakham dee khwaai* as excipient. To be taken or applied, mixed with river water and python's bile.

(3) If that is not effective:

[224] *lin thale*
khong saam yaan
khamin oi
khaao saan khaang khrok

Mix together these 4 ingredients and apply to counteract the poison of *saang fai*.

(4) If ineffective:

[225]	*nam tao*	leaves
	rangap phit	leaves
	krathung maa baa	leaves
	sawaat	leaves
	kaphrao	leaves
	saniat	leaves
	mafueang	leaves
	praai	fruit
	phinlangkaasaa	fruit
	chan	seeds
	chan	arils
	krawaan	
	kaan phluu	
	thian daeng	
	nam prasaan thong	

Equal parts, 15 items. Pills to be mixed with river water with borax added. To be taken to counteract all kinds of poisoning.

(The description of *saang fai* ends here.)

Siddhikāriyaḥ **A summary of the aetiology of *saang nam* follows.** *Saang nam* is the main illness of a child born on Monday. The signs of *saang nam* when the mother is three months pregnant are: headaches, painful breasts, a craving for sweet things, muscular fatigue in both arms, sometimes hardness of hearing, night blindness, fainting, dizziness and discomfort, vomiting and severe thirst continuing until the time of delivery.

Description of *saang nam*. [The patches are] about the size of a leaf of the Chinese date [oval shaped and about 1" across] and the red colour of the almost ripe fruit of Ceylon spinach. They come up on the back and sides or on the arms and chest. There are no major pustules and the baby will not die from this. The doctor should examine it carefully, then first treat it with these medicines.

(1) **Medicine to treat *saang nam*:**

[226] *phak khraat* — leaves
phak pet — leaves
sawaat — leaves
samee — leaves
waan nam
nam prasaan thong
manaao — seeds
phrik Thai
khing — dried

Equal parts, 9 items. Pills to be taken mixed with alcohol. This has often been effectively used.

(2) If ineffective:

[227] *maeng lak* — leaves
bai naat
thian dam
pho baai — bark
dee plee

Equal parts, 5 items. Pills to be taken mixed with alcohol.

(3) If ineffective:

[228] *maduea* — bark
thong phan chang — leaves
chan — seeds
phinlangkaasaa — fruit
saaraphat phit — fruit
prakham dee khwaai — fruit
phrik Thai
khing — dried

Equal parts, 8 items. Pills to be taken mixed with alcohol.

(4) If ineffective:

[229] *praai* — fruit
raatchadat — fruit
saaraphat phit — fruit
phinlangkaasaa — fruit
nam prasaan thong

waan keep raet		
waan ron thong		
chan	seeds	
chan	arils	

Mix together 2 *salueng* of each of these 9 items, add

horaa duai kai	2 *salueng*
phrik Thai	1 *fueang*

A total of 11 ingredients. Pills to be taken mixed with alcohol. Excellent to treat *saang nam* and all kinds of *saang*.

(End of description of *saang nam*.)

Siddhikāriyaḥ **A summary of the origin of *saang daeng* follows.** *Saang daeng* is the main illness of a child born on Tuesday. The signs of *saang daeng* when the mother is three months pregnant are: sharp gastric pain, dizziness, shallow breathing, vomiting, general fatigue and muscular pain, swollen hands and feet and insomnia.

Description of *saang daeng*. There are six major pustules - three in the crown of the head and three in the middle of the spine. There are 72 followers. *Khamao* is not visible while the mother and child are by the fire, because from one to five major pustules of *saang* erupt on the palate, so there is no *khamao* while by the fire. *Khamao*, *taan* and *saang* occur after they leave the fire. When three months have passed [since leaving the fire], one of the major pustules moves from the crown to the spine, where it erupts with two heads. Then red pustules of *saang daeng* appear at the neck, chin, groins, underarms and anus. *Saang daeng* gives the baby a lot of trouble, causing diarrhoea, vomiting, thirst, listlessness and steamy eyes, and its poison produces coughing, with a dry throat and the child becomes thin and yellow, passes mucus and blood and cannot eat or drink.

The doctor should investigate whether it is the male or female form of *saang daeng* and satisfy himself quite definitely whether it is a fatal or mild form. He should give considerable care to his choice of treatment, because the baby will be in great difficulty within nine days if the wrong medicine is given. Whether they have studied the texts or not, doctors should take great care in their deliberations. After three more months, another major pustule of *saang* will appear, another after six months and another after nine to eleven lunar months, each coming from one of the primary pustules in the crown, which are the most virulent ones. These primary pustules have six heads and are poisonous and extremely painful. The doctor should be very careful with his treatment, because the baby will die unless he knows how to cure it. Drastic purgatives and drugs to expel flatus should not be given, otherwise it will be very difficult to cure later. When the baby is a year old, the virulent pustule subsides to re-emerge in and on the navel, joined by another at one year and three months of age, another at one year and six months, one year and eight months, one year and eleven months, and at two years and two months. There are then six major pustules altogether in the navel. Now the 72 followers break out with the major *saang* in the bladder, ileum, colon, supra-pubic area, spine or on the chin; on both sides of the body, in the chest, the throat or on the tongue, hurting all over. If they erupt in the supra-pubic area and bladder, they cause difficulty in urinating and constipation; in the colon, diarrhoea; in the ileum, heavy urination. When they are on the sides of the body, they produce a high temperature; in the long muscles of the back, insomnia; in the stomach, vomiting; in the bladder, extreme thirst; in the throat, dryness and coughing; in the eyes, soreness; in the mouth, redness; and the pustules in the ears produce a foul discharge from the ears.

In order to be able to distinguish between male *saang daeng* and female *saang daeng*, the doctor should know that, if it [unspecified] comes up in the armpits, it withdraws and re-emerges on the right side of a male child and on the left side of a female child. When the female variety of *saang daeng* is finished, the male variety of *saang daeng* develops as one pustule under each arm. Then the baby will die. *Saang daeng* establishes itself at three to nine months of age, continuing until one year and nine months of age, when it enters the body internally, resulting in the child passing blood, mucus and pus in the stools. The spleen hangs down [is enlarged], the child has a high temperature, is thin and yellow, passes yellow faeces and urine, has abdominal colic and excessive mucus/ arises at the left and right and at the centre,[27] and/causes muscular spasms of the hands and feet. When he sees this, the doctor should examine the navel to see if it has dropped down on either side or in the centre. If so, he must take the precaution of treating it. If this is not the case, then this *lom* is called *utthangkhammaawaat.* It will go away by itself if care is taken of the baby from the time it is by the fire until it is three months old. If the doctor gives medicine and exorcises the spirits, and it does not go, then the primary pustule will move down from the navel and along the ribs and chest and will emerge in the navel [sic]. It is then called *lom kong yai*, and it blows from the navel up along the tendons, and blood and mucus travel up close to the spine to the upper chest and the throat, and from there, quickly diffuse to the ears, nose and the crown of the head.

Doctors should understand clearly that the baby will die if it is the time of the waxing moon; if it is the dark of the moon, it will not die. This disease is called *trabong Rāhū, maanthalun, atsawamukkhee* or *taphan fai* - it has many names. It can happen to both boys and girls, there is no difference. To treat it, first prepare this medicine:

(1) Medicine to treat *saang daeng:*

[230]	*boraphet*	
	matuum	bark
	hom daeng	
	kaarabuun	
	phrik Thai	
	khing	dried
	krathiam	

Equal parts, 7 items. Prepare pills to be taken mixed with alcohol.

(2) If ineffective:

[231]	*kot so*	
	kot khamao	
	thian khaao	
	chan hom	
	chum het	leaves

Equal parts, 5 items. Prepare pills using lime water as excipient. To be taken mixed with alcohol or applied mixed with alcohol and *phimsen* to treat *saang daeng* and *saang puang* [possibly cholera].

(3) If ineffective:

[232] *phak waan baan*
thap thim leaves
khamin oi
masaang heartwood
Equal parts, 4 items. Pills to be taken mixed with alcohol.

(4) If ineffective:

[233] *boraphet*
kraphrao leaves
khamin oi
krawaan fruit
kaan phluu
faang
fin
benyakaanee
Equal parts, 8 items. Prepare pills. Before it is to be used, add a small amount of python's bile. To be taken or applied to treat *saang daeng* and all forms of *saang*.

(5) If ineffective:

[234] ***Yaa daeng yai***
kammathan daeng
phimsen
krisanaa
kot thang 5
thian thang 5
chan arils
khrai khruea root
cha-em thet
chaat kon
kamyaan
lot thanong
see siat thet
saan som
sak khee
samo thet
waan rong thong
neraphuusee
tumkaa daeng
Equal parts, 26 items. Prepare pills using alcohol as excipient. To be

taken or applied mixed with alcohol, to treat *saang daeng* and all kinds of *saang*.

(End of description of *saang daeng*.)

Siddhikāriyaḥ **A summary of the origin of *saang sako* follows.** *Saang sako* is the main illness of a child born on Wednesday. When the mother is three months pregnant, the signs of *saang sako* are: severe, griping abdominal pains [colic]; at five months, vomiting; at seven months, swelling of the legs from the feet to the thighs, with great difficulty in moving the hips; she finds the taste of food bitter, has small pustules at the anus and urethra and general fatigue until delivery.

Description of *saang sako*. There are four major pustules in the abdomen. After three days at the fire, the infant has *khamao* accompanied by 42 followers. The four major pustules have ten followers each; four at the anus, five at the spleen and one at the crown of the head. After leaving the fire, the baby has *khamao taan* and *khamao saang*. Three months later, all the followers spread throughout the body and intestines. The four at the anus cause constipation and difficulty in defecation and urinating; the five at the spleen move to the upper chest, then emerge at the throat, tongue and mouth, remaining for three months.

When this happens, the doctor should ascertain whether it is *saang sako* and if so be sure to give the right treatment, otherwise the baby is sure to die within two months. The followers in the abdomen spread, then come together in the chest. Two of the major pustules in the abdomen move up to the lower gums, one appearing on each side, with six or seven followers in front of the teeth and in the upper and lower gums. These cause diarrhoea, vomiting, thirst, fever, and the baby is lethargic, stuporous and restless. The major pustule in the crown of the head moves down to the spine, causing backache and flatulence. This happens once at four months and again at eight months. In time, the *saang* moves inside, then the baby has diarrhoea, passes blood, mucus and pus, has yellow eyes and yellow urine, cannot eat or drink, has abdominal distension and an aversion to food. This recurs at one year, one year and six months, one year and eight months and at two years and ten months, causing colic, thinness and yellowness, stomach ache and inability to eat or drink. In such cases, whenever the major pustules of *saang sako* come together in the abdomen, one in the navel, one above it and one on each side, they cause griping abdominal pains. Also, the 42 followers appear, some on the sides, some in the armpits, some in the tendons, some inside the spine and on the shoulders, elbows and knees, causing various illnesses depending on the age of the patient. It is established that *saang sako* affects all children in this way and doctors should know this. To treat it, have this medicine prepared first, as follows:

(1) **Medicine to treat *saang sako*:**

[235]	*tanot*	root
	maak mia	root
	chum het thet	root
	mafueang	leaves
	khaa	young
	krachaai	

phrik lon

Equal parts, 7 items. Pills to be taken mixed with alcohol.

(2) If ineffective:

[236]	*lep mue naang*	root
	mon ko	root
	(sometimes it is *malako* root) [sic]	
	samun waeng	
	marum	root
	sakhaan	
	waan naang kham	
	khing	
	dee plee	

Equal parts, 7 items. Pills to be taken mixed with alcohol.

(3) If ineffective:

[237]	*chang thang 2*	
	thon dee	root
	phak hom	root
	khrai khruea	root
	phrik Thai	
	krathiam	

Equal parts, 7 items. Pills to be taken mixed with alcohol.

(4) If ineffective:

[238]	*chetta phang khee*	
	phayaa mue lek	
	samo thet	
	kralam phak	
	khing	dried
	khondok	
	kot hua bua	
	kot phung plaa	
	khai nao	bark

Equal parts, 9 items. Pills to be taken mixed with alcohol to treat *saang sako*. This has definitely been used frequently.

(End of description of *saang sako.*)

Siddhikāriyaḥ **A summary of the origin of *saang wua* follows.** *Saang wua* is the main illness of a child born on Thursday. The signs of *saang wua* when the mother is three months pregnant are: inflammation inside the mouth and five or six pustules along each side of the tongue, so that she cannot eat hot-and-spicy food. At six months, the sores spread to the middle of the tongue, then break and are very painful and sting. She has diarrhoea with blood and mucus in the stools continuing until delivery when this clears up.

Description of *saang wua.* There are four major pustules, and 40 followers. *Saang wua* starts with *khamao taan* and *khamao saang* filling the mouth of the baby at the fire, then going away. Next, a rash of small spots covers the body, like a heat rash, and this causes a high temperature and writhing of the body. When this subsides, the child has diarrhoea. The four major pustules erupt when the baby is three months old; one at the tip of the tongue, one on each side of the tongue and one, with three heads, at the root of the tongue. This last is the primary pustule of *saang* and the most virulent.[28] When the child is six months old, the primary pustule goes down into the abdomen, then ten followers enter the stomach and 40 appear in the tongue and cheeks. The primary pustule within produces diarrhoea, vomiting and thirst. At nine months of age, the primary pustule at the tip of the tongue descends within the right side of the abdomen and ten followers go to the bladder, causing diarrhoea, vomiting and thirst. At eleven months of age, the major pustules at the sides of the tongue, together with 30 followers, descend; one major pustule with ten followers to each of the colon and ileum and another ten followers to the supra-pubic area below the abdomen. When the child has reached a year and six months, it passes mucus and blood in the stools. The doctor should make sure that his diagnosis is correct and treat *saang wua* within nine or ten days. First have these medicines prepared according to the stages of the disease.

(1) **Medicine to treat *saang wua*:**

[239]	*ching cho*	fruit
	mo noi	fruit
	yaa tai bai	
	neraphuusee	
	samo thet	
	nom wua khon	
	chan	seeds
	chan	arils
	phrik Thai	

Equal parts, 9 items. Pills to be taken mixed with alcohol.

(2) If ineffective:

[240]	*som saa*	leaves
	makruut	leaves
	mafueang	leaves
	haeo muu	
	khoei taai	fruit
	samo phiphek	
	chaa phluu	root

Equal parts, 7 items. To be taken mixed with alcohol and a small amount of python's bile.

(3) If ineffective:

[241]	*lao lok*	fruit
	krawaan	fruit
	phum riang	fruit
	phrik Thai	
	khamin oi	
	nam prasaan thong	

Equal parts, 6 items. Pills to be taken mixed with alcohol.

(4) If ineffective, use this:

[242] ***Yaa yai***

makok thet	fruit
prakham dee khwaai	fruit
taan khamooi	fruit
matuum	fruit
marum	bark
benyakaanee	
chan	arils
kaan phluu	
hing haai	root
khondok	
chaluut	

Equal parts, 11 items. Prepare pills to be taken mixed with alcohol or to be used, mixed with aromatic water, as an application to treat *saang wua*. Very potent.

(End of description of *saang wua*.)

Siddhikāriyaḥ **A summary of the aetiology of *saang chaang* follows.** *Saang chaang* is the main illness of a child born on Friday. The signs of *saang chaang* when the mother is three months pregnant are: itchy spots like a heat rash at the urethra, which break, become inflamed and suppurate, spreading out around the area, causing severe pain in the supra-pubic region, pain at the loins and difficulty in urinating. She has gastric pain during the fourth, fifth, sixth and seventh months and swollen feet from the eighth or ninth month up to the time of delivery.

After the baby is born and by the fire, it has *khamao* which increases layer upon layer until it becomes very thick. *Saang* comes up from inside the abdomen to the chest and throat, and from the throat, it travels up to the tongue. After nine to eighteen or nineteen days, it comes out all over the tongue and mouth. Three months after leaving the fire, three major pustules erupt in the abdomen, two or three in the palate and three in the chest. Six months after leaving the fire, the two or three pustules in the palate descend to the throat and 80 followers emerge in lines, here and there, on both legs, on both sides of the supra-pubic area, on the arms, on the sides and in the middle of the spine. When these all erupt at the same time like this, the major pustules which have moved from the palate to the throat cause a dry, sore throat, coughing and dry retching, bruises and spots around the throat and suppurating sores and itching all over the body. Nine months after leaving the fire, these sores dry up by themselves. Then, when they have withdrawn internally, the baby has diarrhoea, vomiting and thirst, and is unable to eat or drink. Small pustules next erupt in the cheeks and, each day, five or six major pustules come up somewhere on the body. At one year and three months of age, the major pustules in the throat move down to join those in the chest, making five there. These cause a high temperature from afternoon to midnight, when they subside, but even though the baby is very thirsty, it takes little milk and is lethargic and stuporous.

During the next four months, the five major pustules in the chest go down to the stomach. The child is not hungry. Then these pustules erupt in the intestines causing constipation; next they move to the supra-pubic area where they cause difficulty in urinating.

As the child develops, when it starts to sit and to walk, it passes mucus and blood, because the liver, lungs, intestines and abdomen are swollen. And when it eats fat and meat which are strange and new to the four elements of the body [that is, to which the body is unaccustomed], this *saang* has an opportunity to arise, and it causes aches and pains and many problems.

The doctor should realize that the baby will not die if he knows how to cure it. If he does not know, the baby will die. He should examine the abdomen, neck and chest of the child if it dies, and he will notice that the area around the abdomen looks [speckled] like the egg of a bulbul; the upper chest is as blue as a crow's egg; the neck is blood red; and the body is swollen. Doctors wishing to treat it should understand *saang chaang* and make an accurate diagnosis then use this medicine first.

(1) **Medicine to treat *saang chaang*:**

[243]	*chup het thet [chum het thet]*	leaves
	sawaat	leaves
	phak khuang	leaves
	kaphrao	leaves
	la-ong phrakrit	leaves

Equal parts, 5 items. Prepare pills using as excipient fresh urine of a horse. To be taken mixed with alcohol.

(2) If ineffective:

[244]	*phak khraat*	
	khop chanaang daeng	
	khop chanaang khaao	
	phak sian phee	
	khamin oi	
	prakham dee khwaai	fruit
	phrik Thai	
	rayom	

Equal parts, 7 items. Pills to be taken mixed with alcohol.

(3) If ineffective:

[245]	*yaa sai*		1 *kam mue*
	tao rang	young shoots	1 *kam mue*
	krathue		
	phlai		
	taan sian		

Equal parts, 5 items. Reduce to a powder to be taken mixed with alcohol.

(4) If ineffective, prepare this:

[246].	***Yaa yai***	
	san phraa mon	root

chamot ton	root
phimsen	leaves
chuk rohinee	
sang karanee	
phak chee lom	fruit
phak chee laa	fruit
phak kaat	fruit
phinlangkaasaa	fruit
chan thet	fruit
kralamphak	
waan ron thong	
khing	dried

Equal parts, 13 items. Pills to be taken mixed with alcohol to treat *saang chaang*. Without a doubt, this is a very special and reliable remedy which is highly recommended.

(End of description of *saang chaang*.)

Siddhikāriyaḥ **Next, a summary of the aetiology of *saang khamooi*.** *Saang khamooi* is the main illness of a child born on Saturday. The signs of *saang khamooi* when the mother is three months pregnant are: a craving for raw and undercooked fish and meat, duck, hen and turtle eggs, hot-and-spicy food, sweet and sour flavours and strong salads. She feels restless, her breasts hurt and sores erupt in her mouth, which spread and become inflamed and she passes mucus and blood in the stools. She has a sore throat and severe pain at the waist until the time of delivery.

Saang khamooi has nine major pustules. When the infant is three days old, there are two major pustules in the spine. At three months the *saang* appears in the mouth - one pustule in the upper gums and one in the lower gums. Sometimes these have yellow heads. Sometimes they come up on or beside the navel, resembling broken rice. The centres are black, with a rim, and next to that, yellow. The bases are red. The baby has a pattern on its body like the spiny eel. The major pustules [have spots] like daphnia and make the whole body hurt and sting. When the baby is six months old, inflamed pitted sores appear all over the body causing continual diarrhoea. The major pustules at the crown [not previously mentioned] then descend to the centre of the back where all five pustules merge, then the sores go away. Another major pustule moves down from the crown of the head to the middle of the back, at eight or nine months of age, one year, and one year and six months, increasing the number of pustules in the back, one by one, until there are nine [eight] altogether. These cause diarrhoea and vomiting. When all eight have come together, they erupt in the abdomen, giving the child diarrhoea with offensive smelling, liquid faeces with mucus, blood and pus. When the *saang* has reached the abdomen, one pustule with ten followers moves to the supra-pubic area; a similar group enters the bladder; one major pustule erupts in each eye, with nine followers; one, with six followers, on the right side of the throat; and one, with four lesser ones, on the left side of the throat. When this happens, with the major *saang* spread to the important organs, then the baby is poisoned and this is a sign of death.

From the age of nine, ten or eleven months up to one year and two, three, four, five or six months, the child has blurred vision for fifteen days to a month, because the major pustules of *saang* are in the eyes. Then there is mucus in the eyes and a series of membranes develops at the outer corners of the eyes, encroaching on the eyeballs, making the eyes itchy, because the major pustules and followers spread all over the eyes and the vitreous humour dries up. The doctor must be sure to give the right medicine, otherwise the baby might lose one or both eyes. The five followers around the throat cause a sore throat, coughing and vomiting of water only and enter the stomach, with the result that the baby does not want to eat. When they enter the bladder, the child becomes thirsty, craves fishy and meaty food and sweet things, which are very harmful, and prefers fish to rice. When they enter the liver, the child passes blood and mucus and becomes chicken-chested. When they enter the ileum, the faeces are as green as a leaf and the body is covered with scales, like a cobra. When they enter the colon, the baby has diarrhoea, with faeces like liquor ferment. When they enter the abdomen and the external and internal areas of the spine, diarrhoea and severe, stinging, burning gastric pain follow. When they enter the supra-pubic area, the baby has dysentery, with intestinal pain and prolapsed anus and is averse to water, thin and yellow; and when death approaches, the *saang* in the eyes and on the eyelids moves down to attack both sides of the throat. The major pustules are as large as Chinese dates, and the followers from the eyes erupt all over the tongue and the uvula and around the lips like raw cotton. The child is certain to die if the doctor cannot cure it within four to six days. *Saang khamooi* should not be treated if the major pustules ripen and become as yellow as turmeric, flatten and then move down to the root of the tongue. If you want to know whether or not it is in the throat, as explained, apply some medicine to the finger, and insert the finger into the throat and feel it. If it is as described, the baby will surely die.

To treat this, use the following medicines in sequence.

Medicine to treat *saang khamooi:*

[247] *akkhanee chawaa*

raatchadat	fruit
prakham dee khwaai	fruit
chan	seeds
manaao	seeds
fin	
nguu lueam	bile

Equal parts, 7 items. Prepare gold coated pills. To be taken mixed with alcohol to treat internal poisoning. If the child is unconscious for a whole day and remains so at night time, it will revive if it is able to take this medicine. To treat the poison of *saang khamooi*, *saang daeng* and all kinds of *saang*.

[248] ***Lueang horadaan***

horadaan thong		1 *baht*
rong thong	toasted until cooked	1 *fueang*
khamin oi		1 *fueang*
phimsen		1 *fueang* 2 *phai*

Equal parts, 5 items. Pills to be taken mixed with alcohol to treat *saang lueang* and all kinds of *saang*.

[249] ***Khaao kabang***

kabang		1 *baht*
bia phuu	calcined	1 *salueng*
chan khaao		1 *salueng*
phimsen		2 *phai*
chan	seeds	1 *fueang*
chan	arils	1 *fueang*

6 items. Prepare pills using alcohol as excipient. To treat *saang khaao* and all kinds of *saang*.

[250] ***Khieo khee thong***

yaa khieo khee thong		1 *baht*
chan	seeds	1 *fueang*
chan	arils	1 *fueang*
krawaan		1 *fueang*
kaan phluu		1 *fueang*
kaarabuun		1 *fueang*
horaa duei kai		1 *fueang*

7 items. To be taken mixed with alcohol to treat *saang khieo* and all kinds of *saang*.

[251] ***Dam muek***

muek hom		1 *baht*
chan	seeds	1 *fueang*
thian thang 5	of each	1 *fueang*
horaa duei kai		1 *fueang*

4 items. Pills to be taken mixed with alcohol to treat *saang dam* and all kinds of *saang*.

[252] ***Yaa daeng***

kammathan daeng		2 *salueng*
phimsen		1 *fueang*
kot thang 5	of each	1 *fueang*
thian thang 5	of each	1 *fueang*
chan	arils	1 *fueang*
khrai khruea	root	1 *salueng*
cha-em thet		1 *fueang*
chaat kon		1 *fueang*
kam yaan		1 *fueang*
lot thanong		1 *fueang*
see siat thet		1 *fueang*
saan som		1 *fueang*
krak chee [krak khee]		1 *fueang*
samo thet		1 *fueang*
waan ron thong		1 *fueang*

neraphuusee	1 *fueang*
rangap yai	1 *fueang*
kaarabuun	2 *phai*

27 items. Reduce to powder. To be taken mixed with alcohol to treat *saang yot daeng* [*saang daeng*] and all kinds of *saang*.

Whenever the doctor definitely identifies one of these diseases, then *Yaa lueang, Yaa khaao, Yaa khieo, Yaa dam, or Yaa daeng* [yellow, white, green, black or red medicine] should be prescribed as appropriate. *Yaa dam* and *Yaa daeng* are both used to treat *la-ong phloeng*, but *nam krisanaa* is used as the medicinal vehicle, whether it is to be taken as a mixture or to be used as a throat paint.

(End of description of *saang khamooi*.)

Siddhikāriyaḥ Summary of symptoms of fevers of infants, so that doctors will understand.

First of all, if the tendons of the baby's forefinger look as red as *nam chaat* [vermilion] or fiery red, it has fever caused by *saang daeng* and it has a disorder of the element fire. Prepare medicine for *saang daeng*, and it will counteract the fever and the element fire, and the baby's strength will improve.

And if the fever is due to mucus, the baby will vomit after eating rice or milk. If the fever is due to [the element] wind it always lies quietly, but does not sleep, the chin becomes stiff [lockjaw] and the vision blurred. Examine the eyes carefully.

If it is due to fire and mucus, the eyes are bright and not dull.

If the baby has fever in the first, second or third month of the year do not let the mother eat the white gourd.

If fever occurs in the fourth, fifth, sixth, seventh or eighth month, do not let the mother have sugar cane or palm sugar, bathe in the rain,[29] or eat sweet fruits.

And if fever develops in the ninth, tenth, eleventh or twelfth month, do not let the mother eat raw meat and fish, or strong salads and dishes made from unheated raw fish.

Next follow recipes for medicines for all diseases.

[253] ***Bencha taan*** [cf. no. 92]

taan thang 5	
chan thang 2	
cha-em thang 2	
thian thang 5	
waan keep raet	
waan rong thong	
chan	seeds
benyakaanee	
maklam khruea	

Equal parts, 19 items. Powder together, then add fruit of *prakham dee khwaai*. Make a decoction [by boiling with water], then prepare pills using water as excipient.

If the child is passing mucus and blood, the pills are to be taken mixed with alcohol. If the child is thirsty or vomits, they are to be taken mixed with hot water; if this is ineffective, with *cha-em* and *chan* seeds; if this is ineffective, with *sawaat* leaf sap. If the body is very hot and the child has a fever due to internal heat and wind, mix with aromatic water and *phimsen.* If the crown of the child's head is very cold, the fever is due to mucus combined with wind, and the pills are to be taken with *nam chum het thet.* If the child is vomiting, its body is hot and the skin yellow, the illness is due to mucus combined with bile, and the pills are to be taken mixed with *nam chan.* If a child is ill in any way, the doctor should first treat it with *Yaa bencha taan* as described here, using the medicinal vehicle appropriate to the disease, according to the texts.

Medicine to treat wind affecting a child so that it makes the face blue and the eyes roll up and back, for example:

[254]	*hing yaang pho*	1
	thian dam	2
	thian khaao	3
	krathiam	4
	kraphang hom	8

5 items. Pills to be taken mixed with alcohol to treat abdominal pain, putrid mucus in the abdomen, and stomach ache increasing until vomiting occurs, caused by abnormal elements.

If a baby has fever from morning till noon, it is because of the harmful effects of mucus and internal heat. The *saang* and *khamao* then seize the opportunity to spread inside the body, then the baby cannot eat because of the mucus. Sometimes the mucus is purulent, causing the child to pass mucus and blood in the faeces. To treat this:

[255] *waan keep raet*
waan ron thong
neraphuusee
sang karanee
thian dam
thian daeng
cha-em thang 2
maklam khruea

Equal parts, 9 items. Pills. To reduce the body temperature, to be taken mixed with aromatic water; to treat *saang,* to be taken mixed with alcohol; to treat diarrhoea, it is to be taken mixed with *nam chan.*

Medicine to expel poison of all kinds:

[256]	*khrai khruea ton*	root
	khrai khruea	root
	phitsanaat	
	plaa lai phueak	
	nom maeo	root
	krak khee	
	nguu lueam	bones
	sang	
	muk	
	kammathan daeng	

dee plee		
neraphuusee		
benyakaanee		
waan kleep raet [waan keep raet]		
waan ron thong		
sadao	seeds	

Mix together 1 *salueng* of each of these 16 ingredients, and add

makhaam pom		2 *salueng*
mahaa kaan	rhizome	2 *salueng*
chan khaao		2 *salueng*
raeng	bones	2 *salueng*
plao noi		2 *salueng*
rayom		2 *salueng*
krisanaa		2 *salueng*
kralamphak		2 *salueng*
raet	molar tooth	2 *salueng*
chaang	molar tooth	2 *salueng*
chan	seeds	2 *salueng*
tao lueang	carapace	2 *salueng*
saaraphat phit	fruit	2 *salueng*
yaa dam		12 *baht* 2 *salueng*

32 items. Prepare pills the size of *thong laang* fruit. Dry in the sun, and keep in a bottle to protect it from the air. To counteract the poison of smallpox, boils and severe forms of *saang* which cause unconsciousness from morning to midday, to be taken mixed with rose water. If the medicine comes up as soon as it reaches the stomach, mix with *nam maduea*. If there is acute abdominal pain, add some opium and if the child vomits, add *phimsen*.

Medicine to treat *saang daeng*:

[257]	*benyakaanee*	
	nguu lueam	bones
	kwaang	horn
	cha-em thet	
	samo phiphek	
	khrai khruea	root

Mix together 1 *fueang* of each of these 6 ingredients. Prepare a stick to be mixed with alcohol and taken or used as a throat paint. Before applying to the throat, add *phimsen* to the mixture to counteract *saang daeng* and all kinds of *saang*.

Medicine to dab on the pustules of *saang*:

[258]	*kaphrao*	leaves
	sawaat	leaves
	chum het	leaves
	krathiam	

khamin oi
kluea sinthao
nam prasaan thong
Add a little *chunsee* and prepare a stick using lime juice as excipient. To use in the mouth, mix with alcohol; to use in the throat, mix with lime water and dab on the pustules only.

There is one kind of *saang* in which the pustules cannot be seen, but a red eczematous eruption, which spreads. This is called *saang daeng*. Treat this by applying:

[259] *khon thee so* — powdered root

and give by mouth:

[260] *chik* — root
chaang — molar tooth
powdered together.

There is one kind of *saang* which is smooth and white, and has no pustules. This is called *saang khaao plueak*. To treat it:

[261] *kaang plaa* — powdered root
To be taken and applied. If the child has severe diarrhoea, give by mouth:

[262] *mangkhut* — powdered root

The *saang* which erupts like an expanse of mud puddles, and is slightly yellowish-white, **is called *sang takua*.** To treat this:

[263] *mo noi* — powdered root
To be applied.

And:

[264] *matuum* — powdered root
To be taken.

One very bad kind of *saang* erupts like pimples. **This is called *saang khamooi*.** To treat *saang khamooi:*

[265] *taan dam* — root
taan mon — root
Reduce to a powder to be taken and applied.

One kind of *saang* erupts and then subsides. **This is called *saang khum*.** To treat *saang khum:*

[266] *kaa kathing* — root
Reduce to a powder to be taken and applied.

There is one kind of *saang* **called *saang taan*,** which erupts then shrinks and softens. To treat *saang taan*:

[267] *faai daeng* — root
phak waan — root
Reduce to a powder to be taken and applied.

If *saang* erupts all over the body and affects the soft parts, this is called *saang khamooi* or *saang khum*.

[268]	*nam taan*	granulated	1 cupful
	nam taan mon		1 cupful

	nam taan dam		1 cupful
	nam taan tanot		1 cupful
	nam taan khamooi		3 cupfuls
	nam ching cho		1 cupful
	nam khee khwaii		1 cupful
	nam man ngaa		1 cupful

8 items. Simmer until all of the water has evaporated, leaving only oil remaining. Apply to all kinds of *saang.*

Oil to treat spreading *taan* which causes inflammation all over the body:

[269]	*maphrao*	the cream of three fruits [coconuts]	
	nam man ngaa		1 cupful

Boil down until only oil remains, then add

	thian dam		1 *fueang*
	thian khaao		1 *fueang*
	thian sattabut		1 *fueang*
	fin		1 *fueang*
	see siat		1 *fueang*
	chan takhian		1 *fueang*

6 items. Mix together, reduce to a powder and add the oil. To be applied to *taan* and *saang* which spread and cause inflammation.

Medicine to treat *taan* and *saang* :

[270]	*phrommi*	leaves	
	cha-em		
	maklam khruea		
	kluea		
	khanthatsakon		

Equal parts. Pills to be taken or applied [mixed with a liquid] to counteract the poison of all kinds of *saang.*

Medicine to treat intestinal worms [*sai duean*]:

[271]	*thian yaaowa phaanee*		1 *salueng*
	cha-em		1 *salueng*
	phluu	leaves	1 *salueng*
	krung khamao		1 *salueng*
	mawaeng ton	fruit	1 *salueng*
	phalaan satruu	fruit	5 *salueng*
	sakae	fruit	3 *salueng*
	nam prasaan thong		3 *salueng*
	chik	root	3 *salueng*
	khing khraeng		3 *salueng*
	samo thang 3	of each	2 *salueng*

13 items. Pills to be taken mixed with alcohol, in doses according to the strength of the child, to counteract the flatulence of *taan* and *saang* and to expel intestinal worms. When the child has taken this medicine, all the worms will come away.

Decoction to treat *paang*:[30]

[272]	*taan khamooi*	
	taan sian	
	peep	root
	maklam khruea	root
	lep mue naang	root
	sawaat	root
	kaphrao	root
	samrong	bark
	som sieo	rind

Equal parts, 9 items. Reduce to 1/3 volume by boiling. To be taken to treat *taan* and *saang* in the chest and *paang*.

Another:

[273]	*maklam khruea*	root
	makhuea khuen	root
	som sieo	rind
	samrong	root
	lep mue naang	root
	peep	root
	phinlangkaasaa	fruit

Equal parts, 7 items. Reduce to 1/3 volume by boiling. To be taken to treat *paang*.

Medicine to treat vomiting and hiccoughs:

[274] *khaao tok*
khanthatsakon
priang prakho
kluea thet

Equal parts. Grind down and mix with fruit juice of *yo*. Prepare a decoction to be taken.

To treat the discomfort of bladder obstruction [or inability to urinate]:

[275]	*waan proh*	
	phluu kae	
	nam tao	leaves
	thaan fai paa chaa	

Do not use equal parts of each. (It appears that this should be use equal parts of each.) [sic] Poultice. Apply to the supra-pubic area.

Another, to treat retention of urine:

[276]	*waan proh*	
	phluu kae	leaves
	phrik	
	khing	

Equal parts to be ground together. Apply to the lower abdomen and supra-pubic area.

Application for the abdomen to treat flatulence and hiccoughs:

[277] *phrik Thai*
khing
krathiam
hom
hing
hua phluu
Equal parts to be ground together. Apply to the lower abdomen to counteract flatulence and hiccoughs.

To treat incessant diarrhoea in children:

[278]	*son thet*	
	prakham dee khwai	fruit
	praduu	heartwood
	som poi	root
	chum het	root

Equal parts. Reduce to 1/3 volume by boiling. To be taken.

Decoction to treat *taan khamooi:*

[279]	*taan tanot*	root	5 *tamlueng*
	taan mon	root	5 *tamlueng*
	sanun	bark	5 *tamlueng*
	khamin oi		5 *tamlueng*
	takhrai		5 *tamlueng*

Reduce to 1/3 volume by boiling. To be taken to treat *saang*. To treat the elements fire and wind and to increase the vigour, add *phimsen*, and it will restore the elements to their normal condition.

Medicine to treat *saang daeng, saang khum,* and *saang yuang*:

[280]	*maklam khruea*	leaves	1
	nam prasaan thong		1
	cha-em thet		1
	nam man (which kind of oil is not specified in the original) [sic]		1 cupful

Boil together, then paint the tongue to treat all kinds of *saang* in the throat. It is worth the weight of 10 *baht* in gold.

[281]	***Thepphayaa nimit***		
	khrai khruea	root	2
	phitsanaat		1
	chetta phang khee	root	1
	sang karanee	root	1
	waan keep raet		1
	waan ron thong		1
	neraphuusee		1
	chan thang 2		1
	cha-em		1
	prakham dee khwaii	fruit	1

nguu lueam	bile	1

Equal parts, 11 items. Pills to be taken mixed with alcohol to treat the poison of smallpox and all kinds of *taan* and *saang*.

Cleansing medicine called *Phrom nimit:*

[282]

hing yaang pho	1 *tamlueng*
phrik Thai	1 *tamlueng*
dong dueng	1 *tamlueng*

3 items. Prepare pills the size of kapok seeds. To be taken mixed with alcohol to treat the poison of *saang khamooi* and all kinds of *saang*.

[283] ***Inthachon***

chan daeng	
benyakaanee	
neraphuusee	
kwaang	horn
raet	molar tooth
chaang	molar tooth
kraphrao	root
takhrai	
nam prasaan thong	
proh	fresh
phak sian phee	
cha-em thet	
waai takhaa	
yaa khaao yen	
nguu lueam	bile

Equal parts, 15 items. Prepare pills using ripe areca nut juice as excipient. To be taken mixed with *nam chan*. This is highly recommended to treat the diarrhoea of *taan* and *saang*. [cf. no.131]

[284] ***Mahaa khong khaa***

yaa nguang chaang	leaves
khamin oi	
nam tao	leaves
kathung maa baa	leaves
thao wan priang	leaves
phak waan	leaves
rangap	leaves
prakham dee khwaai	leaves
din prasiu khaao	

Equal parts, 9 items. Pills to be mixed with aromatic water or water used to wash rice, as required, and used as an application to treat the poison of *taan, saang* and all distressing kinds of poison.

[285] ***Mahaa khong khaa*** [same name as above]

muuk man	fruit	1 *salueng*

yaang daeng	bark	1 *salueng*
yaang khaao	bark	1 *salueng*
phak krashet		1 *salueng*
phinlangkaasaa	fruit	1 *salueng*
haeo muu		1 *salueng*
chuk rohinee		1 *salueng*
krung khamao		1 *salueng*

8 items. Pills to be taken mixed with alcohol to treat the poison of *saang* causing the child to pass blood and mucus in the stools, and to treat the *tridoṣa* and painful dysentery; to treat the passage of red faeces resembling water used to wash meat. If this is ineffective add python's bile, and it will cease.

[286] ***Yaa lueang* to treat unconsciousness:**

chan thang 2
benyakaanee
neraphuusee
waan keep raet
waan ron thong
sang karanee
krawaan
kaan phluu
kammathan daeng

1 *fueang* of each of these 10 ingredients to be powdered together, then add some phython's bile and *phimsen.* Soak in water, then prepare pills to be taken mixed with syrup. To treat unconsciousness resulting from the poison of *taan, saang* or smallpox, mix it with alcohol. To treat snakebite, this prescription is to be taken mixed with crocodile's bile.

Application for the abdomen:

[287] *hatsakhun thang 2*	
rong	
hing	
chetta muun phloeng	
waan nam	
bai naat	
phrik Thai	
khing	
krathiam	
phlai	
samae thale	heartwood
phluu kae	leaves
chetta phang khee	root

Equal parts, 14 items. Prepare a stick. Mix with *nam phlai* and use as an application to the abdomen.

Laxative for children:

[288]	*tree katuk*		1 *fueang*
	krathiam		1 *fueang*
	chan	seeds	1 *fueang*
	chan	arils	1 *fueang*
	benyakaanee		1 *fueang*
	kaan phluu		1 *fueang*
	nam prasaan thong		1 *fueang*
	saan som		1 *fueang*
	kluea sinthao		1 *fueang*
	chaang	molar tooth	1 *fueang*
	thian dam		1 *fueang*
	waan ron thong		1 *fueang*
	kot kraduuk		1 *fueang*
	kot kaan phraao		1 *fueang*
	nguu lueam	bile	2 *salueng*
	salot	fruit	1 *baht*

18 items. Prepare pills the size of kapok seeds. [Dose to be taken according to the development of the child as follows:] 3 months, 3 pills; [old enough to be] able to sit up, 5 pills; able to crawl, 7; able to walk, 9. To treat blood and mucus in the stools, the pills are to be given mixed with alcohol. To treat all kinds of *saang*, mix with *kaphrao* leaf sap.

Laxative for children:

[289]	*kaphrao*	leaves	1 *salueng*
	taan mon	leaves	1 *salueng*
	sawaat	leaves	1 *salueng*
	chan	seeds	2 *phai*
	chan	arils	2 *phai*
	dee plee		2 *phai*
	kaan phluu		2 *phai*
	krawaan		2 *phai*
	yaa dam		6 *salueng*
	salot	the seeds of 7 fruits,boiled until cooked	

10 items. Prepare pills the size of peppercorns, using alcohol as excipient. To be taken mixed with goat's milk. If the child is aged 1 month, give 1 pill; 2 months, 2 pills; 3 months, 3 pills; and increase the dose in proportion to the age of the child.

Laxative for children:

[290]	*phak khraat*	leaves
	phak khet	leaves
	chum het thet	leaves
	kaphrao	leaves
	yaa tai bai	leaves

samo thet	leaves
nam prasaan thong	
khamin oi	

Equal parts, 8 items. Add a quantity of *salot* leaves equal to twice the rest of the ingredients. Prepare pills the size of kapok seeds, to be taken mixed with alcohol. Dose according to age: 4 to 5 months, 1 pill and then increase the dose in proportion to the age of the child.

Medicine to treat *taan* and *saang*:

[291]	*nam tao*	leaves
	khop chanaang thang 2	
	taan mon	leaves
	chum het thet	leaves
	rangap	leaves
	muun kaa daeng	leaves
	kathue	
	phlai	
	hom daeng	
	krathiam	
	phrik Thai	
	khing	
	khamin oi	

Equal parts, 14 items. Pills to be taken to counteract the effects of *taan* and *saang*, and mucus and blood in the stools. If the faeces have an offensive smell, add *yaa dam* to the prescription.

Medicine to treat *taan* and *saang*; *saang khamooi*; diarrhoea; flatulence; to use as a laxative; and to treat *saang* on the tongue.

[292]	*kaphrao*	leaves	1 *baht*
	chum het thet	leaves	1 *baht*
	sawaat	leaves	1 *baht*
	taan mon	leaves	1 *baht*
	khop chanaang thang 2	of each	1 *baht*
	phak khraat	leaves	1 *baht*
	khamin oi		1 *baht*
	kathue		1 *fueang*
	phlai		1 *fueang*
	phrik Thai		1 *fueang*
	khing		1 *fueang*
	krathiam		1 *fueang*

13 items. Pills to be taken mixed with alcohol to treat *taan* and *saang khamooi*. If the child has diarrhoea, mix with leaf sap of *taan mon*; to use as a laxative, mix with leaf sap of *kaphrao;* to treat flatulence, mix with leaf sap of *sawaat*. If the *saang* erupts on the tongue add *nam prasaan thong*, and use as a paint.

Medicine to treat *taan* and *saang*:

[293]	*chan*	seeds
	benyakaanee	
	fin	
	khrai khruea	
	prakham dee khwaii	fruit
	see siat thet	

Equal parts. Prepare pills using alcohol as excipient. To be taken mixed with alcohol to counteract the effects of *taan* and all kinds of *saang*, to treat *taan khamooi* and to break up very bad boils and abscesses.

Another:

[294]	*yaa klet hoi*	
	ching chaa chaalee	fruit
	nguu lueam	bile

Equal parts. Prepare pills using alcohol as excipient. To be taken for *taan* and *saang* or applied to abscesses or pustules. Mix with alcohol.

Another:

[295]	*mawaeng ton*	fruit
	kaphrao	leaves
	chum het thet	leaves
	khamin oi	
	phrik Thai	
	khing	
	dee plee	
	phlai	

Equal parts. To be taken mixed with alcohol to treat *taan* and the effects of *saang* in the mouth preventing the child from eating and drinking.

Another:

[296]	*samo thet*	
	makhaam pom	
	horaphaa	fruit
	thian yaowa phaanee	
	kot so	

Equal parts. Pills to be taken mixed with alcohol to treat diarrhoea; to treat dysentery, mix with *nam raatcha phrik*; to treat the effects of *saang* on the tongue, mix with alcohol.

Another:

[297]	*chan*	seeds
	hing	
	phrik Thai	
	khing	
	krathiam	

khon thee so	leaves	
kluea sinthao		

Equal parts. Pills to be taken mixed with alcohol to counteract fever caused by *taan* and *saang*.

Paint for the tongue:

[298] *bai naat*		
raet	eye tooth	
suea	eye tooth	
nam tao khom		
prakham dee khwaai		
samun waeng		

Equal parts. Prepare a stick and use to paint the tongue to treat *saang daeng* and *saang lueang*.

Paint for the tongue:

[299] *kaphrao*	leaves	1 *baht*
bai naat		1 *baht*
khon thee so	leaves	1 *baht*
suea	eye tooth	1 *fueang*
raet	eye tooth	1 *fueang*
nuea	horn	1 *fueang*
kaan phluu		1 *fueang*
chan	seeds	1 *fueang*
khrai khruea		1 *baht*
krisanaa		1 *fueang*
nguu lueam	bones	1 *fueang*
cha-em thet		2 *phai*

Prepare a stick, using lime juice as excipient and paint the tongue to treat the throat.

Paint for the tongue:

[300] *sadao*	bark	2 salueng
sanun	bark	2 *salueng*
phrik Thai lon		3 peppercorns
krathiam		7 cloves
waan haang chaang		1 *salueng*
kraphao	leaves	1 *salueng*
nam prasaan thong		2 *salueng*

Grind together and paint the tongue, then the *saang* will go away immediately.

Paint for the tongue:

[301] *sadao*	bark	
sanun	bark	
kaphrao	bark	
taan mon	leaves	
chaang	tusk	

krathiam
sang
nam prasaan thong

Equal parts. Prepare a stick, using the juice of the pods of *som poi* as excipient. Mix with *nam khram* to treat *saang lueang, saang daeng* and *saang fai.*

Medicine to treat mucus and fever:

[302] *chan hom*
krisanaa
kot so
kot khamao
kot phung plaa
saaraphee pollen

Equal parts. Reduce to powder. Prepare pills the size of peppercorns using a decoction of *lep mue naang (ton mai)* as excipient. [To be taken by children according to age:] 1 to 4 years, 7 pills; 3 to 10 months, 5 pills. To be taken mixed with either cucumber juice, syrup, honey or jasmine flower water. In treating a child of one month of age, add 5 *klam* of *phimsen.*[31] Without a doubt a very potent and reliable recipe.

[303] ***Saeng aathit***

chaat kon
chaat horakhun
kammathan daeng
muun maeng saap
nam prasaan thong

Equal parts. Prepare a stick to be used mixed with alcohol as a paint for the tongue. If this is ineffective, mix with lime juice.

Medicine to treat all kinds of *taan* and *saang*:

[304]	*cham-em thet*	root
	lep mue naang	root
	som poi	root
	phinlangkaasaa	root
	rangap phit	root
	khok kra-om	root
	phitsanaat	
	khrai khruea	root
	samun waeng	
	krachaai	
	chaluut	
	opchoei	
	mawaeng khruea	root
	krathin daeng	
	chan	seeds

	kaan phluu	
	chan thet	
	son	
	krak khee	
	inthanin	heartwood

Equal parts, 20 items. Pills to be taken mixed with alcohol for *taan* and *saang.*

Decoction to treat *taan, saang* and *taan khamooi*. For children who are thin and yellow, and those who are thin and dehydrated:

[305]	*taan thang 5*		
	samo thang 3		
	khamin oi		
	phlai		
	haeo muu		
	samrong	bark	
	phak sian phee		
	hom daeng		
	4 baht of each		
	makruut	3 fruits split into 7 pieces	
	khee kaa khaao	3 fruits	
	khee kaa daeng	3 leaves	
	saan som		2 *salueng*
	yaa dam		1 *baht*

Prepare a decoction with pods of *raatcha phrik.* Reduce to 1/3 volume by boiling. If this causes diarrhoea, add *dee kluea.* To be taken according to whether the elements are heavy or light. Very reliable.

To treat children for *taan* and *saang* of all kinds:

[306]	*kot so*		1 *salueng*
	kot phung plaa		1 *salueng*
	kot chiang		1 *baht*
	kot hua bua		1 *baht*
	kot kaan phraao		1
	khrai khruea	root	1 *salueng*
	phak chee	fruit	1 *salueng*
	horaphaa	fruit	1 *salueng*
	benyakaanee		1 *salueng*
	samo Thai		1 *salueng*
	samo phiphek		1 *salueng*
	makhaam pom		1 *salueng*
	nam prasaan thong		1 *salueng*
	saan som		1 *salueng*
	cha-em		2 *salueng*

15 items. Prepare pills using aromatic water as excipient. To treat diarrhoea, mix with sap of *maduea* bark or of *khae* bark; to treat

dysentery, to be taken mixed with *nam kathue*; to treat vomiting, mix with *nam samo* or honey and add a little *phimsen;* to treat hiccoughs, mix with hot water to which have been added a little *phimsen* and salt. If it is to be used as a laxative, it is to be taken mixed with the sap of *kraphang hom* leaves; to apply, add salt. When there is both flatulence and diarrhoea, the medicine is to be taken mixed with *kaphrao* leaf sap. To treat *taan khamooi* causing swollen intestines, it is to be taken mixed with the sap of *chum het* leaves and *khamin oi.* To treat the effects of *taan* and *saang* on the tongue, mix with n*am khamin oi* and use to paint the tongue. To treat fainting in adults, give this medicine mixed with *nam som saa* to which salt has been added.

[307] ***Ratsawong mahaa thi khun***

thian dam		1
thian daeng		1
thian khaao		1
thian taa tak taen		1
horadaan		1
khrai khruea		1
kaan phluu		1
tree phalaa		1
kot so		1
samon waeng [samun waeng]		1
tree katuk		1
nam prasaan thong		1
cha-em thet		3

17 items. Pills to be taken mixed with syrup and some salt and snake's bile. Dose: 1 *fueang* to treat children who are thin and yellow and unable to eat.

To treat mucus and blood [in the stools], and *saang* in the chest:

[308]

kraphang hom	leaves	
khrai khruea		
krathin daeng		

To be taken mixed with alcohol.

Another:

To treat mucus and blood [in the stools]:

[309]

chan hom		1 *baht*
krisanaa		1 *baht*
cha-em thet		1 *baht*
kot so		5 *salueng*
kot kaan phraao		1 *salueng*
kot hua bua		1 *salueng*
chaang	tusk	1 *salueng*
chan	seeds	2 *salueng*
dee plee		1 *salueng*

chan	arils	2 *salueng*
phimsen		3 *klam*

Pills to be taken mixed with alcohol and snake's bile.

Medicine to treat mucus and blood [in the stools]:

[310]

krathiam		1 *salueng*
thian dam		1 *salueng* 1 *fueang*
kraphrao	leaves	1 *baht*
khamin oi		1 *baht*

Grind together. To be taken mixed with alcohol.

Medicine to treat mucus and blood [in the stools]:

[311]

taan khamooi	
chan daeng	
chan khaao	
benyakaanee	
neraphuusee	
nam prasaan thong	
kaan phluu	
nguu lueam	bile
kaphrao	leaves
sawaat	leaves
maeng lak	leaves

Equal parts, 11 items. Pills to be taken mixed with alcohol. Remedy for mucus and blood in the stools resulting from *taan* and *saang* and for foamy faeces.

Decoction for mucus and blood [in the stools] and prolapse of the rectum:

[312]

yaa khaao yen		3 *baht*
lep mue naang	root	3 *baht*
nguu lueam	bones	3 *baht*

Reduce to 1/3 volume by boiling. To be taken for *taan*, the pot belly of *saang khamooi*, and lymph or mucus and blood in the stools.

Medicine to treat abdominal pain; a laxative and diuretic:

[313]

khon thee so	leaves	4 *baht*
kraphrao	leaves	1 *baht*
taan mon	leaves	1 *baht*
khamin oi		1 *salueng*
satao	leaves	1 *fueang*
krathiam		2 *salueng*
krasaai [krachaai]		2 *salueng*
phrik Thai		2 *salueng*
hom daeng		2 *salueng*
chan	seeds	1 *fueang*
dee plee		1 *fueang*

Powder together then mix with proof spirit [*yat suraa*]. To be taken according to the strength of the child.

Stomach mixture:

[314]	*taan mon*		2 *salueng*
	kraphrao	leaves	2 *salueng*
	sawaat	leaves	6 *salueng*
	dee plee		1 *fueang*

Equal parts to be taken mixed with alcohol.

Stomach mixture:

[315]	*sawaat*	leaves	1 *baht*
	kaphrao	leaves	2 *salueng*
	taan mon	leaves	1 *salueng* 1 *fueang*
	phak khraat	leaves	2 *salueng*
	chan	seeds	1 *fueang*
	chan	arils	1 *fueang*
	kaan phluu		1 *fueang*
	dee plee		1 *fueang*
	kameng	leaves	2 *salueng*
	yaa dam		3 *salueng*

To be taken morning and evening mixed with alcohol.

Medicine to treat insomnia:

[316]	*chan hom*		2 *salueng*
	kot thang 5	of each	1 *fueang*
	saaraphee	pollen	1 *salueng*
	bua luang	root	1 *fueang*
	mai see suk	skin	1 *fueang*
	kaarabuun		2 *klam*
	bia phuu		1 *fueang*
	lin thale		1 *salueng*

Mix together with coconut milk. Give to the child to cheer him up and enliven him, to make him sleep and to quench his thirst.

Medicine to treat *la*:

[317]	*malaeng saap*	faecal matter
	phimsen	
	chan khaao	
	maklam taa chang	
	thian khaao	
	krisanaa	

Equal parts. Prepare pills the size of peppercorns to be applied [mixed with a liquid] to the *la*.

Medicine to expel the poison of all kinds of *taan* and *saang*:

[318]	*neraphuusee*	
	saaraphat phit	fruit
	raatchadat	fruit

Equal parts. Add an amount of aloes equal to the whole. Prepare pills the size of peppercorns using bark sap of *marum* as excipient. Dose, 7 pills to sedate the child.

Medicine to contain the liver and to counteract poison:

[319]	*neraphuusee khao*		
	neraphuusee daeng		
	waan keep raet		
	waan ron thong		
	waan proh		
	waan naang kham		
	yaa klet hoi		
	haang chorakhe		
	chan thang 2		
	krisanaa		
	prakham dee khwaai	fruit	
	khrai khruea	root	
	kammathan daeng		
	nam prasaan thong		

Equal parts, 14 items. Pills to be taken mixed with alcohol.

Medicine to contain the liver and to counteract poison:

[320]	*waan keep raet*		1 *salueng*
	waan ron thong		1 *salueng*
	sang karanee		1 *salueng*
	kot so		1 *salueng*
	kot khamao		1 *baht*
	chan daeng		1 *salueng*
	chan khaao		1 *salueng*
	chaang	tusk	1 *salueng*
	waai takhaa		1 *salueng*
	neraphuusee		1 *salueng*
	thao yaa naang		1 *salueng*
	nguu lueam	bile	1 *salueng*

12 items. Prepare pills using alcohol as excipient. To be taken mixed with alcohol to contain the liver, to counteract poison and for mucus and blood [in the stools] resulting from *taan khamooi*.

Medicine to contain the liver and to counteract poison:

[321]	*samo Thai*		1 salueng
	chaang	tusk	1 *salueng*
	raet	molar tooth	1 *salueng*
	chaang	molar tooth	1 *salueng*
	mee	eye tooth	1 *salueng*
	suea	eye tooth	1 *salueng*
	chorakhe	eye tooth	1 *salueng*
	kui	horn	1 *salueng*

faan	horn	1 *salueng*
chan thang 2		1 *salueng*
khrai khruea	root	1 *salueng*
ngoh	bark	1 *salueng*
khee aai	bark	1 *salueng*
haang kraai		1 *salueng*
waan keep raet		1 *salueng*
maak	ripe	1 *salueng*
saan som		2 *salueng*
tabuun	fruit	2 *salueng*
maphuu	leaves	7 *salueng*
mamia	leaves	1 *baht*
faai daeng	leaves	2 *salueng*
thian	leaves	3 *baht*
thap thim	leaves	3 *baht*
mafueang	leaves	2 *salueng*
khamin oi		1 *salueng*
krisanaa		1 *salueng*
saluut [chaluut]		1 *fueang*
opchoei		1 *salueng*
kamyaan		1 *salueng*
benyakaanee		1 *salueng*
kaan phluu		1 *salueng*
neraphuusee		1 *salueng*
waan proh		1 *salueng*
see siat thet		1 *salueng*
chan	seeds	1 *salueng*
phrik hom		1 *salueng*
chan takhian		1 *salueng*
khrang		1 *salueng*

38 items. Pills to be taken mixed with alcohol to treat *taan, saang,* smallpox and boils. This is a very special medicine to contain the liver and counteract poison.

Medicine to treat *taan khamooi:*

[322]	*sawaat*	leaves	6 *salueng*
	taan mon	leaves	3 *salueng*
	khon thee so	leaves	1 *baht*
	kaphrao	leaves	1 *baht*
	krathiam		1 *salueng*
	hom daeng		2 *salueng*
	khamin oi		2 *salueng*
	yaa dam		1 *baht*
	phrik hom		1 *salueng*
	dee plee		1 *salueng*

chaa phluu	fruit	1 *salueng*
boraphet		1 *salueng* 1 *fueang*
chetta phang khee	root	1 *salueng*
krachaai		1 *baht*
kaan phluu		1 *salueng*
chan	seeds	1 *salueng*
plaai	fruit	1 *salueng*
raet	blood	1 *baht*

18 items. Pills to be taken mixed with alcohol for *taan* and *saang* and to treat children who are thin and yellow - just skin and bones - [as a result of] *taan khamooi*, with red faeces like *khonong nuea*,[32] caused by *taan khamooi* attacking the liver. If the child can take this, it will recover.

Medicine to treat *taan khamooi*:

[323]	*sawaat*	leaves	1 *baht*
	kameng	leaves	2 *salueng*
	faai daeng	leaves	2 *salueng*
	nam tao	leaves	2 *salueng*
	taan mon	leaves	1 *baht*
	khee kaa daeng	leaves	2 *salueng*
	khop chanaang		2 *salueng*
	kaphrao	leaves	2 *salueng*
	yaa dam		1 *baht*

9 items. Prepare pills using alcohol as excipient. To be taken mixed with alcohol.

Throat paint to overcome [an infant's] inability to suck at the breast:

[324]	*khrai khruea*	
	chueak thao muak [chueak khao muak]	
	krisanaa	
	nguu lueam	bones
	suea	eye tooth
	raet	eye tooth
	kwaang	horn
	cha-em thet	
	nguu lueam	bile

Mix together with alcohol and apply to the throat. Highly recommended.

Medicine for an infant who cannot suck:

[325]	*nom phichit*	leaves	1 *baht*
	kraphrao	leaves	1 *baht*
	krathiam		2 *salueng*
	chamot		1 *fueang*
	phimsen		1 *fueang*
	lin thale		2 *salueng*

	nam prasaan thong		2 *salueng*

Mix with ghee and apply to the tongue. It may also be taken, mixed with alcohol, to treat all kinds of *saang.*

Application for the abdomen:

[326]	*khee thao luuk wua*		2 *salueng*
	chetta phang khee		1 *salueng*
	muuk man	fruit	1 *salueng* 1 *fueang*
	masaang	heartwood	1 *salueng*
	nuu ring	faecal matter	1 *salueng* 1 *fueang*
	khai nao	bark	1 *salueng*
	phlai		1 *salueng*

Mix with alcohol and apply beneath the navel, then the bowels will function.

Application for the abdomen to treat diarrhoea:

[327]	*faai daeng*	leaves
	samee	leaves
	krathue	
	krathum khee muu	leaves
	takuu	leaves
	khamin oi	
	fin	

Equal parts, 7 items. Mix with river water and apply to the lower abdomen.

Application for the abdomen:

[328]	*thon dee*	root
	khaa kae	
	hing	
	yaa dam	
	rong	

Reduce to a powder and apply when the bowels and bladder do not function.

Application for the abdomen, to treat flatulence:

[329]	*waan nam*	
	chetta phang khee	root
	phlai	
	sabaa Thai	fruit
	malaeng saap	faecal matter

Mix together and apply to the abdomen.

Decoction to cleanse breast milk [galactagogue]:

[330]	*tree katuk*	
	tree phalaa	
	chetta muun phloeng	
	chaa phluu	root
	sakhaan	

	chan thang 2		
	phanom sawan	root	
	kannikaa	root	

Equal parts, 13 items. Reduce to 1/3 volume by boiling. To be taken.

To cleanse breast milk:

[331]	*taan mon*		1 *salueng*
	taan khamooi		1 *salueng*
	chetta muun		1 *salueng*
	khing	dried	1 *salueng*
	dee plee		1 *salueng*
	chaa phluu	root	1 *salueng*
	sakhaan		1 *salueng*
	khrai bok		1 *salueng*
	mai praduu		1 *salueng*
	mai sak		1 *salueng*
	chum het		1 *salueng*
	thao yaa naang		1 *salueng*
	som poi	root	1 *salueng*
	kraphang hom	root	1 *salueng*
	phum riang paa	root	1 *salueng*
	chong kho	root	1 *salueng*
	prakham dee khwaai	fruit	2 *salueng*

18 items. Reduce to 1/3 volume by boiling. To be taken [by the mother] as medicine to purify bad milk, and to treat *taan, saang* and *taan khamooi* when they attack the bones, making the child thin and yellow, and to treat hiccoughs, hunger with nausea, and to treat mucus.

Throat paint to treat *saang daeng*:

[332]	*neraphuusee*	
	hom daeng	
	khem daeng	root
	phimsen	

Prepare a stick, [mix with a liquid] and apply to the throat, for *saang daeng.*

Throat paint to treat *saang daeng* and *khamao*:

[333] *mercuric sulphide*
carcass of a spider
faecal matter of a cockroach
uric acid salts obtained from human urine
Borneo camphor

Prepare a stick and use to paint the mouth.

Throat paint to treat *saang fai:*

[334] *yaa tai bai*

	chan daeng		
	raet	molar tooth	
	chaang	molar tooth	

Grind finely with alcohol or honey and paint the tongue of a child who has a red mouth, a hot body and red palms and soles caused by *saang daeng* and *saang fai.*

Medicine to treat 12 kinds of *saang*:

[335]	*faai daeng*		2 *salueng*
	kraphrao	leaves	2 *salueng*
	phak khraat	leaves	2 *salueng*
	thian	leaves	2 *salueng*
	sawaat	leaves	2 *salueng*
	thap thim	leaves	2 *salueng*
	khamin oi		2 *salueng*
	phlai		2 *salueng*
	khaa		2 *salueng*
	khing		2 *salueng*
	dee plee		2 *salueng*
	yaa tai bai		2 *salueng*

Prepare pills. To treat diarrhoea, to be taken mixed with *nam chan.* To evacuate the bowels 1 to 4 times, to be taken mixed with lime juice. For the stomach, to be taken mixed with alcohol. If it is to be used as a mouth paint, it should be mixed with salt water or the juice of the rind of ripe areca nuts. Without a doubt, this is very reliable.

To treat poison in the mouth and throat becoming worse:

[336]	*nam prasaan thong*	2 *salueng*
	din prasiu khaao	2 *salueng*
	hin fan maa	2 *salueng*
	chaat horakhun	2 *salueng*
	krabaang	2 *salueng*
	saan som	2 *salueng*
	phimsen	1 *fueang*

Powder together, then boil with salt water. Swab the throat, then paint the mouth of an infant who cannot suck. Also use for any form of poisoning which is getting worse.

[337] ***Sapaathikhun***

	phak khraat	
	kaphrao	leaves
	nam prasaan thong	
	din prasiu khaao	
	saan som sat	
	lin thale	
	yaa yong fai	
	phrik Thai	11 peppercorns

8 items. Prepare a stick and mix with lime juice to paint the tongue for *saang daeng*, *saang fai* and *saang khamoi*. Also give this to an infant who cannot suck.

[338] ***Prasa dam***

prakham dee khwaai	fruit	1 *baht*
khamin oi		1 *baht*
raatchadat	fruit	1 *baht*
khrai khruea		1 *baht*
nguu lueam		2 *salueng*

5 items. Prepare pills the size of cotton seeds. To be taken mixed with lime juice to treat dysentery; mixed with *sakae* leaf sap to treat mucus and blood in the stools; and mixed with *nam khaa* to treat diarrhoea. To be taken mixed with alcohol to treat all poisons. Very reliable.

[339] ***Chakara naaraai***

faai daeng	leaves
kraphrao	leaves
sawaat	leaves
tree katuk	
nam prasaan thong	

Equal parts, 7 items. To be taken mixed with alcohol. Dose, according to strength: aged 1 month, 1 pill; aged 4 months, 2 pills. If the tongue is affected, mix with lime juice and apply.

[340] ***Hom chakara naaraai***

kot so	
kot khamao	
kot kaan phraao	
kot chulaa lamphaa	
kot nam tao	
thian dam	
thian daeng	
thian khaao	
thian khaao plueak	
thian taa tak taen	
thian yaowa phaanee	
thian taa kop	
chan	seeds
chan	arils
krawaan	
kaan phluu	
chan thang 2	
krisanaa	
kralamphak	
chaluut	

khondok	
cha-em thang 2	
opchoei	
khrai khruea	root
waan keep raet	
waan ron thong	
chaa phluu	fruit
en	fruit
samo thet	fruit
samo Thai	fruit
makhaam pom	fruit
chamot	
phimsen	
bunnaak	flowers

Equal parts, 36 items. Prepare pills using rose water as excipient. To be taken mixed with juice of *raatcha phrik* pods when required as a laxative. To be taken with bark sap of *maduea* to treat diarrhoea. Mix with *kaphrao* leaf sap to treat flatulence. To treat swollen intestines caused by *taan khamooi* it may be taken mixed with any of the following: *taan mon* leaf sap, *chum het* or *khamin oi*. Mix with *nam khamin oi* and *phimsen* to paint the tongue if it is affected by *saang*. If *saang* affects the chest, the mixture may be taken with *maklam khruea* leaf sap and a small quantity of python's bile. To treat poisoning from *saang*, it should be taken mixed with rose water.

[341] ***Hom noi***

kot so	
kot phung plaa	
kot chulaa lamphaa	
thian yaowa phaanee	
cha-em thet	
nam prasaan thong	
saan som	
horaphaa	fruit
phak chee	fruit
samo Thai	fruit
samo phiphek	fruit
makhaam pom	fruit

Equal parts, 12 items. Mix together with alcohol, and leave to macerate for three days. Prepare pills. To be taken mixed with *maduea* bark sap or *khae* bark [sap] to treat diarrhoea; mixed with lime water or *nam krathue* to treat mucus and blood in the stools; and mixed with honey or *nam samo* and *phimsen* for vomiting. If the *saang* affects the tongue, paint with this mixture after adding *nam khamin oi* and *phimsen*. To be taken mixed with *nam maklam khruea* to treat a dry throat. To treat poisoning from *saang*, this mixture should be taken with aromatic water and *phimsen*.

[342] ***Hom yai***

kot thang 5	
thian thang 5	
chan	seeds
chan	arils
krawaan	
kaan phluu	
chan daeng	
chan khaao	
krisanaa	
kralamphak	
chaluut	
khondok	
cha-em thang 2	
neraphuusee	
en	fruit
waan proh	
son	
kamyaan	
phimsen	leaves
kham	flowers
lam chiak	flowers
phikun	flowers
bunnaak	flowers
saaraphee	flowers
mali son	flowers
mali laa	flowers
kannikaa	flowers
kradang ngaa	flowers
champaa	flowers
bua luang	pollen
sattabongkot	pollen
sattabut	pollen
bua phuean	pollen
bua khom	pollen
kaarabuun	
chamot sot	
chamot chiang	
phimsen	

Equal parts, 47 items. Prepare pills using aromatic water as excipient. To be taken mixed with alcohol to treat *saang*, Mix with water used to wash rice or *nam thao yaa naang*, rose water or *nam chan* to treat fever; mix with rose water, or jasmine flower water and coarse sugar and granulated sugar to treat delirium causing restlessness. This is strong medicine. Do not give it if the child is not very ill, because it is not necessary in that case. Use this only as an application, then if that is ineffective, it can be taken. Highly recommended.

[343] ***Mahaa chakara noi***

kot so		2 *salueng*
kot phung plaa		2 *salueng*
thian thang 5	of each	2 *salueng*
chan	seeds	2 *salueng*
krawaan	flowers	2 *salueng*
kaan phluu		2 *salueng*
samo thang 3	of each	2 *salueng*
makhaam pom		2 *salueng*
phak chee lom	fruit	2 *salueng*
horaphaa	fruit	2 *salueng*
cha-em thet		2 *salueng*
yaa dam		2 *salueng*
phrik Thai		2 *salueng*
khing		2 *salueng*
dee plee		2 *salueng*
krathiam		2 *salueng*
nam prasaan thong		2 *salueng*
saan som		2 *salueng*
din prasiu khaao		2 *salueng*

25 items. Pills. If required to be used as a laxative, to be taken mixed with *kaphrao* leaf sap or *kraphang hom* leaf sap; to treat diarrhoea, it may be mixed with the bark sap of *maduea*; to treat flatulence, to be taken mixed with *nam krathue*; to treat vomiting, to be taken with a decoction of *nam samo*. To treat *saang* which has developed in the mouth, mix with *nam khamin oi* and use as a paint, then it will go away.

[344] ***Thong naep nuea***

nam prasaan thong		1 *klam*
chaat horakhum		3 *klam*
hoi sang	calcined	3 *klam*
chan daeng		1 *fueang*
kralamphak		1 *fueang*
chamot chiang		2 *phai*
phimsen		2 *phai*

7 items. Pills. Spread out to dry in the sun on palmyra palm leaves. To be taken mixed with fresh jasmine flower water or rose water. It is very good for infants who cannot suck or eat if a little *thong ngoen* is added. It is considered to be worth a *tamlueng* of gold.

To treat the putrefaction caused by *saang*:

[345]	*phrik Thai*		1 *salueng* 1 *fueang*
	khing	dried	2 *salueng*
	krathiam		1 *baht*
	dee plee		1 *salueng*
	khamin oi		2 *salueng*
	phlai		2 *salueng*
	utta phit		1 *fueang*
	buk		1 *fueang*

Grind together. To be taken or applied, mixed with alcohol.

To treat cough:

[346]	*matuum*	fruit peel
	dee plee	
	naat	root

To be taken mixed with honey.

Application to treat swollen feet:

[347]	*nguu lueam*	bones
	khamin oi	
	khaao nieo kanyaa	

To be applied mixed with aromatic water. If this is ineffective, use *saniat* leaf sap. If this is ineffective, use *naat* leaf sap.

[348] ***Nam dap fai***

mamuang kalon	leaves
mali	leaves
samee	leaves
tamlueng tua phuu	leaves
phak khuang	
sadao	leaves
nam tao	leaves
khok kra-om	leaves
khamin oi	

Prepare a stick, mix with fresh jasmine water and use as a lotion to counteract poison.

Medicine to apply to the crown of the head to treat insomnia:

[349]	*horadaan thong*		1 *salueng*
	lamphong kaa salak	flowers	2 *salueng*
	kanchaa thet		3 *salueng*
	kho	dung	2 *salueng*
	phimsen	leaves	

Mix with aromatic water and apply to the crown of the head, for insomnia.

Throat swab and mouth paint to treat inflammation in the mouth caused by *saang*:

[350]	*takhian*	bark

see siat thet
kon mo kaeng
nam prasaan thong sat
Equal parts. Prepare pills, using alcohol as excipient. To be applied mixed with good quality oil for sores in the mouth resulting from *saang.*

To treat ***saang daeng*** and ***saang fai***:

[351]	*kwaang*	horn
	raet	horn
	raet	eye tooth
	suea	eye tooth
	mee	eye tooth
	chaang	molar tooth
	kraben	baked skin
	waai takhaa	
	kaphrao	leaves
	sawaat	leaves
	cha-em thet	
	faek hom	
	neraphuusee	
	chan thang 2	
	dee plee	
	fin	

Equal parts, 17 items. Prepare pills using the bile of a python as excipient. [Make the sacrifice] to buy an equivalent amount, because it is worth its weight in gold. For all 7 kinds of *saang* and for fevers.

[352] ***Mahaa rangap phit***

phrik Thai		1 *baht*
khing		1 *baht*
dee plee		1 *baht*
sak	charcoal	6 *salueng*
manaao	seeds	1 *fueang*
phluu kae	leaves	2 *salueng* 1 *fueang*
fin		1 *fueang*

8 items. Pills to be taken mixed with lime juice to counteract poisons; for headache, mix with river water to be taken or applied.

[353] ***Suraamrit***

kaphrao	leaves
katang muut	
nam prasaan thong	
muun malaeng saap	
lin thale	

Equal parts, 5 items. Pills to be taken mixed with river water or alcohol to counteract the poison of all severe forms of *saang.*

[354] ***Mahaa nin***

nguu thap thaang	bones	1 *salueng*
phak phaeo daeng		1 *salueng*
sahatsakhun thet		1 *salueng*
khaa taa daeng		1 *salueng*
phrik lon		1 *salueng*
khing	dried	1 *salueng* 1 *fueang*
dee plee		1 *salueng*
krawaan		1 *salueng*
tumkaa daeng	fruit	1 *salueng*
khamin oi		1 *salueng*
lin thale		1 *salueng*
nam prasaan thong		1 *fueang*
din prasiu khaao		1 *fueang*
saan som		1 *fueang*
raak din	roasted	1 *baht*
chorakhe	bile	2 *phai*
nguu lueam	bile	2 *phai*
nguu hao	bile	2 *phai*

18 items. Pills to be taken mixed with alcohol to counteract the poison of *saang daeng* and all kinds of *saang*.

[355] ***Mahaa nin tua phuu***

borax	
Indian ink	
snake-head fish	burnt scales
stingray	burnt skin
black cat	burnt head
reticulated python	burnt bones
many banded krait	burnt bones

Equal parts, 7 items. Pills to be taken mixed with alcohol for smallpox and boils. To treat *taan* and *saang*, mix with aromatic water. To paint the mouth, mix with Borneo camphor. If this is ineffective, mix with *chaat horakhun thet*, syrup and arsenic disulphide and paint the mouth or dab on the pustules of bubonic plague.

[356] ***Sommit***

kot so
kot khamao
kot chiang
kot phung plaa
kot chulaa lamphaa
kot hua bua
kot kraduuk
kot kakkran
kot kakling

chang thang 2	
krisanaa	
kralam phak	
krak khee	
chaluut	
opchoei	
phikun	flowers
bunnaak	flowers
champaa	flowers
kradang ngaa	flowers
saaraphee	flowers
bua luang	pollen
sattabut	pollen
amphan dok mai	
amphan thong	
amphan khee plaa	
chamot	fresh
chamot chiang	
phimsen	
khondok	

Equal parts, 30 items. Mix together, then add crocodile's bile and soak in aromatic water. Pills to be taken mixed with rose water to treat all diseases resulting from internal heat associated with the three seasons and to cheer up and enliven the child.

[357] ***Mahaa wong***

ngaa chaang kamchat		1 *baht*
ngaa chaang kamchaai		1 *baht*
ngaa chaang dee		1 *baht*
chaang	molar tooth	1 *baht*
raet	molar tooth	1 *baht*
raet	eye tooth	1 *baht*
raet	horn	1 *baht*
suea	eye tooth	1 *baht*
mee	eye tooth	1 *baht*
chorakhe	eye tooth	1 *baht*
plaa phayuun	eye tooth	1 *baht*
kui	horn	1 *baht*
faan	horn	1 *baht*
liang phaa	horn	1 *baht*
chum phaa	horn	1 *baht*
sing	horn	1 *baht*
phae	horn	1 *baht*
kae	horn	1 *baht*
kwaang	horn	1 *baht*

krabue phueak	horn	1 *baht*
krabue dam	horn	1 *baht*
wua phueak	horn	1 *baht*
wua dam	horn	1 *baht*
hin kaa rang daeng		1 *baht*
neraphuusee		1 *baht*
benyakaanee		1 *baht*
chan	seeds	1 *baht*
chan	arils	1 *baht*
kaan phluu		1 *baht*
waai takhaa		1 *baht*
kot hua bua		1 *baht*
opchoei		1 *baht*
sang karanee		1 *baht*
phimsen		1 *baht*
cha-em thet		1 *baht*
chan thang 2	of each	2 *baht*
nguu lueam	bile	2 *baht*
krung khamao		1 *salueng*
amphan thong		1 *salueng*
kaphrao	leaves	2 *salueng*
sawaat	leaves	2 *baht*
maklam khruea	leaves	8 *baht*
khrai hom	leaves	2 *baht*
maeng lak	leaves	4 *baht*
krathuep yop		4 *baht*
kraphang hom	leaves	4 *baht*
phak sian phee	leaves	4 *baht*

48 items. Prepare pills using alcohol as excipient. To treat *saang* and poisonous boils and abscesses, to be taken mixed with alcohol and *phimsen.* To treat throat abscesses, to be taken mixed with alcohol and a little *cha-em thet* and *khrai khruea* root. To treat snake-bite, to be taken mixed with alcohol, python's bile and *phimsen.* To treat hiccoughs in both children and adults, to be taken mixed with hot water and a little *waai takhaa* and *phimsen.* For poisonous boils and abscesses, add horn of an albino buffalo. To treat *saang daeng* and *la-ong phrabaat,* mix with *nam maklaam khruea* and borax. If the child is unable to eat, mix with *nam cha-em.*

If you want to rid the child of *saang* in the throat and chest, when the faeces are like bitter gourd seeds [crinkled like walnuts, and livid green], mix with *nam phak sian phee* and alcohol, equal parts, and add a little borax. To treat diarrhoea, to be taken mixed with *nam chan thang* 2. If *saang* affects the tongue mix with *nam chan khaao* and a little nut gall and paint the tongue. For flatulence, to be taken mixed with *nam phak sian phee*. Without a doubt, this medicine can be relied upon.

[358] ***Chan pit ruea***

bencha thap thim	
maak	dried
waai takhaa	
makhaam	shells of roasted seeds
kammathan daeng	
nam prasaan thong	
faang	
mai sak	
waan keep raet	
waan ron thong	
kraphrao thang 2	
neraphuusee	
chan thang 2	
krabue	burnt horn
thian dam	
krathiam	bulb

Equal parts, 23 items (actually 18 items) [sic]. Prepare pills, using *nam saaraphat khieo ngaa* as excipient. To be taken mixed with lime water or *nam chan*. If ineffective, use *maduea* bark sap or *khae daeng* bark sap. If that is ineffective, use *nam kluai taanee*.

Medicine to obtain relief from *taphan, tabong Rāhū* and *akkhamukkhee*:

[359] Place finely powdered pepper in the fresh gall bladder of a crocodile. Bake dry over a fire, then apply to the palms of the hands, soles of the feet and armpits.

Poultice to apply to the child's abdomen to obtain relief from *taphan*:

[360]

chetta muun	leaves
hing	
kammathan	
banlangsinlaa	
lin thale	

Mix with a child's urine and apply to the abdomen as a poultice.

[361] ***Naak phot***

bai naat	
phrik Thai	
bia chan	calcined
khing	
rang maaraa	burnt
malaeng mum	carcass
lamphan	

Equal parts, 7 items. Pills to be taken or used as a lotion [mixed with a liquid] to treat all kinds of *saang*, for *la-ong phrabaat* and for *taphan.*

Medicine to treat *la-ong phrabaat*:

[362] *nom phichit* leaves
nam prasaan thong
horadaan thong
krathiam
khing
dee plee
nguu lueam bile
phimsen

Equal parts. Pills. To use as a laxative, add *kaphrao* leaves, 3 parts; before it is taken, mix with *kaphrao* leaf sap; to treat any kind of *saang*, mix with *krathiam* leaf sap and paint the tongue. Reliable.

Application to encircle the wrists and ankles.[33]

[363] *bai naat*
phlap phlueng
khing
dee plee
krathiam
phlai
waan nam
hing

Mix with lime juice and encircle the wrists and ankles, using alcohol.

Book II of *Prathom chindaa* ends here.

NOTES

1 *paksee:* a winged creature; a bird; a class of children's diseases. *Theppheepaksee* is a form of children's disease characterized by disordered digestion, cold hands and feet, and feverish head. *Mc,* p.422.

2 Cf. Book I, p.40.

3 *athitsaruup:* meaning obscure. *ruup* means 'form' or 'figure'.

4 *haritathaat:* possibly one of the body elements.

5 Kinds of children's diseases.

6 Comments on the excellence, potency or reliability of prescriptions continue throughout the text, but, from this point, are omitted from the translation in most cases.

7 *phutsaa* seed: about the size of a cherry seed.

8 Cf. Book I, note 13.

9 *la-ong:* a mouth disease. Fur on the tongue. *So,* p.815.

10 *to:* corneal ulcers or corneal opacities. *Mc,* p.347.

11 *siddhikāriyaḥ* (Pāli): may success be achieved; so be it.

12 Not given in 1961 edition.

13 Meaning 'the smell of vultures and the smell of crows', listed as separate improbable ingredients. The plant *saap raeng saap kaa* is no doubted intended. The *paksee* are winged animals, such as mosquitoes, which it is hoped will be repelled by the smells of the fumigants. Similarly, the smell of camphor and asfoetida in the previous receipe should keep insects away.

14 To share bad luck with anyone who saw it floating on the canal or river.

15 *sangyot* (*saṃyojana* , Skt): the text, *Khampee sangyot,* mentioned previously and below.

16 See Book I, note 31.

17 The word '*yot*' , translated here as 'pustule', might also be translated 'abscess', 'boil', 'pimple' or anything similar. Unless the context suggests otherwise, the word 'pustule' will be used, with the understanding that 'abscess' or 'boil' or another word denoting a 'head' could have been intended. Pustules are differentiated in several ways: '*mae*', translated here as 'major'; '*ek*', primary, synonymous with '*pathommakan*' (see pp.73,152,234) and '*boriwaan*', 'minor pustules' or 'followers' (see note 20 below).

18 This comment in parentheses occurs in the 1961 edition, but not in the 1871 text. Evidently the compilers questioned this apparent error, but were not prepared to alter the text as they received it.

19 This phrase in brackets occurs in other editions, but not in the 1961 edition.

20 *boriwaan:* in this context has been translated as 'followers' or 'minor pustules'. It appears to suggest the existence of a rash that breaks out on various parts of the child's body during the course of many forms of *saang*. (See note 17.)

21 This phrase in brackets occurs in other editions but not in the 1961 edition.

22 This phrase in brackets occurs in other editions, but not in the 1961 edition.

23 *kwaat:* a common method of administering medicine to children. The finger, coated in the medicine, is inserted into the child's throat and the medicine is quickly applied.

24 *mafai: Baccaurea sapida* Muel.-Arg. Euphorbiaceae. The fruit looks almost the same as the *langsat*. (VJ) The *langsat* is creamy yellow, like a pale loquat. *Mc*, p.637, mentions this tree and other species, but none as having red fruit. Perhaps the word 'red' should have been 'yellow', or else the tree now known as *mafai* is not the tree known by that name when the text was composed.

25 *sadue:* the navel. The terms *naaphee* and *sadue*, the navel or abdomen, appear to be used interchangeably and in most cases the precise meaning is unclear. Whether it is the external abdomen or the abdominal cavity that is meant can often be determined from the context.

26 Literally, 'like liquor ferment, water used to wash meat, fishy smelling water (or amniotic fluid, depending on one's interpretation), and rotten eggs'.

27 This is unclear and also contains a misprint, '*fuuk*' for '*fuum*'. The words for 'left, right or centre' are repeated in the following statement in this edition and the 1871 text, suggesting an error in the compilation of the 1871 text. If these words are omitted here, we have 'excessive mucus causes muscular spasms ...'.

28 See note 17 above.

29 She may bathe in rainwater kept in a jar or pouring from a roof, but she should not get caught in the rain in case she gets chilled. (VJ)

30 *paang:* hypertrophy of the spleen due to chronic malarial poisoning. *Mc*, p.523.

31 The 1871 text has *phimsen* 1 part, and 2 parts if the child is 1 year old.

32 *khonong nuea:* meaning obscure. *khonong* means 'eyebrows' and *nuea*, 'flesh' or 'meat' or an animal of the deer kind.

33 Possibly for magical purposes, as when the wrists are tied with cotton to prevent the *khwan* (spirit or vitality) leaving the body.

[Book III]

Phrakhamphee prathom chindaa, Book III, Part 1.

Summary. Children born on Sunday have the symptoms of *saang phloeng* as the predominant illness, *saang kraai* is the minor *saang*; the *la* is called *utthayakaan* and the *la-ong* is called *pleo fai faa*.

Here we explain. Jīvaka Komārabhacca came to the place of the ascetic Nālayadābasa and asked him about diseases. Phra Nālayadābasa replied that various diseases occur in new-born infants. There are three [main] kinds of *saang*, which are subdivided into fourteen types. The three [main] kinds are *saang* of birth, minor *saang*[1] and *saang* of the *mae sue*. The fourteen types are the *saang* of the seven days [of the week], which are the birth *saang*, plus seven kinds of minor *saang*, making a total of fourteen types. As for the *mae sue*, there are seven types of *mae sue* of birth and another 24 types of minor *mae sue*, altogether 31 types. There are twelve kinds of *saphan* of birth and another seven kinds of minor *saphan Rāhū*,[2] a total of nineteen types. And these are the diseases which occur in all infants as has been explained.

Birth *saang* affects all infants while in the womb, three months after conception, when the foetus has become differentiated to have the five parts. At that time, one pustule of birth *saang* will develop, the type depending on the day of birth. If it is the time of the waxing of the moon, the pustule will be above the navel; if the moon is waning, it will be below the navel. If it is a girl, the pustule will be on the left side; if a boy, on the right side, and it will grow there until delivery. To diagnose which kind of *saang* the foetus has, the mother's symptoms should be investigated, as described previously.

Here the masters will go into the details, in turn, of the origin of each form of *saang* of the seven days - which affects all infants - to enable doctors to examine the signs and symptoms critically and to make an accurate diagnosis, as follows.

First, the description of children born on Sunday and the development of *saang phloeng*, the main illness of those children. (*Saang phloeng* is described on p. 177 of this volume,[3] but some of the details are different. These are repeated here to enable the student to decide for himself [which version to accept].) [sic]

Saang phloeng has four major pustules and 40 followers. *Khamao* develops when the baby is born and remains for seven days while the mother and child are by the fire, before it disappears. Then, if the baby is a boy, one major pustule will appear on the sole of the right foot and one on the left. If it is a girl, there will be three pustules on the sole of the left foot and one on the right. There are 40 followers on each of the shins (this should be 20 on each) [sic]. Three months after leaving the fire, one major pustule moves up from the foot to the abdomen. A month later, the baby has slight bruising on top of the feet, sore ankles and difficulty in swallowing and takes a long time to wake up. After six months, another pustule erupts with two heads together forming a small [purple] spot on the skin, the colour of jambolan fruit. After six to ten days it is gone. After eight months, one major pustule with three heads comes up in the abdomen and the followers erupt between the ankles and knees. After nine months, one major pustule with four heads develops in the abdomen, then the forty followers spread out, some in the middle areas of the upper and lower legs and on the knees. The heads of these minor pustules are at first as red as *mafai* fruit, then they turn black and rough, with red edges like burns. The skin blisters and the blisters merge together, since they all ripen at the same time, making the baby ache from the feet up to the hips or the waist.

Doctors should definitely not treat this condition because the four major pustules of *saang* in the abdomen will become a sore like a tuber of elephant yam, becoming inflamed and spreading to the supra-pubic area, anus and rectum, then up to the liver, lungs, large and small intestines, and after that, around the abdomen. Then the child will pass mucus and pus and offensive smelling liquid faeces, because the major *saang* has passed through the ileum and colon and affected the liver, lungs and heart before emerging at the anus. The followers then hurt and sting and feel as hot as burns. If the palms of the hands and the soles of the feet are blood red, this is the sign of death. Whenever the symptoms of *saang phloeng* all occur together like this, the baby is sure to die within eight to eleven days. But even if the *saang phloeng* is very severe, since the pustules come up only one at a time, though it is still very painful for the child, it can be cured with the right medicine. The critical period for *saang phloeng* is during the first nine months. If the child survives, then *saang phloeng* will recur at eighteen months of age. And the primary pustule of *saang* which the baby has had since it was in the womb will come up at the base of the tongue and cause diarrhoea. This is called *pathommakan.* It will make the uvula swollen and later this will make the baby cough, but it will subside if the right medicine is applied. If it affects the eyelids, it will make the liver hang down. If the whole liver is affected, it will swell and become compressed within the rib-cage. In this case, it is very difficult to cure, and even if the baby survives, one must beware of the complications caused by the minor form of *saang* which will follow. This is also fatal. To treat it, first prepare this medicine:

To treat *saang phloeng*:

[364] *waan keep raet*
waan ron thong
neraphusee
thian dam
thian daeng
cha-em thang 2
maklam khruea leaves

Equal parts, 8 items. Boil together until reduced to 1/3 volume. To be taken to reduce body heat and for all kinds of *taan* and *saang*. If pills are required, mix with alcohol to treat mucus and blood in the stools.

To treat *saang phloeng*:

[365] *yaa klet hoi*
san phraa hom leaves
phung kho leaves
chueak khao fai

Equal parts, 4 items. Mix with decoction of *prakham dee khwaai.* Prepare pills, to be taken or applied, mixed with river water and python's bile.

If that is ineffective:

[366] *lin thale*
khong saam yaan
khamin oi
khaao saan khaang khrok
Equal parts, 4 items. Grind together and apply to counteract the poison of *saang phloeng.*

If that is ineffective, prepare this:

[367]	*nam tao*	leaves
	rangap phit	leaves
	kathung maa baa	leaves
	sawaat	leaves
	kaphrao	leaves
	saniat	leaves
	mafueang	leaves
	kraai	fruit
	phinlangkaasaa	fruit
	chan	seeds
	chan	arils
	krawaan	
	kaan phluu	
	thian daeng	
	nam prasaan thong	

Equal parts, 15 items. Pills to be taken mixed with river water and borax to counteract all kinds of poison.

(The description of *saang phloeng* ends here.)

Siddhikāriyaḥ **Here we will describe *saang kraai*,** which is the minor *saang* of *saang phloeng*, together with a description of the *la* called *la utthayakaan* of the days [of the week] and the *la-ong phrabaat* called *la-ong pleo fai faa. La utthayakaan* is explained with *saang daeng* in Part 3. *La-ong pleo fai faa* is described with *saang chon* in Part 7. Here, in Part 1, on *saang phloeng,* we will discuss only *saang kraai,* the minor *saang.* Whenever these three - the minor *saang, la* and *la-ong* - occur together with or following *saang phloeng,* they might continue until the child is twelve years of age. Sometimes *saang phloeng* and the minor *saang* or *la* and *la-ong* might even then not be finished. Doctors should understand, likewise, that it is not necessarily so.

The description of *saang kraai,* the minor *saang* of *saang phloeng,* the *saang* of those born on Sunday, states: When the mother has been pregnant for eight, nine or ten [lunar] months, the infant is born. This child is easy to rear. While the mother and child are by the fire, only *khamao* develops. The *khamao* subsides after nine or ten days and after fourteen or fifteen days, *saang phloeng* first begins. When the *saang phloeng* has finished, *saang kraai* erupts. This *saang* comes from the spine.

Saang kraai has four major pustules - two in the supra-pubic area and two in the abdomen - and 40 followers. When the baby is a year and six months old, the followers spread over the skin like a heat rash. For about three days the child writhes and starts in its sleep, then the rash subsides and the followers enter the colon. At three months of age,[4] one of the major pustules moves up from the supra-pubic area to the abdomen, joining the two there to make a total of three. When the child is eight months old, the remaining major pustule in the supra-pubic area joins those in the abdomen, making a total of four altogether. This results in the child's having a high temperature with diarrhoea, vomiting and thirst, and it cannot eat or drink. At one year and seven or eight months of age, ten of the followers spread to the supra-pubic area, ten to the abdomen, ten to the stomach and ten to the tongue. If the doctor treats this disease with medicine which does not successfully counteract it, the disease will become stronger. Consequently, when the child is two years and three months old, it will pass mucus and blood and the symptoms will keep changing. Doctors are strongly warned that it is very difficult to cure this disease if they do not understand fully that minor *saang* follows or occurs with birth *saang*, and that *saang kraai* is the minor *saang* of *saang phloeng*, which is in the spine from the time when the baby was in the womb.

Medicine to treat saang phloeng and saang kraai:

[368]	*raang daeng*	root
	raang dam	root
	samo phiphek	bark
	phak waan	root
	thua phuu	root
	prakham kai	bark
	mamuang khan	bark
	mawaeng thang 2	fruit
	maduea	bark
	khae daeng	bark

11 items. Use one cupful of juice of each ingredient, then boil until only oil remains. Prepare next

chan	seeds
chan	arils
thian dam	
thian khaao	

mixed with 3 brown eggs and combine with the oil. To be taken according to the strength of the child, to treat *saang phloeng* and the minor *saang* which is *saang kraai.*

Medicine to treat *saang phloeng* and *saang kraai*:

[369]	*kaang plaa daeng*	root
	lep mue naang	root
	chum het thet	root
	chum het Thai	root

salot nam	root
taan dam	root
taan mon	root
maduea	bark
thaeng thuai	bark
phutsaa	bark
krathum khee muu	bark
chan thang 2	
prakham kai	leaves
ching chaa chaalee	leaves
khamin oi	

Equal parts, 16 items. Pills to be taken mixed with river water to counteract [the effects of] *saang phloeng, saang kraai* and other forms of *saang* which cause severe diarrhoea. When other medicine fails, this prescription will ensure that the diarrhoea ceases.

The masters say do not treat the disease called *bencha taan* with medicine called *Bencha taan!*

The masters have set forth in the description of the characteristics of those born on Sunday that *saang phloeng* is the major cause of illness, *saang kraai* is the minor cause, and *la utthayakaan* and *la-ong pleo fai faa* are complications of *saang phloeng.*

End of summary.

Phrakhamphee prathom chindaa, Book III, Part 2.

Summary. Children born on Monday have the symptoms of *saang nam* as the predominant illness, *saang faai* is the minor *saang*, the *la* is called *saeng prachan* and the *la-ong* is called *kaeo witchian.*

Siddhikāriyaḥ Next, the masters describe children born on Monday and the development of *saang nam,* the main illness of those children, so that doctors can diagnose it.

(*Saang nam* has already been described once on p. 180 [108], but some of the details are different. These are here repeated [for you] to decide [which version to accept].) [sic]

Description of *saang nam.* It has nineteen major pustules. When the mother is three months pregnant she tends to have headaches and painful breasts, a craving for sweet things, muscular fatigue in both arms, difficulty in hearing, night blindness, fainting, sometimes dizziness and discomfort, vomiting, and severe thirst continuing until the time of delivery.

The nineteen major pustules of *saang nam* are about the size of Chinese date leaves, and the red colour of the almost ripe fruit of Ceylon spinach. The pustules appear on the legs, in the centre of the back, on the shins and on both cheeks, erupting one at a time until the child is two and a half years old. Then they break, suppurate and form sores all over the body, after which they dry and withdraw inside the body. As a result, the child's head and body become hot and it has abdominal pain. The doctor should first give medicine to expel the *saang* completely, then give a dose of the medicine four or five times to help it recover. *Saang nam* produces no followers. The doctor should be on the alert for the minor *saang* and *saang la-ong,* as it is very serious if they both come at the same time because the *saang nam* will then be severe too. If *saang faai,*[5] *la saeng phrachan,* which is the *la* of *saang nam,* and *la-ong kaeo witchian,*[6] which is its form of *la-ong phrabaat,*[7] all affect the child, then it is as if it were under the influence of Rāhū.

The description of *saang nam* ends here.

(For prescriptions for *saang nam* see p.180 [108])

Siddhikāriyaḥ We now give a brief description of **the origin of *saang faai,*** the minor *saang* of *saang nam* so that doctors will understand.

Saang faai has no pustules. It appears thick and white, like cotton fibres, on the palate, inside the cheeks, at the roots of the teeth and on the tongue. This makes the baby sick; the whole body is hot, the mouth is hot and dry and there is no saliva. The child cannot close its mouth - it just opens its mouth and cries - it cannot eat, vomits copiously and has diarrhoea and the faeces smell foul like rotten eggs.

When the doctor sees this, he should be able to make an accurate diagnosis of *saang faai.*

Medicine to treat *saang faai:*

[370]	*nam tao*	leaves	1
	khop chanaang thang 2		1
	taan mon	leaves	1
	chum het	leaves	1
	rangap	leaves	1
	khee kaa daeng	leaves	1
	kathue		1
	phlai		1
	hom daeng		1
	phrik Thai		1
	krathiam		3
	khing	dried	1
	khamin oi		1

Equal parts, 14 items. Pills to be taken to treat *saang faai,* all *taan* and *saang;* and mucus and blood in the stools. If the faeces smell offensive, add aloes.

To treat *saang faai:*

[371]	*kaphrao*	leaves	
	chum het	leaves	
	sawaat	leaves	
	taan mon	leaves	
	khop chanaang thang 2	leaves	
	phak khraat	leaves	
	khamin oi		
	1 *baht* of each		
	kathue		1 *baht,* 1 *fueang*
	phlai		

phrik Thai	
khing	dried
krathiam	

1 *fueang* of each

12 items. Prepare pills to be taken mixed with alcohol to counteract the effects of *saang faai, saang daeng, saang chon* and *saang phloeng.* To treat diarrhoea, mix with *taan mon* leaf sap; when used as a laxative, mix with *kaphrao* leaf sap; to treat flatulence, mix with *sawaat* leaf sap. If *saang* affects the tongue, add borax and apply.

[372] ***Thep nimit***

san phraa hom	leaves
muek hom	
chan	seeds
dee plee	
kammathan daeng	
saan som	
chamot	
phimsen	

Equal parts, 8 items. Pills. If *saang nam, saang faai* or any type of *saang* affects the tongue, the medicine is to be taken or applied to the tongue, mixed with lime juice. If it affects the chest, it should be taken mixed with alcohol; if the *saang* affects the throat, add some snake's bile and swab the throat.

Mouth paint to treat *saang faai*:

[373]

khamin oi		
phlai		
marum	bark	
thong laang bai mon	bark	
manaao	seeds	
saan som		
hom		
kammathan daeng		
1 *salueng* of each		
krathiam		
dee plee		
1 *fueang* of each		
nam prasaan thong		2 *salueng*
phrik Thai		3 peppercorns

12 items. Prepare a stick. To treat *saang nam, saang faai* and all *saang* which affects the chest and intestines, and for pain, mucus and blood in the stools, *khamao* on the tongue, and *saang* encroaching on the mouth causing inflammation and offensive smelling faeces. Rub down [a little of the stick] to powder, add a little *yaa yong fai* and apply [to the mouth]. Without a doubt, this is highly recommended.

[374]	***Mahaa prakaan***		
	sang karanee		
	nguu lueam	bile	
	prakham dee khwaai	fruit	
	tumkaa daeng		
	reesee phasom laeo		
	raatchadat	fruit	
	krathiam		

Equal parts, 7 items. Prepare pills the size of cotton seeds, using a decoction of *nam tumkaa daeng* as excipient. Give dry pills to the child to treat the poison of *saang* which makes the child lose its voice.

Stomach mixture to treat *saang faai* and all *saang:*

[375]	*phrik Thai*	
	khing	
	dee plee	
	krathiam	
	saan som	
	din prasiu khaao	
	kluea sinthao	
	khamin chan	an amount equal to all the other ingredients

8 items. Prepare pills using lime juice as excipient. To be taken mixed with lime juice.

To treat *saang nam* and *saang faai:*

[376]	*kraphrao*	leaves
	taan mon	leaves
	faai daeng	leaves
	kraphang hom	leaves

Equal parts, 4 items. Pills to be taken mixed with alcohol.

Oil to treat inflammation caused by *saang nam:*

[377]	*fin*	decoction of bark sap	1 cupful
	nam dee nguu [8]	decoction	1 cupful
	thua phuu	bark sap	1 cupful
	ngaa	oil	1 cupful

Boil down until only oil remains, then mix together

benyakaanee		5 galls
see siat thet		1
nguu lueam	bile	1

Combine these three items with the oil and apply to the inflammation of *saang nam* all over the body. If this is to be taken, add *kaarabuun.*

Mouth paint to treat *saang nam* and *saang faai:*

[378]	*kaarabuun*	
	mafai	leaves
	nam prasaan thong	

Equal parts, 3 items. Prepare a stick to be used to make a mouth paint to counteract the effects of *saang nam.*

The masters warn doctors treating *saang nam* and *saang faai* not to give the medicines called *Benchataan* and *Prasakaphrao.*

Here ends the description of *saang faai,* the minor *saang* of *saang nam.*

Here the masters discuss ***la saeng phrachan,*** which is associated with *saang nam.*

La saeng phrachan occurs not only with *saang nam,* but also with other kinds of birth *saang.* Doctors must understand this. The diagnosis of *la saeng phrachan* is made clear in the description of *saang* [*chaang*] in Part 6.

In the description of *saang nam* here in Part 2, the masters next give the remedies for *la saeng phrachan* when it is associated with *saang nam,* as follows:

Mouth paint for *la saeng phrachan*:

[379]	*thian dam*		
	saan som		
	mawaeng thang 2	fruit	
	dee plee		

Equal parts, 5 items. Prepare a stick using alcohol as excipient and use to make a paint to apply to *la saeng phrachan.*

Paint to dab on *la saeng phrachan*:

[380]	*nam prasaan thong*		
	tuk kae	faecal matter	
	malaeng saap	faecal matter	
	2 *klam* of each[9]		
	manaao		7 seeds

Prepare a stick from these 4 items using alcohol as excipient. Add some *chamot* and *phimsen* and dab on the *la saeng phrachan.*

Another:

[381]	black dog	head
	crow	bones
	vulture	bones
	python	bones
	Burn until charred, then add	
	cuttle fish	bone
	borax	
	cloves	
	Borneo camphor	

using equal parts of each of the 8 ingredients. Then add an equivalent amount of burnt earthworms. Prepare a stick, using alcohol as excipient. Mix with alcohol and paint the mouth to counteract the effects of *la saeng phrachan.*

Another:

[382]	*chaat horakhun cheen*	
	malaeng saap	faecal matter

lin thale	
som poi	roasted pods
nam prasaan thong	
saan som sat	
chun see sat	

Equal parts, 7 items. Prepare a stick, mix with salt water and paint the mouth affected by *la saeng phrachan.* If a child does not respond to these 4 prescriptions, then it will be impossible to cure *saang nam* later.

Here ends the description of *la saeng phrachan.*

Here we speak briefly of the *la-ong phrabaat* **called *la-ong kaeo witchian***, which comes from *saang nam*; for the information of doctors.

Description of *la-ong kaeo witchian.* Examine the palate, tongue and inside the mouth on both sides. If it looks like the shiny white surface of coconut meat before it is touched, it is called *la-ong phrabaat.* It results from *la saeng phrachan* and causes continuous diarrhoea which prevents the baby from sleeping. At the same time there is a great deal of flatulence, as if [the abdominal contents] are both rising and falling. Doctors will find this condition difficult to cure. If it resembles coconut cream on the palate and tongue, it is called *la-ong kaeo witchian* and comes from *saang nam.* This affects the whole mouth, making it impossible for the child to eat or drink. If the doctor gives the right treatment, this condition will go and never return, but it will continue if the medicine is not appropriate. If medicine is applied to the throat in the evening the *la-ong* might go, only to reappear in the morning or, if treated in the morning, it might go then reappear in the evening. The baby will then feel hot and be unable to sleep. It will start in its sleep and sometimes have diarrhoea, or it will have flatulence and constipation and the eyes will roll back, then the child will have a constant cough. This *la-ong kaeo witchian* is a very serious condition in children. It will be impossible to cure if the doctor gives medicine which is not effective within three days. Doctors should be aware that the throat paint should be applied at sunset and then the *la-ong* will go. It should never be done in the morning for *la-ong kaeo witchian* or any kind of *saang, la* or *la-ong.* Doctors should understand what has been stated here!

Medicine to treat *la-ong kaeo witchian*:

[383]	*makruut*	root
	manaao	root
	mangua	root
	phut son	root
	mali	root
	anchan khaao	root
	rayom	root
	phitsanaat	root
	chetta phang khee	root
	kraam [khraam] daeng	root
	kraam chaang [plant]	root

khraam dee	root
khaa kae	

Equal parts, 13 items. Prepare a stick. Mix with proof spirit [*nam yat lao*], both to apply and be taken to counteract the effects of *la-ong kaeo witchian.*

Another:

[384] *puu chao loi thaa*

som kop	root
haang krakok	root

Equal parts, 3 items. Pills to be taken mixed with alcohol to treat *la-ong kaeo witchian.*

Mouth paint to treat *la-ong kaeo witchian* and *la-ong phrabaat* resulting from *la saeng phrachan:*

[385]	*mai ruak*	skin
	proh hom	
	lin thale	
	nam prasaan thong	

Equal parts, 4 items. Prepare a stick, mix with lime water and paint the child's mouth.

Mouth paint to make *la-ong kaeo witchian* subside:

[386]	*chaat horakhun*	
	phimsen	
	nom phichit	leaves
	mara	leaves
	malaeng saap	faecal matter
	nguu lueam	bile
	kluea	

Equal parts, 7 items. Prepare a stick, mix with lime juice and paint the mouth. Recommended.

[387] ***Fon saen haa***

bua luang	root
puu thale	claws
lin thale	
khong saam yaan	leaves
thua phuu	root
din so phong	

Equal parts, 6 items. Prepare a stick, mix with water used to wash rice and apply to the *la-ong kaeo witchian* and *la-ong phrabaat* resulting from *la saeng phrachan.*

Astringent mouth paint to treat *la-ong kaeo witchian* which causes inflammation:

[388] *phimsen*

nam prasaan thong

chaat horakhun

Equal parts, 3 items. Prepare a stick and make a paint. For inflammation in the child's mouth.

The masters have set forth, in the description of children born on Monday, that *saang nam* is the main illness, *saang faai* is the minor intervening disease, and the *la* called *saeng phrachan* and *la-ong* called *kaeo witchian* are complications of *saang nam*. It ends here.

Phrakhamphee prathom chindaa , Book III, Part 3.

Summary. Children born on Tuesday have the symptoms of *saang daeng* as the predominant illness, *saang kranae* is the minor *saang,* the *la* is called *utthayakaan*, the *la-ong* is *kaeo morakot* and the *lom* is called *utthonwaat.*

(*Saang daeng* has already been described on p.109, but it differs [from the following] towards the end and in the prescriptions. These particular sections are therefore presented here.) [sic]

Examine the middle ribs of the right side. If the tendons are still sound, there is no paralysis. Otherwise, the baby is affected by *lom utthonwaat* [the wind of the womb], which has been present since it was in the womb. This makes the infant cry from the time it is still by the fire until it is three months old, when *lom utthonwaat* goes away of its own accord. Treatment has no effect. When the *lom* moves down from the head to the chest and then to the abdomen, it is called *lom kong yai.* It moves [literally, blows] up through the abdomen, along the tendons next to the spine into the chest and throat and up to the orifice of the right ear and to the crown of the head.[10] If this occurs during the waxing of the moon, the baby will die; if during the waning of the moon, it will not die. Some say this disease is caused by *tabong Rāhū,* some say *kumaatthasang* or *akkhamuukkhee.* These seven kinds of demons affect boys and girls in the same way.

If the male form of *saang daeng* occurs in the chest, the baby has difficulty in breathing; if it occurs in the shoulder, there is pain and stiffness in the back; if it is in the throat, the child cannot eat or drink. The sign of death from *saang daeng* is the development of an abscess in each armpit. These are the size of lotus seeds in the flesh, and the skin is the colour of candle smoke. Then a pustule or abscess comes up in the crown of the head and moves down to the forehead. It is like *champaa* petals [orange or yellow], then changes to the colour of candle smoke. If it reaches the space between the eyebrows, it makes the baby blind and deaf. Then it spreads to the tip of the nose and at first the lips curl back, and when the child is about to die, [the *saang*] appears all over the body. On the forehead there are round, yellow, red and white spots like seals [stamps]. Whether it is male or female *saang daeng,* this is the sign of death. If the doctor cannot cure it the baby will die, without a doubt.

The masters then bring together all the recipes for medicine to treat the male and female forms of *saang daeng,* as follows.

Mouth paint for *saang daeng*

[389]	*raak din*	burnt
	nam tao khom	burnt bark
	plaa chon	burnt scales
	nam prasaan thong sat	

Equal parts, 4 items. Powder finely and mix with lime juice to paint the mouth.

Another:

[390] *lahung daeng* root
prakham dee khwaai fruit
manaao seeds
yaa fin
1 part of each
chaat horakhun 2 parts
5 items. Prepare a stick and mix with lime juice to paint the mouth to counteract the effects of *saang daeng.*

Another:

[391] *sang*
nam prasaan thong
lin thale
manaao seeds
khai fak shell
phimsen flakes
Equal parts, 6 items. Prepare a stick and mix with lime juice to paint the mouth or apply to the throat to treat *saang daeng.*

Another:

[392] *faek hom*
plaa chon tail
nam prasaan thong
samo rong raeng
manaao leaves
nam tao leaves
Equal parts, 6 items. Prepare a stick. To treat *saang daeng,* mix with river water and paint the mouth. To use as a laxative, mix with *nam makhaam piak* and python's bile and apply to the throat; if the child has a temperature [if its body is hot], use water which has been used to wash rice; for hiccoughs, use *matuum* fruit juice or *som saa* juice; for diarrhoea with red faeces, mix with *benyakaanee* gall juice; for cough, use lime juice and salt and add a small amount of the tail feathers of a peacock scorched brittle; and to treat *saang daeng,* mix with lime juice and *phimsen* and apply to the throat.

To treat *saang daeng* and *saang lueang:*

[393] *chaang* tusk
mahaatsadam
nun bark
kaphrao leaves
taan mon leaves
krathiam bulb
nam prasaan thong

Equal parts, 7 items. Reduce to a powder, then use a decoction of *som poi* seed pods as excipient to make a stick. To treat *saang daeng*, mix with lime juice and apply to the throat; to treat *saang phloeng*, mix with *nam khram*.

Another:

[394]	*benyakaanee*	galls	1 part
	prakham dee khwaai	fruit	2 parts
	nam prasaan thong		3 parts

3 items. Prepare a stick and mix with *nam som saa* and paint the tongue to treat *saang daeng* on the tongue.

Another:

[395]	*lin thale*	toasted
	raak din	burnt
	nam prasaan thong sat	
	boraphet	
	kon mo kaeng	

Equal parts, 5 items. Prepare a stick, mix with *nam mangua* and apply to the throat. Before using this, first apply salt water, then this throat application will be very effective.

Mouth paint to treat *saang daeng*, *saang faai* and *saang kraduuk*:

[396]	*hoi phimphakaarang*	shell
	kraben	burnt skin
	lin thale	toasted
	nam prasaan thong	
	malaeng saap	faecal matter
	manaao seeds	
	benyakaanee	galls
	chaat horakhun thet	
	chaat horakhun cheen	
	chaat cho sae	
	hoi khong	calcined shell
	maaraa nest	
	krathiam	bulb
	nguu lueam	bile
	phimsen	flakes

Equal parts, 14 items. Prepare a stick, mix with lime juice and apply to the throat to counteract the effects of all types of *saang*.

If the previous prescription is ineffective, the doctor should quickly prepare this stronger medicine, then the child's life will be saved.

[397] ***Pakhaao kwaat wat***

malaeng saap	faecal matter
chaat horakhun	
thian yaowa phaanee	
phak chee raa [laa]	

samo Thai	
saan som	
kot so thet	
one part of each	
khrai khruea	root
cha-em thet	root
kammathan daeng	
nam prasaan thong	
lin thale	
bia chan	calcined
banlangsinlaa	
yaa tai bai	
katang muut	
raak din	burnt
horaphaa thet	fruit
maklam khruea	root
som kung noi	fruit
2 parts of each	

20 items. Prepare a stick. To treat vomiting, mix with a decoction of *nam samo Thai* and apply to the throat; to treat *saang* on the tongue, and all seven kinds of [birth] *saang*, mix with *nam khamin oi.*

[398] ***Thep mongkhon***

malaeng saap	faecal matter
yaa yong fai	
bunnaak	flowers
bua luang	pollen
krisanaa	
kralam phak	
khondok	
waai takhaa	
thian dam	
nam prasaan thong	
chan thang 2	
suea	eye tooth
chorakhe	eye tooth
chaang	tusk
kot phung plaa	
chaat horakhun	
nguu lueam	bile
chorakhe	bile
chamot	
phimsen	
thong kham pleo	

Equal parts, 22 items. Prepare a stick to use to make an application for the throat. To treat *saang daeng*; stiff tongue and lockjaw; loss of sensitivity to the eyes [*taa khaeng*], with no tears; and unconsciousness.

To treat white coloured *la-ong phrabaat*, mix the previous medicine with aromatic water and apply to the throat; to treat blue-green coloured *la-ong phrabaat*, mix with *nam khram* and alcohol; to tread red coloured *la-ong phrabaat*, mix with *nam hua hom*; to treat yellow coloured *la-ong phrabaat*, mix with *nam khamin oi*, and apply to the throat.

Mouth paint for *saang daeng*:

[399]	*hoi sang*	calcined
	chaat horakhun Thai	
	banlangsinlaa	
	raet	molar tooth
	chaang	molar tooth
	faan	horn
	suea	eye tooth
	chorakhe	eye tooth
	bua luang	pollen
	phimsen	

Equal parts, 10 items. Prepare a stick. To be applied with aromatic water to treat *saang daeng*.

Another:

[400]	*nguu hao*	head
	raeng	head
	kaa	head
	hoi sang	
	raak din	
	bunnaak	flowers
	din thanam	
	nam prasaan thong	
	muek hom	
	raet	horn
	kui	horn
	nuu thuean	droppings
	krisanaa	
	kralam phak	
	chan	seeds
	chan	arils
	suea	eye tooth
	chorakhe	eye tooth
	raet	eye tooth
	muu	eye tooth
	raet	molar tooth

chaang	molar tooth

Equal parts, 22 items. Prepare a stick, mix with lime juice and apply to the throat for all kinds of saang.

Another:

[401] *kammathan daeng*
phimsen
krisanaa
kot thang 5
thian thang 5
chan arils
khrai khruea
cha-em thet
chaat kon
kamyaan
lot thanong
see siat thet
saan som
krak khee
samo thet
waan keep raet
waan ron thong
neraphuusee thet
tumkaa daeng

Equal parts, 27 items. Prepare a stick using alcohol as excipient and mix with lime juice. To be taken, used as a [mouth] paint or applied to the throat to treat *saang daeng* and all kinds of *saang*.

In treating *saang daeng*, doctors should never give medicine containing croton or oil or hot-and-spicy medicine. Use only mild medicine and treat as for poisoning from *khai sannibaat* with a high temperature. Do not use the medicine called *Benchataan* [no. 92], then the baby will escape from Phrayaa Matchuraat and be saved.[11]

[402] ***Prasaan thong***

chamot	fresh	
chamot chiang		
1 *fueang* of each		
phimsen		1 *salueng*
krung khamao		
amphan		
bunnaak	flowers	
nam prasaan thong		
lin thale	toasted	
2 *salueng* of each		
tree katuk		
kot thang 5		
thian thang5		

chan	seeds
chan	arils
krawaan	
kaan phluu	
chan [*thang*] 2	
krisanaa	
kralam phak	
chaluut	
khondok	
proh hom	
raatchadat	fruit
saaraphat phit	fruit
phayaa raak khaao	
plaa lai phueak	
tumkaa thang 2	
khukha	
mahaatsadam	
mahaa lalaai	
rayom	root
khrai khruea	root
waan keep raet	
waan ron thong	
waan nam	
saen prasa ton	
saen prasa khruea	
suraamrit	
omchoei [*opchoei*] *thet*	
1 *baht* of each	
thong kham pleo	20 sheets

61 items. Grind finely together, then add these 7 [6] kinds of bile

python	bile
crocodile	bile
soft-shelled turtle	bile
wild boar	bile
serpent-headed fish	bile
peacock	bile

Prepare pills, using water as excipient. To treat the poison of *saang* and *khai sannibaat*, this is to be taken mixed with aromatic water. To treat the poison of smallpox; boils and abscesses; and of venomous snakes, to be taken mixed with alcohol.

[403] ***Sommit kumaan noi***

son	heartwood
chan	seeds
chan	arils

krawaan		
kaan phluu		
opchoei		
samun waeng		
chan chamot		
krisanaa		
kralam phak		
chaluut		
khondok		
chamot chiang		
yaa faran		
phak chee raa [*laa*]	fruit	
sang karanee		
1 *salueng* of each		
kot thang 5		
phimsen		
amphan thong		
2 *salueng* of each		
thian thang 5		
1 *baht* of each		
kamyaan		5 *salueng*

33 items. Grind together finely. To treat the poison of *saang* affecting the heart, and *saang* affecting the liver, lungs and upper chest, causing mucus and blood in the stools, listlessness, weakness and exhaustion, prepare pills using aromatic water as excipient. To be taken mixed with aromatic water and *nam chan* to treat agitation; to treat vomiting, use a decoction of *yo* fruit; to treat breathlessness, with debility and weakness, use a decoction of *thua phuu* root sap; to treat delirium, mix with a decoction of sap from the heartwood of *son*; to treat inability to eat, it is to be taken mixed with syrup; to treat listlessness, mix with a decoction of *nam cha-em*; and to treat diarrhoea, mix with a decoction of bark sap of *marum*. This has been used and found very effective for all these purposes.

The masters say that all people, whether male or female, born into this world have diseases and parasites. It depends on the four elements [of the body]. If the elements are not in a satisfactory condition, first they will change, then diseases will develop later.

Doctors should prepare this tonic for the elements:

[404]	*taan dam*	root
	taan khamooi	root
	san phraa naang ae	bark
	khamin oi	
	phlai	
	tree phalaa	
	yaa tai bai	

thian yaowa phaanee
takhop bark
nam prasaan thong
saan som
chan thang 2
Equal parts, 13 items.
kaphrao an amount equal to the whole
Grind together finely and prepare pills to be taken mixed with alcohol to treat the stomach and all four elements.

[405] ***Patshannathaat***
tree katuk
krathiam
5 *salueng* of each
thian thang 5
1 *baht* of each
waan proh
haeo muu
muuk man bark
2 *baht* of each.
12 items. Pills. To treat diarrhoea, mix with *kaphrao* leaf sap, to be taken; to treat cough, mix with *nam mawaeng khruea*; to treat pain, this is to be taken after boiling with juice of *benyakaanee* galls and pomegranate fruit or *nam khrang,* and adding python's bile.

Medicine to treat the elements:

[406]	*yaa dam*		1
	kaphrao	leaves	2
	taan mon	leaves	2
	sawaat	leaves	3

4 items. Pills to be taken mixed with alcohol, in the mornings only. This medicine should not be taken in the afternoon. For children from one month to one year old. Dose according to the strength of the child.

Medicine to treat the elements:

[407] *chan* seeds
chan arils
krawaan
kaan phluu
khamin oi
1 *baht* of each
krachaai 2 *salueng*
kaphrao leaves
khon thee so leaves
taan mon leaves
2 *baht* of each

9 items. Prepare pills using proof spirit as excipient. To be taken, mixed with alcohol, in the evening. It should not be taken in the morning. For children from one month to one year old. Dose according to age and strength.

Medicine to counteract the effects of poor quality milk:

[408]	*cha-em thet*	
	chan thet	
	nam taan	granulated
	1 *salueng* of each	
	kot so thet	
	kot khamao	
	kot phung plaa	
	kot kaan phraao	
	kot chulaa lamphaa	
	2 *salueng* of each	

8 items. Prepare pills using aromatic water as excipient. To be taken mixed with a combination of lime juice, honey and river water. Give to children to counteract the effects of poor quality milk, the poison of *saang* in the throat and upper chest, and for coughs, hiccoughs and vomiting.

Another recipe to treat *saang daeng* when it affects the duct of the liver, first causing diarrhoea with blood for four to five days, then a severe cough, yellow eyes, and regular fever; and the liver is enlarged [literally, hangs down below the ribs on the right side].

[409]	*benyakaanee*	galls	
	krathiam		2
	faang sen		3

3 items. Pills to be taken according to the strength of the child, mixed with lime water.

Next, prepare this poultice to apply to the ribs to contract the liver.

[410]	*no mai*
	khamao lek
	puun khaao

Apply this poultice to the ribs for three days.

If the liver does not contract completely, use this:

[411]	*tree phalaa*		1
	makhaam pom		1
	aai nieo	root	1
	lep mue naang	root	1
	khai nao	bark	1
	haeo muu		1
	boraphet	a piece of stem 3 inches long	
	muun kaa	cut one fruit in halves and use one half	
	thian dam		2 *salueng*
	thian khaao		2 *salueng*

nam prasaan thong		2 *salueng*
yaa dam		1
matuum	fruit	1
bua luang	pollen	1
bunnaak	flowers	1
raatcha phrik	pods	1
khamin oi		3 pieces
saan som		1
kaphrao	leaves	an amount equivalent to all the other ingredients combined

Mix with equal parts of alcohol and water. Reduce to 1/3 volume by boiling. To be taken.

The description of *saang daeng* ends here.

Siddhikāriyaḥ **Next a summary is given here of the development of *saang kranae,*** the minor *saang* of *saang daeng*. Doctors must know [this].

Saang kranae has three major pustules and 30 followers. It develops as one or two pustules together, with yellow, indented centres. One pustule comes up on the tip of the tongue, with ten followers; one on the tip of the chin, with ten followers; and there is one major pustule with ten followers at either the root of the tongue or in the upper chest. When the followers spread out around the major pustules they form the shape of a flame and make the baby sick, so that it cannot suck at the breast, the tongue and chin are stiff and it has spasms of the hands and feet. When the child is five months old, the three major pustules at the tip of the tongue, on the chin and at the root of the tongue or in the chest all move down together to the abdomen. Then the baby has diarrhoea with mucus and blood and the faeces look like water used to wash meat [or amniotic fluid], or spittle from a quid of betel and areca; and the baby passes purulent mucus and blood, is emaciated, cannot eat and is in severe pain. If a doctor intends treating it, he should be quite certain that his diagnosis of *saang kranae* is accurate.

[412] ***Chian nai phet*** throat paint

malaeng saap	roasted faecal matter	1
raak din	roasted	1
kraben	burnt skin	1
nam prasaan thong	anhydrous	1
nok yuung	the eyes of the tail feathers, scorched until brittle	1
nguu hao	head	1
puu thale	carapace	1
puu naa	carapace	1
katang muut		1
khai fak	shell	1
lin thale		1
benyakaanee	galls	1
kammathan daeng		1

bia phuu	calcined	1
muek hom		1
chaat kon		1
chamot chiang		1
amphan thong		1
thong kham pleo		10 sheets

Equal parts, 19 items. Prepare a stick, mix [some of this] with lime juice and apply to the *saang kranae* .

[413] ***Tree phalaa tret***

samo Thai
samo phiphek
makhaam pom
1 *salueng* of each

chan	seeds
chan	arils
krawaan	
kaan phluu	
tree katuk	
phak chee	fruit
horaphaa	fruit

2 *salueng* of each

benyakaanee	galls
see siat thet	

1 *baht* of each

12 items. Prepare pills using river water as excipient. To be taken mixed with a little opium, *din*[?] and *khamin oi* added. To treat the poison of *saang kranae* which enters the body and affects the abdomen; and the *saang* which affects the intestines, liver and lungs, causing painful dysentery with foul smelling blood and mucus in the faeces.

[414] ***Sangkha mutthathai***

sang nam
fun
chaat phong
chan thang 2

bua luang	pollen
saaraphee	flowers
phikun	flowers
bunnaak	flowers

Equal parts, 8 items. Pills to be taken mixed with the root sap of *bua luang* or *makok* to relieve the thirst of *saang kranae.*

Astringent for an inflamed tongue:

[415]	*waa*	juvenile leaves placed in the mouth of a cooking pot and steamed until cooked
	benyakaanee	galls

kho	dried dung
nam prasaan thong	
see siat thet	

Equal parts, 5 items. Prepare a stick. Mix with areca nut juice and paint the mouth and tongue of the child.

The description of *saang kranae*, the minor *saang* of *saang daeng* ends here.

Next, a summary is given here of the characteristics of the ***la* called *utthayakaan*** which results from *saang daeng*.

When *la utthayakaan* develops it causes convulsions with spasms of the hands and feet, kicking and crying, and neither the bowels nor the bladder function.

Medicine to treat *la utthayakaan*:

[416] *phimsen*
kluea sinthao
sakhaan
krathiam
Prepare a stick. Mix with cow's milk and paint the child's mouth.

Medicine to dab on the *la* of *saang kraduuk*:

[417]	*nguu lueam*	bones
	nguu thap thaang	bones
	chaat horakhun cheen	
	khaao	roasted
	malaeng saap	roasted faecal matter
	nuu ring	roasted droppings
	waai takhaa	

Equal parts, 7 items. Prepare a stick to be mixed with lime juice and dabbed on [the *la*].

Medicine to dab on *la*:

[418] *faang*
chan thang 2
phimsen
Mix with *nam makluea* and dab on.

Medicine to dab on *la*:

[419]	*kapee*	paste, partially burnt
	benyakaanee	galls
	phrik Thai	7 roasted peppercorns
	kaan phluu	
	chan thang 2	
	chamot	
	phimsen	

Equal parts, 8 items. Prepare a stick. Mix with water and dab on the *la*.

Here ends the description of *la utthayakaan* which results from *saang* [*daeng*].

A description of *la-ong kaeo morakot* is given here. It is very bad when this develops. The face is blue and black; [the child] has convulsions, spasms of the hands and feet, the mouth is open but makes no sound and the tongue and chin are stiff. The child will certainly die if the treatment is unsuccessful. Treat it with:

[420]	*chan thang* 2	
	neraphuusee	
	khrai khruea	
	dee nguu ton	
	rayom	
	phitsanaat	
	nguu lueam	bones
	waai takhaa	
	waai tamoi	

Equal parts, 10 items. Pills to be mixed with aromatic water to be taken or used as a lotion for *la-ong kaeo morakot.*

Medicine for *la-ong kaeo morakot*:

[421]	*puu chao phung kae*	
	tap tao thang 2	
	see huat noi	
	shat phra in	
	puu chao saming kui	
	khrai khruea	
	rayom	
	phitsanaat	
	neraphuusee	
	chan thang 2	
	nguan muu	
	yaa naang	root
	phrakham dee khwaai	root
	mai phai paa	decayed root-stock
	phak phaeo daeng	

Equal parts, 19 items. Pills to be taken mixed with aromatic water or water used to wash rice, to treat *la-ong kaeo morakot.*

Medicine to treat *chap* and *mua*:[12]

[422]	*chan chamot*	
	chan thanaa	
	phak chee	fruit
	phan phak kaat	
	yaa naang	root
	phlai	
	krachaai	
	cha-em thet	

Equal parts, 8 items. Pills. To treat *khlang,* to be taken mixed with aromatic water; to treat *chap,* mix with a decoction of *samo* juice; to treat breathlessness, mix with a decoction of *thua phuu* root sap; to treat vomiting, mix with a decoction of *yo* fruit juice, and add a little honey.

Saang daeng is worse than any other type of *saang*. The masters explain that the skilled doctor should notice the way the symptoms of this disease change, and adjust the treatment accordingly. The masters have described the symptoms of children born on Tuesday whose predominant illness is *saang daeng* and whose minor *saang* is *saang kranae*; the development of the *la* of *saang daeng*, called *la utthayakaan*, and of the *la-ong phrabaat* of *saang daeng* called *la-ong kaeo morakot*.

The summary ends here.

Phrakhamphee prathom chindaa, Book III, Part 4.

Summary. Children born on Wednesday have the symptoms of *saang sako* as the predominant illness, *saang kratang* is the minor *saang*, the *la* is called *niarakanthee* or *niaraphloeng*, the *la-ong* is called *saeng phloeng* and the *lom* is called *sunthonwaat*.

(*Saang sako* has already been described on page 111 of this volume.) [sic]

Note: when *saang sako* has finished, beware of the *la-ong phrabaat* and minor *saang* of *saang sako* which follow.

Here we give a brief description of *saang kratang*, the minor *saang* of *saang sako*. Doctors should understand this.

Now *saang kratang* has three major pustules and 30 followers. The baby has no *khamao* while by the fire; this comes at one month of age, after leaving the fire. When the *khamao* has gone, the major pustules of *saang* erupt one at a time - one in the abdomen, with ten followers; one in the throat, with ten followers; [and one in the chest, with ten followers].[13] When the baby is a month and a half old, the ten followers in the abdomen spread out and emerge in the ileum, the colon and up as far as the chest. The ten in the chest move down to the bladder and stomach, and the ten followers in the throat spread, some to the palate, some to the lips and tongue and some inside the cheeks, three layers thick, like filaments of soot clinging like cobwebs over a fireplace. If they appear in these three places at the same time, then the *saang* in the intestines causes dysentery, the *saang* in the bladder causes difficulty in urinating, the *saang* in the stomach causes colic and the baby does not feel like eating and cannot sleep. The *saang* in the throat causes a dry throat and the child makes no sound when it cries. The *saang* in the palate causes headache and breathing difficulties and the baby cannot suck at the breast. Doctors should not give laxatives to babies with *saang kratang*. This minor *saang* which sometimes arises with the main *saang* and sometimes follows it, can continue until the child is thirteen years old. They say that *saang kratang* is resistant to medicine. Sometimes, if medicine is smeared on the throat in the morning the symptoms abate until the following morning, when the *saang* reappears causing flatulence, a high temperature and goose-flesh. When the baby is three months old, all the major pustules and the followers which have spread all over the body move to the abdomen and two or three pustules enter the intestines, making the baby cry and twist and turn. When the child is six or seven months old, the doctor should apply a poultice and then the *saang* will go. The child will have diarrhoea, flatulence, thirst and other disorders at eleven months of age; and when it can walk, the abdomen is shaken up, causing mucus and blood in the stools once more. If a doctor is to treat this, he should prepare a lotion to be applied to the body to reduce the temperature. This *saang* is not incurable. If the doctor gives the wrong medicine, he might lose the battle, so he should be quite certain of his diagnosis of the disease before treating it.

Medicine for *saang sako* and *saang kratang*, the minor *saang*:

[423]	*yaa naang*	leaves
	khamin oi	
	neraphuusee	leaves
	krop kraep	leaves
	san phraa naang ae	leaves
	maak phuu	leaves

Equal parts, 6 items. Prepare a stick, using *nam yaa paak khwaai* as excipient. To be applied, mixed with water used to wash rice, to treat both external and internal heat.

Another:

[424]	*mara*	leaves	1
	faai thet	leaves	1
	phak khuang	leaves	1
	rangap phit	leaves	1
	nam tao	leaves	1
	chum het thet	leaves	1
	phekaa	leaves	1
	kaa ron	leaves	3
	fak khaao	leaves	1
	khamin oi		1

Equal parts, [sic] 10 items. Prepare a stick. To be applied mixed with water used to wash rice.

To treat the poison of this *saang*, first give *Yaa benchataan*. [no. 92]. If this is ineffective, *Yaa lueang sapphakhun* should be given next.

[425]	***Lueang sapphakhun***	
	khon thee so	leaves
	naat	leaves
	kaphrao	leaves
	phak khraat	leaves
	yaa tai bai	leaves
	khong saam yaan	leaves
	haang chorakhe	leaves
	waan nam	leaves
	waan haang chaang	leaves
	waan keep raet	
	waan ron thong	
	khamin oi	
	phlai	

kathue	
krachaai	
tree katuk	
khaa ling	
khaa hom	
khaa taa daeng	
kammathan lueang	
lin thale	
khrang	
horaa thao sunak	
horaa ammarit	
malaeng saap	faecal matter
chan	seeds
chan	arils
thian dam	
thian daeng	
neraphuusee	
din prasiu khaao	
saan som	
nam prasaan thong	
som poi	pods
hom	
krathiam	
khrai hom	
manaao	seeds
thian	leaves
thap thim	leaves

Equal parts, 41 items. Grind together. To be taken mixed with *saaraphat dee*, soaked in water, to counteract the poisonous effects of *saang sako* and *saang kratang*.

Medicine to treat listlessness [or stupor]:

[426]

chan thang 2	
krisanaa	
chaluut	
khondok	
bunnaak	flowers
bua luang	pollen
sattabut	pollen
chaat cho sae	
chamot	

Equal parts, 11 items. Grind together and mix with dew, spread out to dry on lontar palm leaves, then mix with aromatic water. Prepare pills to be taken to treat *saang sako*, *saang kratang* and *saang chon* affecting the upper chest and causing listlessness and restlessness, thirst, and breathlessness.

[427] ***Phat waan wichannee***

yaa sai	leaves	
chan thang 2		
krak khee		
khao nao	heartwood	
cha-em thet		

Equal parts, 6 items. Prepare a stick using aromatic water as excipient. Mix with water used to wash rice and apply.

Another:

[428]

khon thee so	leaves	
sadao	leaves	
khamin oi		
son	heartwood	
krak khee		
din prasiu khaao		
khot so thet		

Equal parts, 7 items. Prepare a stick. To be applied mixed with water used to wash rice or *nam thao tamlueng.*

To treat children who have flatulence at night:

[429]

thian khaao		
krawaan		
kaan phluu		
chan	seeds	
chan	arils	
1 *salueng* of each		
yaa tai bai		2 *salueng*
taan mon	leaves	
sawaat	leaves	
yaa dam		
1 *baht* of each		
mahaa hing		2 *baht*
neraphuusee		
dee plee		
chum het thet	leaves	
kaphrao		
4 *baht* of each		

14 items. Prepare pills, the size of kapok seeds, using water used to wash rice as excipient. Give one pill to infants one month old and increase the dose according to the age of the child.

Throat paint for *saang sako*:

[430]

mawaeng khruea	fruit	
tree katuk		

	krathiam	
	kammathan daeng	
	makruut	skin
	khamin oi	
	manaao	seeds
	saan som	
	din prasiu khaao	

Equal parts, 11 items. Grind together and add an equivalent amount of borax. Prepare a stick. To use as a throat paint for *saang*, mix with lime juice, salt and a little *phimsen*; to treat vomiting, it is to be taken with a decoction of *yo* fruit juice; to treat a dry throat, it is to be taken mixed with *nam cha-em*; and to obtain relief from bladder obstruction, inability to urinate, or bladder stones, the medicine is to be taken mixed with cucumber juice.

Throat paint for *saang sako* and *saang kratang*:

[431]	*waeo nok yung*	the eyes of the tail feathers, scorched brittle
	plaa chon	burnt tail
	maleang saap	burnt faecal matter
	takhrai	root-stock
	maeng daa	shell
	tree katuk	
	yaa yong fai	
	din prasiu khaao	
	kluea sinthao	
	phak khraat	flowers
	krathiam	
	lin thale	

Equal parts, 14 items. Prepare a stick using lime juice as excipient. To be used to apply to the throat [to counteract the effects of] *saang sako* and *saang kratang.*

Here ends the description of *saang sako* and its minor *saang, saang kratang.*

This is a brief description of **the *la* called *nerakanthee* or *ninlaphloeng*.** This *la* results from *saang sako.* Doctors should understand this.

When *la nerakanthee* or *ninlaphloeng* first develops it looks as green as a fresh leaf, then blood vessels can be seen. This passes, and in five days the child will have diarrhoea and very dry lips as well as a dry throat.

Medicine to treat *la nerakanthee* or *ninlaphloeng:*

[432]	*nam tao*	leaves
	phak hai	leaves
	praduu	leaves
	prakham dee khwaai	fruit
	fak khaao	leaves
	chan hom	leaves

Equal parts, 6 items. Prepare a stick, mix with alcohol and apply.

Medicine to treat *la nerakanthee* or *ninlaphloeng*:

[433]	*thian dam*	
	bai naat	
	din prasiu khaao	
	phrik Thai	
	chan	arils

Equal parts, 5 items. Prepare a stick. Mix with alcohol and paint the child's mouth.

Another:

[434]	*malaeng saap*	carcass
	nam prasaan thong	
	kaphrao	leaves
	krawaan	

Equal parts, 4 items. Prepare a stick. Mix with alcohol and paint the child's mouth.

Here ends the description of the *la* called *nerakanthee* or *ninlaphloeng*.

Here we give a brief description of ***la-ong saeng phloeng***. Doctors should understand this.

La-ong saeng phloeng results from *saang sako*. At first, the inside of the cheeks is white for a day and a night, then it turns as green as a leaf. The baby next becomes listless and stuporous, and has diarrhoea with leaf-green faeces, because the *la-ong* has moved down to the ileum and the neck of the gall bladder. To treat this kind of *la-ong*:

[435]	*manaao*	fruit, leaves and roots
	mai phai	buds
	boraphet	
	faang	
	hom	
	rayom	
	phitsanaat	
	chetta phang khee	

Equal parts, 10 items. Prepare a stick. Mix with lime water and paint the mouth, or mix with alcohol if it is to be taken.

If that is ineffective, prepare:

[436]	*khraam thang 3*	leaves	
	rak khaao	leaves	
	phluu kae	leaves	
	kaphrao	leaves	
	phak phaeo daeng		
	manaao	seeds	roasted until crisp
	makruut	seeds	roasted until crisp
	mangua	seeds	roasted until crisp
	raak din	burnt	
	som poi	toasted pods	

tree katuk	
krathiam	
raet	horn
chaang	tusk
kwaang	horn
nguu lueam	bile
fin	

Equal parts, 21 items. Prepare a stick using alcohol as excipient, then mix with river water and paint the child's mouth.

If the medicine is not effective, the doctor will be sorely pressed to cure this, because the whiteness of the tongue will extend to the base of uvula, causing emaciation, and the child's body will become as yellow as if painted with turmeric. When the baby is going to die, its body changes from yellow to white. Doctors should understand this!

Here ends the description of the *la-ong* called *saeng phloeng.*

Next is a brief description of the *lom* called *sunthonwaat* which results from *saang sako,* so that doctors will understand.

Now *sunthonwaat* starts in the vicinity of the navel and the lower abdomen, causing stomach ache and flatulence. Then the child has severe diarrhoea, sleeps continually, has convulsions with spasms of the hands and feet, its abdomen is distended and its face is blue.

Cleansing medicine to treat the seven kinds of *lom:*

[437] *phimsen*	leaves	
kaarabuun		
makruut	skin	
1 *salueng* of each		
mahaa hing		2 *salueng*
bai naat		1 *baht*
krathiam		1 *baht*
phrik Thai		1 *baht*
khing	dried	1 *baht*

8 items. Grind together. To be taken mixed with lime juice to counter the effects of *lom chuk siat, lom khop thaeng* and *lom arit;* and all the seven *lom* associated with *saang* of the seven days.

Decoction to treat *lom sunthonwaat,* causing diarrhoea:

[438] *yaa luuk khlao*	
thaeng thuai	bark
thian leaves	
thap thim	leaves
kathue	
phlai	
khaa	
khamin oi	
hom	

Equal parts, 9 items. Boil with a mixture of equal parts of alcohol and water, until reduced to 1/3 volume. To be taken.

(For two other recipes for medicine to treat *lom sunthonwaat*, see page 70, line 3 of this volume.)[sic]

The masters have explained the symptoms of children, born on Wednesday, resulting from *saang sako* as the predominant illness, *saang kratang* the minor *saang*, the *la* called *nerakanthee* or *ninlaphloeng*, the *la-ong* called *saeng phloeng* and the *lom* called *sunthonwaat*, associated with *saang sako*.

The end.

Phrakhamphee prathom chindaa, Book III, Part 5.

Summary. Children born on Thursday have the symptoms of *saang kho* as the predominant illness, *saang khaao plueak* is the minor *saang*, the *la* is called *ninlakaan*, the *la-ong* is called *mahaamek* and the *lom* is called *hatsakhinee*.

Medicine to treat *saang kho*:

[439]	*neraphuusee*	
	chan daeng	
	yaa dam	
	wua	dung found near a granary
	thian sattabut	
	benyakaanee	galls

Equal parts, 6 items. Grind together and mix with alcohol. To be taken or applied.

Another:

[440]	*bia phuu*	7 calcined shells
	thong laang naam	root

Mix with alcohol. To be taken or applied.

Another:

[441]	*khing*	dried
	chan	seeds
	chan	arils
	krathiam	

Mix with coconut cream, to be taken or applied to counteract the effects of *saang kho* and *saang kraduuk*.

[442]	***Pancha khong khaa***	
	hoi khraeng	calcined
	tamlueng tua phuu	leaves
	saan som	
	nam prasaan thong	
	din prasiu khaao	
	din so phong	

Equal parts, 6 items. Prepare a stick. Mix with lime juice to apply to the throat. Mix with water used to wash rice to apply as a lotion to treat *saang kho*.

Application for a dry throat:

[443] *cha-em*
tree katuk
krathiam
kluea
Equal parts, 6 items. Prepare a stick, mix with lime juice and a little shallot and paint the mouth if the throat is dry and there is no saliva.

Another:

[444]	*raatchadat*	fruit
	neraphuusee	
	sang karanee	
	chang daeng	
	prakham dee khwaai	6 fruits
	saaraphat phit	fruit
	taeng cheen	fruit
	tumkaa daeng	

Equal parts, 8 items. Prepare a stick. To be taken mixed with alcohol to treat a dry throat.

Throat paint for *saang kho*:

[445]	*nguu lueam*	burnt bones
	nguu thap thaang	burnt bones
	kho	burnt horns
	malaeng saap	roasted faecal matter
	chaat horakhun cheen	
	waai takhaa	burnt

Equal parts, 6 items. Prepare a stick and apply to the throat to treat *saang kho.*

Medicine to treat internal poison:

[446]	*kot so*	
	kot khamao	
	kot phung plaa	
	chan daeng	
	krisanaa	
	saaraphee	pollen

Equal parts, 6 items. Prepare pills the size of peppercorns, using a decoction of *nam lep mue naang* as excipient. Mix with aromatic water and a little *phimsen.* To be taken to counteract the effects of the poison of *taan* and *saang.* To treat listlessness, thirst and breathlessness, add granulated sugar. It may also be used to treat mucus and the seven kinds of *sang.* Highly recommended.

Here ends the description of *saang kho.*

Next is a brief description of *saang khaao plueak*, the minor *saang* which intervenes as a complication of *saang kho.* Doctors should understand this.

Saang khaao plueak has five major pustules and 50 followers. There is one major pustule at the crown of the head, one in the middle of the back, one in the abdomen, one under each arm and ten followers with each. This *saang* results from internal heat [one of the body elements]. Before the *saang* appears, the baby's mouth feels hot and it has diarrhoea. Then the *saang* develops, the child has cold hands and feet and is ill for the first time.[14] The major pustule in the crown of the head then moves down to the abdomen, making two pustules together and this makes the baby sick again. This is repeated when the pustule in the middle of the back moves to the abdomen, then those from the underarms, by which time five pustules have erupted in a row like this:

o o o o o

from beneath the navel to the supra-pubic area and the 50 followers have spread all over the body. Sometimes slightly itchy spots resembling rice-husks appear, which could be mistaken for measles [*hat*]. Sometimes they look like red and black birth-marks. Sometimes there are weals, as if the baby has been beaten with a rattan; sometimes there are red, black or blue marks, as if the child has been slapped with the fingers. The baby vomits, has diarrhoea, flatuence, spasms of the hands and feet, a stiff tongue and chin, and cannot suck at the breast. This continues for three to seven days, then the symptoms go.

If a doctor intends treating it, he should use the medicine ***Phrasuriyachanthanang*** as follows:

[447]	***Phrasuriyachanthanang***	
	salot nam	root
	thong laan naam	root
	phum riang baang [*baan*]	root
	tamlueng	root
	fak khaao	root
	mong	root
	lamduan	root
	lep mue naang	root
	suraamrit	root
	khong khaa dueat	root
	mueat khong	root
	plaa lai phueak	root
	thao yaa naang	root
	phayaa raak khaao	
	phayaa raak dam	
	chueak khao muak thang 2	
	yaa phraek	
	yaa paak khwaai	
	phrommi	
	bua luang	pollen
	chan thang 2	
	chaang	tusk

kwaang	horn
raet	horn
suea	eye tooth
chorakhe	eye tooth

Equal parts, 28 items. Mix these 28 ingredients with 20 fruits of *prakham dee khwaai* soaked in water. Prepare pills to be taken or applied, mixed with aromatic water. To treat heat and thirst and both *saang kho* and *saang khaao plueak.*

Throat paint for *saang kho* and *saang khaao plueak:*

[448]

nom maeo noi	root
lot thanong	
tumkaa daeng	
song baadaan	root
kradaan phon	root
khai nao	root
taeng nuu	root
hatsakhun	root
plao noi	
salot kin long	root
ching chee	root
taan sian	root
taan dam	root

Equal parts, 13 items. Prepare a stick. Mix with lime juice and paint the throat when *saang kho* and *saang khaao plueak* affect the throat and the root of the tongue. Also for the poison of *la* which causes a stiff tongue, lockjaw and inability to suck. To treat smallpox, this medicine is to be taken mixed with alcohol. And to treat the throat, poisoning, *saket* and *khlang*, and to prevent *kaan*[15] entering and developing internally.

To treat a child who has a shrivelled tongue, a dry throat, and cannot make a sound:

[449]

neraphuusee thang 2	
chuk rohinee	
cha-em thet	
waan nam	
thian dam	
phrik lon	
khing	dried
nguu lueam	
khanthatsakon	

Equal parts, 10 items. Prepare a stick, mix with alcohol and paint the mouth.

[450] ***Sommit kumaan yai***

chamot	fresh

chamot chiang	
phimsen	
kot chiang	
kot hua bua	
thian dam	
thian khaao	
thian daeng	
thian yaowa phaanee	
thian sattabut	
chan	seeds
chan	arils
krawaan	
kaan phluu	
chan daeng	
chan khaao	
krisanaa	
kralam phak	
khondok	
faek hom	
amphan	
phung men	
tree katuk	
chetta muun phloeng	
haeo muu	
proh hom	
opchoei thet	
chuk rohinee	
neraphuusee thet	
sadao	leaves
phimsen	leaves
kham Thai	flowers
saaraphee	flowers
phikun	flowers
bunnaak	flowers
champaa	flowers
mali	flowers
bua phuean	pollen
bua khom	pollen
lin chong	pollen
chong konlanee	pollen
sattabut	pollen
chaluut	
nguu lueam	bile
fin	

Equal parts, 47 items. Prepare pills using aromatic water as excipient. To be taken mixed with aromatic water to treat fevers of the three seasons, of *taan*, *saang* and *taan khamooi.*

[451] ***Klom naang noi***[16]

kot so
kot khamao
kot chiang
kot phung plaa
kot chulaa lamphaa
thian dam
thian daeng
thian khaao
thian khaao plueak
thian yaowa phaanee
thian sattabut
thian taa tak taen
bua phuean pollen
bua khom pollen
lin chong pollen
chong konlanee pollen
sattabut pollen
khrai khruea root
sang karanee
khondok
cha-em
nam prasaan thong
chamot
phimsen

Equal parts, 24 items. Powder finely and mix with aromatic water, then stick it on the underneath part of a bronze bowl, hold the bowl upright over a candle, and let it smoke and heat the entire bottom of the bowl. Prepare pills. Mix with aromatic water, to be taken for agitation and restlessness. To treat listnessness, this medicine is to be taken mixed with *nam krisanaa*; to treat mucus and blood in the stools, to be taken mixed with fresh areca nut juice; to treat mucus, mix with *nam mawaeng khruea*; and if [the child's] body is hot, mix with aromatic water and give by mouth or apply as a lotion.

The description of *saang khaao plueak*, the minor *saang* of *saang kho* ends here.

Next is a brief statement on the *la* called *ninlakaan.* This kind of *la* results from *saang kho.* Doctors should understand this.

When *la ninlakaan* arises, it paralyses half the body and [the baby] cannot cry. If this condition lasts more than a day or two, it changes to *mahaaninlakaan* which is very serious and the whole body turns blue.

Medicine to treat *la ninlakaan*:

[452]	*peep*	bark
	saaraphat phit	seeds
	naat	root
	makruut	bark
	khon thee so	leaves
	phak hom hin	root
	kaarabuun	
	thap thim	bark
	phimsen	

Equal parts, 9 items. Prepare a stick, mix with cow's milk and paint the mouth.

If that is ineffective:

[453]	*thua rae*	leaves
	tamlueng tua phuu	stem
	kluai teep	root
	kaan phluu	
	nam prasaan thong	

Equal parts, 5 items. Prepare a stick, mix with buttermilk 3 parts and water 1 part and paint the mouth.

If this is ineffective:

[454]	*horaphaa*	seeds
	maeng lak	seeds
	kaphrao	seeds
	manaao	seeds
	phak khraat	flowers
	nam prasaan thong	

Equal parts, 6 items. Prepare a stick, mix with lime juice and paint the child's mouth and tongue. To treat *saang fai*, *saang khamooi* and *saang khaao*, mix with alcohol and some snake's bile and apply to the throat.

Here ends the description of *la ninlakaan*, which results from *saang kho.*

Next is a brief description of the *la-ong phraabaat* called **(*la-ong*) *mahaa mek*** which results from *saang kho.* Doctors should understand this.

Now, when *la-ong mahaa mek* first develops, [it is the purple colour of] bruised *tabaak* flowers. This causes severe poisoning, a blue face, convulsions with spasms of the hands and feet and the eyes rolling back, and neither the bowels nor the bladder function.

Medicine to treat *la-ong mahaa mek*:

[455]	*naat*	root
	taeng thuean	root
	waai takhaa	
	waai tamoi	
	rayom	

phitsanaat	
khrai khruea	root
chan thang 2	
neraphuusee	
cha-em	

Equal parts, 11 items. Prepare a stick [and mix some of the powdered stick with liquid]. To be taken or applied.

If *saang, la-ong* or *la* affecting the tongue do not clear up after using these prescriptions, but return to their original sites, [looking] like the bottom of a rice pot, treat as follows:

[456]	*khlai samao chai*	
	khlai phrachedee	
	thian dam	
	thian daeng	
	thian khaao	
	thian khaao plueak	
	chan	seeds
	kot chulaa lamphaa	
	raet	burnt horn
	chaang	burnt tusk
	kwaang	burnt horn
	kui	horn
	phae	horn
	makruut	roasted skin
	phak som poi	roasted
	raak din	roasted
	kluea kratang	
	2 *salueng* of each	
	chaat kon	
	nam prasaan thong	
	1 *baht* of each	

Mix together these 18 items, prepare a stick, mix with alcohol and paint the tongue, whether it is black, red or green; whether the tongue is coated, *kratang* [meaning obscure] or covered in spots or pustules.

Here ends the description of *la-ong mahaa mek* which results from *saang kho.*

Next is a brief description of the *lom* called *hatsakhinee* which results from *saang kho.* Doctors should understand this.

Lom hatsakhinee starts with convulsions, spasms of the hands and feet, the back stiff, sweating and flatulence. If it happens in the morning, beware, the baby might die at midday. If it happens between noon and night, the child will not die. Do not bathe the baby in the morning or evening. Do not give medicine containing alcoholic liquor. This *lom* of *saang kho* begins from the third month of pregnancy, thus it affects the infant. This statement of the masters occurs in *Phrakhamphee prathom chindaa*, Book I, which discusses ante-natal care and states that only cool and mild medicine is suitable [to treat] this kind of *lom* as follows.

Medicine to treat *lom hatsakhinee*:

[457]	*taeng mo*	seeds
	oi daeng	buds
	yaa naang	root
	yaa paak khwaai	root
	krameng	leaves
	phak pet	leaves
	waan nam	
	tree katuk	
	krathiam	
	phak sian phee	leaves
	yaa luuk khlao	

Equal parts, 13 items. Pills. To be taken with [suitable] fluid; to apply, mix with water used to wash rice. To counteract *lom hatsakhinee*.

Medicine to treat *lom hatsakhinee*:

[458]	*phak chee*	fruit
	waan nam	
	phak khraat	flowers
	nam tao	leaves
	yaa tai bai	
	yaa paak khwaai	
	oi daeng	buds
	thua khieo	
	tree katuk	
	krathiam	

Equal parts, 12 items. Prepare a stick using water used to wash rice as excipient. To be taken mixed with hot water; to be applied to the crown of the head mixed with water used to wash rice; to treat *lom hatsakhinee*, *lom phutthayak* and *lom kumphanthayak*.

[459] ***Mahaa chak (yai)***

kot so
kot khamao
kot phung plaa
kot kaan phraao
kot kraduuk
thian dam
thian daeng
thian khaao
thian khaao plueak
thian yaowa phaanee
tree phalaa

yaa faran		
chan	seeds	
chan	arils	
krawaan		
kaan phluu		
cha-em		
horaphaa	seeds	
phak chee	fruit	
saan som		
din prasiu khaao		
khamin oi		
krathiam		
nam prasaan thong		
2 *salueng* of each		
yaa dam		2 *baht*
kraphang hom	leaves	15 *baht*

28 items. Pills. To be taken with juice of the Chinese date to treat the *lom* of each of the *saang* of the seven days. Undoubtedly reliable.

The masters have described the symptoms of children born on Thursday. *Saang kho* is the main disease, *saang khaao plueak* is the minor complication, the *la* called *ninlakaan* and the *la-ong phrabaat* called *mahaamek* are associated with *saang kho.* It ends here.

Phrakhamphee prathom chindaa, Book III, Part 6.

Summary. Children born on Friday have the symptoms of *saang chaang* as the predominant illness, the *la* is called *saeng phrachan* and the *lom* is called *lom arit.*

Siddhikāriyaḥ Next, the masters describe the symptoms of children born on Friday. **Saang chaang is the main illness of these children.** Doctors should recognise it by the symptoms.

Medicine to treat *saang chaang*:

[460]	*song baadaan*	leaves
	yaa sai	

Of each, one cupful of juice. Prepare pills, adding some snake's bile. To be taken or applied.

Medicine to treat the diarrhoea of *saang chaang*:

[461]	*son*	heartwood
	prakham dee khwaai	fruit
	praduu	heartwood
	som poi	root
	song baadaan	root

Equal parts, 5 items. Boil down to 1/3 volume. To be taken to treat the diarrhoea of *saang chaang.*

Decoction to treat *saang chaang*:

[462]	*çhum het*	leafy tips of new shoots
	thap thim	leafy tips of new shoots

phutsaa leafy tips of new shoots
khamin oi
Equal parts, 4 items. Reduce to 1/3 volume. To be taken.

Throat paint for *saang chaang:*

[463] *nam tao khom* bark
hoi khom calcined
khon thee so leaves
takhrai root-stock
khamin [*oi*] rhizome
Remove the contents of the *khamin oi* rhizome and replace with 1 *baht* of borax. Heat on a slow fire of rice husks until cooked. Mix with the other ingredients and add a little *phimsen.* Prepare a stick and mix with the juice from the fruit rinds of fresh areca and paint on. If that is ineffective, mix with lime juice and paint the throat or mouth.

[464] ***Malaeng pong* throat paint** to get rid of *saang chaang* quickly:
thua phuu root
thua rae leaves
phak bung thet
prakham dee khwaai fruit
hatsakhun leaves
waan keep raet
waan ron thong
7 items. Of each 1 *salueng.*
nguu taboi phalam bile 1 *fueang*
Prepare pills using alcohol as excipient. To be taken or applied to the throat or mouth to treat *saang chaang.* If this is ineffective, add a little *waan keep raet, waan ron thong* and python's bile. To make it go away quickly, add *chan daeng* and *neraphuusee* and apply to the throat.

Throat paint for *saang chaang*:

[465] *raet* burnt horn
kwaang burnt horn
kraben burnt skin
khon singed hair
waai takhaa roasted
mawaeng thang 2 roasted root
tree katuk
Equal parts, 8 items. Prepare a stick, mix with alcohol and apply to the throat.

[466] ***Hingkhuwatchaa***
tree katuk
mahaa hing
neraphuusee
chan seeds
chan arils

krawaan	
kaan phluu	
kot khamao	
kot so	
thian dam	
thian khaao	
chan thang 2	
benyakaanee	galls
1 *salueng* of each	
krathiam	
sawaat	leaves
thian	leaves
phak khraat	leaves
kaphrao	leaves
kraphang hom	leaves
samee	leaves
kathue	
phlai	
hom	
khamin oi	
2 *baht* of each	
fin	
chorakhe	bile
taphaap nam	bile
nguu lueam	bile
2 *phai* of each	

31 items. Prepare pills using alcohol as excipient, to be taken mixed with alcohol. Stomach mixture to prevent the poison of *saang*, to treat *taan* and *saang* when they affect the liver causing fresh blood to appear in the faeces, *saang* at the anus and urethra, in the mouth, throat or on the tongue, causing severe thirst or listlessness.

[467] ***Inthachak***

thian dam	
thian daeng	
thian khaao	
thian yaowa phaanee	
thian sattabut	
chan	seeds
chan	arils
krawaan	
kaan phluu	
mahaa hing	
yaa dam	
kaarabuun	

phrik Thai
krathiam
2 *salueng* of each

dee plee	1 *baht*

15 items. Pills. To treat back rigidity, insensitivity of the eyes, and lock-jaw, mix with *nam makruut* and some opium and apply to the affected area. If the child is listless because of *lom* or has diarrhoea with mucus and blood, the medicine is to be taken mixed with alcohol. Without a doubt, this is very effective against all [these].

[468] ***Inthon banchop khuu kan***

chamot	
phimsen	
chan thang 2	
krisanaa	
kralam phak	
khondok	
waan keep raet	
waan ron thong	
makhaam pom	fruit
yaa dam	
mahaa hing	
krathiam	
nguu lueam	bile

1 *salueng* of each

thian dam	
thian khaao	
thian daeng	
thian yaowa phaanee	
thian sattabut	
chan	seeds
chan	arils
kaan phluu	
krawaan	

2 *salueng* of each. 23 items. Grind together, then add

nguu hao	bile
chorakhe	bile
thaphaap nam	bile
plaa chon	bile
plaa lai	bile

1 *salueng* of each. Soak in water, then make pills. To be taken mixed with aromatic water to treat extreme distress. If this is ineffective, then mix it with alcohol to counteract the effects of all types of *taan* and *saang*, and to treat convulsions with spasms of the hands and feet.

[469] ***Nanthakraiwaat***	
nguu lueam	bones
nguu thap thaang	bones
chaang	tusk
raet	molar tooth
plaa chon	the underside of the fish's jaw
kot so	
kot kraduuk	
thian dam	
horaphaa	fruit
phak chee	fruit
nam prasaan thong	
phimsen	leaves
san phraa hom	leaves
phak waan baan	leaves
thong laang naam	root
salot nam	root
fak khaao	root
tamlueng	root
thua phuu	root
manaao	seeds
waai takhaa	
saaraphat phit	fruit
khrai khruea	
saaraphee	pollen
phikun	pollen
bunnaak	pollen

Equal parts, 27 items. Prepare pills using aromatic water as excipient and use for convulsions in both children and adults. For listlessness, add some snake's bile and *phimsen*. For thirst, breathlessness, a stiff tongue and lock-jaw, mix with aromatic water or water used to wash rice. To be taken or applied.

Here ends the description of *saang chaang*.

Next is a brief description of the *la* called *saeng phrachan*. This *la* results from *saang chaang* (and *saang nam*). Doctors should understand this.

La saeng phrachan starts with yellow pustules the size of maize kernels on either side of the jaw, giving the baby diarrhoea, loss of sensitivity to the eyes, a stiff tongue and chin, and when it cries it produces no tears. Its forehead is pinched and its body is cold.

Medicine to dab on *la saeng phrachan*:

[470] *thian dam*	
saan som	
kammathan daeng	
benyakaanee	galls

kaan phluu	
dee plee	
nam prasaan thong	
makruut	skin
phrik Thai	roasted
kluea	roasted

Equal parts, 10 items. Prepare pills using *mawaeng* fruit juice as excipient. Mix with lime juice and dab on *la saeng phrachan* which results from *saang chaang.*

Medicine to be taken for *la saeng phrachan*:

[471]

puu chao phung kae	
puu chao samung kui	
shat phra in	
nom maeo noi	
see huat yai	
see huat noi	
tap tao noi	
tap tao yai	
rayom	root
khrai khruea	root
phitsanaat	
neraphuusee	
chan daeng	
chan khaao	
nguan muu	
yaa naang	root
prakham dee khwaai	root
mai phai paa	decayed root-stock
phak phaeo daeng	

Equal parts, 18 items. Pills to be taken and applied as a lotion mixed with aromatic water.

Throat paint for *la saeng phrachan*:

Use the paint recommended for *la ninlaphloeng* caused by *saang sako.* See *Prathom chindaa* [Book III], Part 4.

End of description of *la saeng prachan.*

Next is a brief description of **the *lom* called *lom arit*** which results from *saang chaang.* Doctors should understand this.

When *lom arit* first develops, it makes the neck blue and causes convulsions, with spasms of the hands and feet. Sometimes the convulsions affect only part of the left side, sometimes part of the right side; sometimes [the whole of] the left or the right side, so that the chin stiffens and the baby cannot cry and dribbles, the eyes roll, the eyebrows twitch, he looks with one eye only, and mucus in the throat makes the child make a sound like *krok-krok.* If a child is affected in this way, *lom arit* is the offender. When the baby dies, its body is as yellow as if it had been sprayed with fresh turmeric water, because this *lom* comes from *la-ong phrabaat kaan singkhalee* as explained.[17]

Medicine to treat *lom arit*:

[472]	*khukha*	
	yaa naang	root
	chueak khao muak	
	nam tao taek	bark
	saaraek khaat	
	khaan hua duan	
	tree katuk	
	kaarabuun	
	mahaa hing	
	waan nam	
	makruut	skin
	krathiam	

Equal parts, 14 items. Pills to be taken mixed with hot water, to treat *lom arit, lom sunthonwaat, lom waattaphak, lom akkhamukkhee,* and *lom baa muu.* This is an excellent remedy which can be relied upon to get rid of all these kinds of *lom.*

Another:

[473]	*nam oi daeng*		1 *thanaan*
	kho dam	urine	1 *thanaan*
	ma-uek	root sap	1 *thanaan*
	anchan thang 2	leaf sap	1 *thanaan* of each
	krachao khaao	leaf sap	1 *thanaan*
	krachao daeng	leaf sap	1 *thanaan*
	phak hom hin	leaf sap	1 *thanaan*
	phak hom hat	leaf sap	1 *thanaan*
	nam manaao		2 *thanaan*
	krawaan		
	kaan phluu		
	samun waeng		
	thian yaowa phaanee		
	phak phaeo daeng		
	1 *salueng* of each		
	kot so		2 *salueng*
	dee plee		
	khing	dried	
	waan nam		
	1 *baht* of each		
	mahaa hing		
	phlai		
	2 *baht* of each		

Mix together, and put on a fire in a wide mouthed cooking pot, and stir until well enough done to make pills. To be taken for *lom arit* and all kinds of *lom.*

[474] ***Prasa lom***

phimsen	leaves
kaarabuun	
makruut	skin
1 *salueng* of each	
krathiam	bulb
phrik Thai	
khing	dried
bai naat	
1 *baht* of each	

7 items. Prepare pills with lime juice as excipient. To be taken mixed with *nam makruut*, lime juice or *nam som saa* to counter the effects of *lom chuk siat khop thaeng, lom arit* and all the *lom* of *saang.*

Medicine to treat the convulsions of *lom arit*:

[475]

kaarabuun		1 *baht*
waan nam		1 *baht*
yaa dam		2 *baht*
hing yaang pho		2 *baht*
chan	seeds	2 *baht*
proh hom		2 *baht*
hua hom		2 *baht*
phimsen		9 *salueng*

8 items. Pills. Give one pill at 1 month of age, two at 2 months, and increase according to the age and strength of the child, or use as a lotion. For the convulsions of *lom arit* and all forms of *lom* of *saang.* Highly recommended.

Phrakhamphee prathom chindaa, Book III, Part 7.

Summary. Children born on Saturday have the symptoms of *saang chon* as the predominant illness, *saang naangrin* is the minor *saang,* the *la* is called *mahaaninlakaan,* the *la-ong* is called *pleo fai faa thap thim* and the *lom* is called *lom kumphan, lom baatthayak* and *lom champraap.*[18]

(The description of the birth *saang* of Saturday has been given on page 116 of this volume.)[sic]

Medicine to treat mucus and blood of *saang chon*:

[476]

thap thim	root
maphraao	root
taan dam	root
taan mon	root

4 items, equal parts. Reduce to 1/3 by boiling. To be taken.

[477] ***Chomphuu thaweep***

phekaa	leaves
phutsaa	leaves
phak plaap	leaves
phak pet	leaves
krameng	leaves
chum het Thai	leaves
thong laang bai mon	leaves
waa	leaves
lamphong	leaves
kaphrao	leaves
maduea	leaves

11 items. Use a cupful of juice from each ingredient, and a cup of sesame oil. Boil until only oil remains. To be taken or applied to treat *taan* and mucus and blood in the stools, caused by *saang chon.* If pills are made use equal parts. The pills should be taken mixed with alcohol.

Medicine to treat *saang chon:*

[478] *phak khuang*

mara	leaves
kaa ron	leaves
thum maraatchaa	leaves
thum theng	leaves
makhwit	leaves
khok kra-om	leaves
chabaa	leaves
khaa taa daeng	
khamin oi	

Equal parts, 10 items. Pills to be taken mixed with alcohol to counteract the poison of *taan* and *saang chon.*

[479] ***Saeng phrachan***

krung khamao	
kot so	
benyakaanee	
neraphuusee thang 2	
chan thang 2	
khrai khruea	root
makhaam khop	bark
khrang	
tabuun	fruit
makluea	bark
sadao	leaves
tree katuk	

	boraphet		
	sakae	seeds	
	haang kraai	bark	
	fin thang 2	bark	
	thap thim	under-ripe fruit	
	krathiam	bulb	

Equal parts, 23 items. Prepare pills using python's bile soaked in water as excipient. To be taken mixed with alcohol to treat *taan* and *saang chon* causing painful diarrhoea, and mucus with putrid pus and blood in the faeces, loss of appetite, listlessness, breathlessness, thirst and a high temperature. This medicine should clear it up.

Medicine to treat dysentery due to the poison of *saang chon*:

[480]	*benyakaanee*	galls	
	chan	seeds	
	chan	arils	
	thian thang 5		
	neraphuusee		
	saaraphat phit	fruit	
	waan keep raet		
	waan ron thong		
	chan thang 2		
	krathin daeng		
	khrai khruea	root	
	tabuun	fruit	
	one part of each of these 17 items		
	san phraa naang ae	bark	3 parts
	talum phuk	fruit	4 parts
	tumkaa thang 2	fruit	5 parts of each

Prepare pills using alcohol as excipient. To be taken mixed with lime water to treat diarrhoea with pus and blood in the faeces; restlessness and agitation; diseases of the *tridoṣa* and all kinds of *atisaan*.

[481] ***Thip sup* [*suup*] *suwan***

	kammathan thang 2	
	kaarabuun	
	chan thang 2	
	krisanaa	
	kralam phak	
	kot kraduuk	
	kot khamao	
	chan	seeds
	chan	arils
	see siat thang 2	
	benyakaanee	galls
	khrang	

makhaam khop	bark	
sadao	leaves	
praai	leaves	
cha-em thet		
kanchaa		
fin		
nguu lueam	bile	
khamin oi		
tree katuk		
1 *salueng* of each		
krathiam	bulb	2 *salueng*
kaan phluu		1 *baht*
haang kraai	bark	2 *baht*

Mix together these 29 ingredients, then add

khae daeng	bark	
phekaa	bark	
faang	bark	

Boil with alcohol, mix with water and make pills. To treat diarrhoea, to be taken mixed with a decoction of the bark sap of *maduea*; to treat dysentery, mix with *nam kathue* or lime water. To treat *taan*, *saang* and *saang chon*; and to be taken by adults who have *ritseeduang* causing diarrhoea, with putrid mucus and blood in the faeces.

Cooked medicine to treat *taan chon*:

[482]	*krathiam*		7 cloves
	khamin oi		7 pieces
	phrik Thai		7 peppercorns
	khing		7 pieces
	thian	leaves	1 *kam mue*
	fin thang 2	bark	1 *kam mue* of each
	kraphang hom	leaves	3 *kam mue*

9 items. Bruise, then add to a mixture of equal parts of alcohol and water and cook in a joint of bamboo. Then prepare pills, adding python's bile. To be taken to treat *taan chon* affecting the intestines and causing diarrhoea, mucus and blood in the stools, leaf green faeces or putrid mucus and blood.

Medicine to treat mucus and blood [in the stools resulting] from *saang chon*:

[483]	*kaphrao*	leaves
	phluu kae	leaves
	fin	

Equal parts, 3 items. Prepare pills using alcohol as excipient. To treat mucus and blood in the faeces causing abdominal pain.

Medicine to treat mucus and blood [in the stools resulting] from *saang chon*:

[484]

khee aai	bark	
masaang	bark	
khamin oi		
neraphuusee		
chan	seeds	
chan	arils	
krawaan		
kaan phluu		
khing		

Equal parts, 9 items. Prepare pills using *nam marun* as excipient. To be taken mixed with alcohol. If there is severe diarrhoea, this medicine is to be taken mixed with the bark sap of *khae daeng*, *maduea* or *makok*.

[485] ***Sitthisaan*** to treat diarrhoea:

tree katuk	
phak phaeo daeng	
waan keep raet	
waan ron thong	
see siat thang 2	
kaphrao	leaves
boraphet	
khwaai albino	burnt horn

Equal parts, 10 items. Add horn of an albino buffalo, an amount equivalent to the rest of the ingredients combined. Pills to be taken mixed with alcohol to treat *taan* and *saang chon*.

[486] ***Hing suraa***

bunnaak	flowers	
bua luang	pollen	
mali	flowers	
haang kraai	bark	
chan	seeds	
chan	arils	
benyakaanee	galls	
en	fruit	
kaan phluu		
maak khaao nieo		
see siat thang 2		
2 *salueng* of each		
krathiam	bulb	1 *baht*
khwaai albino	burnt horn	
kaphrao	leaves	

2 *baht* of each. 15 items. Pills to be taken mixed with alcohol to treat painful dysentery, with mucus and blood; bleeding from all the nine body orifices and to treat *lakkapit*.[19]

Medicine to treat *taan chon*:

[487] *chan* seeds
chan arils
dee plee
krathue
phlai
hom daeng
krathiam
din thanam
one part of each
maat lueang half a portion
9 items. Mix with *saaraphat dee*, soaked in water, then stick it on the underneath part of a bronze bowl, hold the bowl upright over a candle, and let it smoke and heat the entire bottom of the bowl, then prepare pills. To be taken mixed with alcohol and rock sugar, to treat *taan chon* affecting the anus and urethra causing prolapse or very painful diarrhoea with mucus and blood. To treat listlessness, this mixture is to be taken mixed with aromatic water or *nam chan* and a little *phimsen*. To treat *saang* in the throat, it is to be mixed with lime juice and salt and applied to the throat. To be taken mixed with *nam makruut* and snake's bile for flatulence. To treat snake-bite, it is to be taken and applied mixed with alcohol. To be taken mixed with juice of unripe areca and a little opium to treat *ritseeduang* and *saang* affecting the nine body orifices, causing prolapse. To treat anything from diarrhoea to *atisaan*, to be taken mixed with *khae daeng* bark sap, *son*, *thian* leaves and pomegranate leaves boiled together until reduced to 1/3 volume. 9 pills to be taken, also apply this mixture to the anus.

[488] ***Nawa thawaan yaa chak hai hot***[20]
chan seeds
benyakaanee galls
mafo root
Equal parts, 3 items
san phraa naang ae bark, an amount equal to all the rest combined.
Pills to be mixed with alcohol and a mixture of equal parts of river water and lime water and taken twice a day, morning and evening, for seven days.

Then prepare this laxative to treat the prolapsed tissues caused when the bowels are evacuated:

[489] *bencha lamphong*
bencha maatsalaa
maat lueang
sadao bark
phekaa bark

kluea

Equal parts, 10 items. Reduce to 1/3 volume by boiling, then put aside until cool. Bathe the affected parts until they retract and the damaged tissues heal also. This is a special prescription to prevent all danger.

If a child has *taan chon* resulting from any kind of *saang*, and bowel evacuation produces prolapse of the bowel, prepare this oil to be taken:

[490]	*khon thee so*	leaf sap	1 *thanaan*
	sadao	leaf sap	1 *thanaan*
	tamlueng tua phuu	leaf sap	1 *thanaan*
	khrai nam	leaf sap	1 *thanaan*
	khrai bok	leaf sap	1 *thanaan*
	taan mon	leaf sap	1 *thanaan*
	taan khamooi	leaf sap	1 *thanaan*
	phutsaa	bark sap	1 *thanaan*
	phekaa	bark sap	1 *thanaan*
	maduea din	root sap	1 *thanaan*
	makhuea khuen	fruit juice	1 *thanaan*
	thua phuu	root sap	1 *thanaan*
	nam khamin oi		1 *thanaan*
	nam maphrao fai		1 *thanaan*

Boil down until only oil remains, then grind together and add *chetta muun* root, python's bile and opium, 1 *salueng* of each. Mix with the oil. This is to be taken. Then use the oil sediment to apply to the prolapsed tissues. If all nine orifices are affected, then apply accordingly.

If any *saang* or *saang chon* changes and diarrhoea with mucus, fresh blood an offensive smell and severe pain develops, and the doctor prepares medicine to prevent this, the pain will increase. The child will then be forced to strain. Whenever this happens, the bowel will protrude. To treat this, prepare medicine to cleanse internally, and to contract the bowel as well as to cause it to be retracted.

[491]	*raatchadat*	fruit
	saaraphat phit	fruit
	2 *salueng* of each	
	sakae	root
	makluea	root
	kraphang hom	root
	yaa dam	
	1 *baht* of each	
	yaa nguang chaang	both roots and aerial parts
	khee kaa daeng	3 fruits, divide each fruit into quarters and use 3 quarters of each of the 3 fruits

makruut	3 fruits; divide each fruit into quarters and use 3 quarters of each of the 3 fruits
boraphet	wrap around the head of the patient
khamin oi	the length of the patient's span[21]

Boil these 11 items with a mixture of equal parts alcohol and water. If this is taken, it will give relief and put things right.

Medicine to contract and retract the prolapsed bowel:

[492] *nam nom raatchasee khruea* — a full *kam mue*

Trim the tops and bottoms while holding the breath.

khamin oi — a large rhizome

Slice it into 32 rings to represent the 32 parts of the body. Boil with lime water. To be taken.

The description of *saang chon* ends here.

Next is a brief description of *saang naangrin*, the minor *saang* of *saang chon*, so that doctors will be able to recognise the symptoms.

Saang naangrin has four major pustules and 56 followers. It starts after the baby leaves the fire, either with *saang chon* or after it has finished. There is one pustule with eight followers at the navel; one, with twelve followers at the chest [throat]; one pustule on the tongue, with sixteen followers which spread down the throat to the chest; and one at the chest, with 20 followers spreading over the supra-pubic area, the ileum and the colon. When the baby is three months old, the major pustule in the throat makes the throat dry and the tongue white and it cannot suck at the breast. At six months of age, three followers at the uvula give the baby a severe cough. Then all the small pustules spread out and combine with the major pustule in the chest, with the result that the baby is thirsty, has a dry throat, is listless and keeps closing its eyes. The followers in the chest spread to the sides of the body and the edge of the liver and combine with the major pustule of *saang* at the navel, causing the child to pass mucus and fresh blood, sometimes mucus and purulent blood; and the liver hangs down to the edge of the rib-cage. There is fever at regular intervals and the eyes are reddened with blood vessels. The baby will die if given the wrong medicine, but will recover with the right treatment. When the child is a year and six months old, *saang* in the bladder causes difficulty in urinating, sometimes the urine is like rice water or like chalky water or pus. This is painful and the baby is restless and tosses about and has incontinence of the bladder. Sometimes there is bruising at the tip of the penis, sometimes bruising and pus in the supra-pubic area and the pus becomes as hard as a cyst. This results from *saang naangrin* and the child will die in three years time. If the baby has reached a year and seven months of age, it will survive, because *saang naangrin* will have started after the *saang chon* has finished and three years later the child will be four years and seven months old, by which time the recognized period for this combination of birth *saang* and minor *saang* will have elapsed. After the time for both *saang chon* and *saang naangrin* has passed, *saang chon* might affect a child until it is seven years old, after which time it will be saved from death. *Saang chon* does not affect only children born on Saturday, it might occur with or follow any other *saang*. Similarly, *saang naangrin* does not occur as a complication of *saang chon* only, but might occur with all forms of *saang*. Whenever a doctor is to treat *saang naangrin*, he should treat it in accordance with the previously existing birth *saang*.

Here ends the description of *saang naangrin*.

Next is a brief description of the *la* called *mahaaninlakaan* which is associated with *saang chon*. Doctors should understand this.

La mahaaninlakaan starts with black pustules like sapphires. After a day, they change to fiery brightness and after two days, change to the brilliance of diamonds on both sides. If a child has *la mahaaninlakaan*, it develops hemiplegia and cannot cry.

Medicine to treat *la mahaaninlakaan*:

[493]	*fin*	bark
	makruut	bark
	saaraphat phit	fruit
	naat	root
	khon thee so	leaves
	phak hom hin	root
	thap thim	leaves
	kaarabuun	
	phimsen	

Equal parts, 9 items. Prepare a stick, mix with cow's milk and paint the mouth.

If this is ineffective, prepare:

[494]	*thua rae*	leaves
	kaan phluu	
	nam prasaan thong	
	tamlueng tua phuu	
	kluai teep	root

Equal parts, 5 items. Prepare a stick, mix with 3 parts buttermilk and 1 part water and paint the mouth.

[495] ***Thep mongkhon***

(The ingredients and method of dispensing have been given on page 159 of this volume. Here we discuss only the way to use the medicinal vehicles not previously mentioned.)[sic][22]

Thep mongkhon medicine is used to treat the eight kinds of *la*. For red *la*, mix with *nam faang* and apply to the throat; for yellow *la*, mix with *nam khamin khruea*; for flame red *la*, mix with shallot juice and a small amount of snake's bile; if the *la* is the [purple] colour of bruised *tabaek* flowers, mix with fresh fruit juice of *thao khan* and a little salt and apply.

Application to counteract the poison of *la*:

[496]	*rangap thang* 2	leaves
	tamlueng tua phuu	leaves

khok kra-om	leaves
chan hom	leaves
chabaa	leaves
fak khaao	leaves
din prasiu khaao	
din see phong	

Equal parts of each ingredient. Prepare a stick and apply as a lotion, mixed with water used to wash rice, for the eight kinds of *la*.

Medicine to counteract the poison of *la* affecting the heart:

[497]

saang karanee	
neraphuusee	
chan	seeds
chan	arils
kaan phluu	
krawaan	
waan keep raet	
waan ron thong	
phrik Thai	
khing	dried
khaa kae	
hom daeng	
khamin oi	
krachaai	
kathue	
phlai	
khrai khruea	root
rayom	
phitsanaat	
raatchadat	fruit
nam nom raatchasee	
phan phak kaat	
plaa lai phueak	
saniat	leaves
nam tao	leaves
phluu kae	leaves
maklam khruea	

Equal parts, 27 items. Prepare pills using alcohol as excipient. To be taken or applied mixed with alcohol, to treat a stiff tongue and lockjaw and to counteract the poison of *la* affecting the heart and causing breathing difficulties or restlessness and agitation. It will be effective without a doubt.

Another:

[498]

muek hom	
kaphrao	leaves

san phraa hom	leaves
phimsen	leaves
khaa kae	
dee nguu	
phimsen	
chamot	

Equal parts, 8 items. Prepare pills using aromatic water as excipient. To be taken or applied to the chin.

Medicine for breathing difficulties:

[499]	*malaeng saap*	faecal matter
	krisanaa	
	chan thet	
	san phraa naang ae	bark
	phan nguu daeng	
	phak chee	fruit
	raet	horn
	chaang	tusk
	kwaang	horn

Equal parts, 9 items. Prepare pills using lime juice as excipient. If the illness results from fever, this is to be taken mixed with aromatic water or the boiled sap of pomegranate leaves to treat a stiff tongue, lock-jaw and difficulty in breathing.

Here ends the description of *la mahaaninlakaan* which is associated with *saang chon.*

Next is a brief description of the ***la-ong phrabaat*** **called** ***la-ong pleo fai faa*** **or** ***la-ong thap thim*** which is associated with *saang chon.* Doctors should understand this.

La-ong phrabaat pleo fai faa or *la-ong thap thim* starts with pustules as red as vermilion, not unlike the colour of the leaf tips of young shoots of the pomegranate tree. This is poisonous; the child's tongue is stiff, it has lockjaw and the eyes lose their sensitivity. The child has convulsions with spasms of the hands and feet and the body feels very hot. If it cannot be treated in time, that is, between morning and midday, the child will die. Do not treat it with medicine that is hot or medicine containing alcoholic liquor, oil or vinegar. Use cool and fragrant, astringent, and bitter tasting medicine,[23] then the child will survive. The same applies to all seven kinds of *la-ong phrabaat.*

Medicine to treat *la-ong pleo fai faa* *la-ong thap thim:*

[500]	*puu chao phung kae*	
	puu chao samung kui	
	tap tao thang 2	
	see huat thang 2	
	nom maeo thang 2	
	shat phra in	
	khrai khruea	root
	rayom	

	phitsanaat		
	neraphuusee		
	chan thang 2		
	nguan muu		
	prakham dee khwaai	root	
	mai phai paa	decayed root-stock	
	phak phaeo daeng		

Equal parts, 19 items. Prepare a stick, mix with aromatic water or lime water and paint the child's mouth.

Another:

[501]	*thong laang naam*	root	
	phung kho	root	
	maklam khruea	root	
	krisanaa		
	chan thang 2		
	benyakaanee	galls	
	see siat thet		

Equal parts, 8 items. Prepare a stick, mix with *nam thalaai maak dip* and use to paint the mouth or apply to the throat.

Medicine to place in the mouth to prevent [*la-ong pleo fai faa*]:

[502]	*khlaa*	bark	1 *kam mue*
	phak bung khan	bark	1 *kam mue*
	waa	leaves	3 leaves

Reduce to 1/3 volume by boiling, add a little sodium sulphate. Decant and allow to cool, then add a little opium and place in the child's mouth.

[503] ***Suwan thaaraa***

	khong khaa dueat		
	samut kluean		
	rangap	leaves	
	nam dap fai	leaves	
	phum riang paa	root	
	yaa naang	root	
	phung kho	root	
	thao yaai mom	leaves	
	salot nam	root	
	maduea	root	
	naang nuun	root	
	ching cho	root	
	nom phaa		
	ngiu	root	
	faang	root	
	khee takran lek		
	din see phong		

fun cheen
din prasiu saao [khaao]
Equal parts, 29 items. Prepare a stick. Mix with water used to wash rice, to be applied as a lotion or taken for thirst or internal poisoning of any kind.

[504] ***Bencha kot*** (*yai*)

kot thang 5	
thian thang 5	
samo thang 3	
chan	seeds
chan	arils
krawaan	
kaan phluu	
bua nam thang 7	pollen
champaa	flowers
kradang ngaa	flowers
saaraphee	flowers
phikun	flowers
bunnaak	flowers
mali son	flowers
mali laa	flowers
salit	flowers
kham Thai	flowers
dee plee	
haeo muu	
ching cho	fruit
nguu lueam	bile
fin	
amphan thong	
chamot	
phimsen	

Equal parts, 41 items. Mix together in the middle of the night, then within one day, prepare pills, and after three days, leave in the sun just long enough to dry, then put in a bottle. To counteract the poison of the *la-ong phrabaat* of all of the *saang* of the seven days which causes irritation of the heart, restlessness or unconsciousness. To treat *saang* affecting the eyes, mix with lime juice and use as eye drops; then apply to the crown of the head and to both jaws and chest, to treat air hunger, restlessness and agitation. To treat listlessness and thirst, to be taken mixed with aromatic water. This is effective in treating both children and adults.

The description of *la-ong pleo fai faa* associated with *saang chon* ends here.

Next, *lom kumphan* and *lom baatthayak* which are associated with *saang chon*, are described together. Doctors should understand this.

When *lom kumphan* and *lom baatthayak* start, the eyes roll back, the face is blue, the child has convulsions, with spasms of the hands and feet, the back is arched and the baby grinds its teeth. This happens when the child is poisoned in some way, and these *lom* seize the opportunity to attack. It results from an injury due to an abrasion or cut, or from a thorn or splinter anywhere in the body. This causes *khai phikhaat* and then *lom kumphan, khom* [*lom*] *baatthayak* and *lom champraap* follow.[24]

To treat this:

[505]	*sabaa*	roasted seeds
	khon thee so	roasted fruit
	phring [*phrik*] *Thai*	roasted
	kameng	leaves roasted
	sahatsakhun	leaves

Equal parts, 5 items. Powder together, mix with leaf sap of *krameng* and give it power with this *gāthā*: *'Sakkatvā buddharatanaṃ buddharatanaṃ thammaratanaṃ thammaratanaṃ saṃgharatanaṃ saṃgharatanaṃ osathaṃ uttamaṃ varaṃ hitaṃ devamanussānaṃ parilāhupasamanaṃ āhuneyyaṃ pāhuneyyaṃ buddhatejena buddhatejena thammatejena thammatejena sotthinā nassantupaddavā sabbe dukkhā sabbe dukkhā sabbhe bhayā sabbe bhayā sabbe rogā vūpasamentu te'*, 180 [times then] stop.[25]

Then prepare pills to be taken to counteract the effects of *lom kumphan* and *lom baatthayak* which cause convulsions with spasms of the hands and feet, a stiff tongue and lock-jaw, as stated previously, and all will go. This has been used 180 [times] and is very potent. This medicine is called *Muun chit.*

Medicine to treat [*lom*] *kumphanthayak*:

[506]	*oi daeng*	buds	1
	phak khraat	flowers	1
	makruut	skin	1
	manaao	skin	1
	mai phai paa	skin	1
	mai see suk	skin	2
	krathue		1
	phlai		1
	taeng kwaa	seeds	1
	phak chee	fruit	1
	fak	tendrils	1
	nam tao	tendrils	1
	mai bong	skin	1
	hua khuun		1
	thua kai	root	1

Equal parts, 16 items. Prepare pills, using water used to wash rice, as excipient. To be taken mixed with aromatic water to treat *lom kumphan* and *lom baatthayak.*

Medicine used to treat convulsions and muscular tremor:

[507]	*maklam khruea*	root	
	yaa naang	root	
	krung khamao	root	
	khaa kae		
	bia phuu	calcined	

Equal parts, 5 items. Pills to be taken with water.

Application for the body to treat convulsions:

[508]	*maeng lak thang* 2	leaves	
	horaphaa	leaves	
	krachaai		
	phak pet	leaves	
	krameng	leaves	

Equal parts, 6 items. Prepare a stick, mix with *som saa* juice or any citrus juice and apply. This has often been used very effectively.

[509]	***Prathaan phit***		
	mahaat	heartwood	
	chan thang 2		
	bua luang	pollen	
	chaluut		
	krak khee		
	kot thang 9		
	cha-em thet	fruit	
	kaan phluu		
	benyakaanee		
	neraphuusee		
	19 items, of each 7 *salueng*		
	kaarabuun		3 *baht*
	chamot		
	phimsen		
	1 *fueang* of each		

22 items. Prepare pills the size of *thua phuu* seeds using aromatic water as excipient. 7 pills to be taken to counteract the poison of boils and abscesses, *khai sannibaat, taan* and *saang* causing convulsions, *lom* which makes the body hot [a raised temperature], causes restlessness and agitation, and to treat a raised temperature causing convulsions on one side of the body or on both sides. This medicine should counteract all these.

If the child does not respond to treatment with this medicine, and the disease becomes worse, as explained previously, the doctor should next treat it with the medicine called *Phrasuryamonthon.*

[510] ***Phrasuriyaamonthon*** [sic]		
chamot chiang		
phimsen		
amphan thong		
1 *salueng* of each		
kot thang 9		
waan keep raet		
waan ron thong		
sang karanee		
neraphuusee		
saaraphat phit	root	
prakham dee khwaai	fruit	
dee nguu ton		
chan	seeds	
proh hom		
krathin daeng		
phrik hom		
phrik haang		
phrik lon		
2 *salueng* of each		
plaa lai phueak	root	1 *baht*
chan thet		
krisanaa		
kralam phak		
khondok		
khrai khruea	root	
rayom		
phitsanaat		
kaan phluu		
nam nom raatchasee		
2 *baht* of each		
thong kham pleo		108 sheets

37 items. Prepare pills using *nam dok mai thet* or rose water as excipient. [sic] To be taken to treat convulsions, with a stiff tongue and lock-jaw; and to treat the poison of *khai nuea, taan* and *saang*; and *lom kumphan* and *lom baatthayak*. This is a very special remedy highly recommended to counteract all of these conditions.

There remains the description of the *lom* called *lom champrap*. ***Lom champrap* is extremely bad.** It is as poisonous as snake venom. At first, the baby is restless and tosses and turns, then it has convulsions, arching the back from the hips, and the body is cold and covered in goose-flesh. If the doctor does not know how to cure this, the child is sure to die and blood will exude from every pore.

Medicine to treat *lom champraap*:

[511] *kot thang 5*

thian thang 5	
phutsaa	bark
takhro	bark

Equal parts, 12 items. Reduce to 1/3 by boiling. To be taken.

Medicinal bath to prevent [*lom champraap*]:

[512]	*makhaam piak*	
	phak chee lom [lon]	fruit
	phak chee laa	fruit
	krachao daeng	fruit
	krachao khaao	root

Equal parts, 4 items. Boil together and use as a medicinal bath. Bathe the whole body, then massage and the child will recover.[26] Do not have it too hot. Use it both to be taken and to be sprayed on the child [by squirting from the mouth], then empower it by reciting these magic words seven times: *'Om champraap champleo. Om bang phrakhlang kraphong savāha.'* Then spray the body again with bark of the Chinese date and *takhrong* bark. Do not spray with alcohol or oil. Do not purge with croton, or the child will die. Use either *Yaa benchammarit* or *Yaa mahaa-ammarit.*

Lom champraap is very difficult to cure. The doctor should make sure of his diagnosis by observing the symptoms, then give medicine. The symptoms are the same as *puang nguu hao*,[27] but the latter causes diarrhoea and vomiting first. Then the body becomes red and is covered in goose-flesh, and the child gets restless and tosses and turns, then loses consciousness. *Lom champraap* is just the same as this, but the body then turns black. The sign of death is the same. The doctor should be sure about it. It is the same in both children and adults.

[513]	***Benchammarit***	
	mahaa hing	
	yaa dam	
	1 part of each	
	rong thong	2 parts
	makruut yai	3 fruits

Stuff each of these three - *mahaa hing, rong thong, yaa dam* in one of the *makruut* fruit, cover with layers of fresh cow dung, then warm over a slow fire of paddy husks until completely cooked. Mix together *tong taek* root, 4 parts and *dee kluea* 16 parts, then combine with the contents of the *makruut* fruit. Prepare pills each weighing 1 *salueng*, to be taken mixed with a triturate of ripe fruit pulp of the tamarind in water. Then the child's bowels will function satisfactorily. It is just as good for children 3 or 4 years old.

[514] ***Mahaa-ammarit***

thian thang 9

tree katuk

samo Thai

yaa dam	best quality
makruut	skin
tong taek	root
1 part of each	
mahaa hing	
matuum	under-ripe fruit
waan nam	
4 parts of each	
kot nam tao	ten and a half parts

16 items. Prepare pills using a triturate of the ripe fruit pulp of tamarind in water as excipient. To be taken with hot water to treat the *lom* of *saang*. To get rid of mucus and blood in the stools, mix with a decoction of *thian* leaf sap, and pomegranate leaf sap.

[515] ***Thaeng thong***

kot so	
kot chiang	
kot hua bua	
thian dam	
krisanaa	
kralam phak	
chaluut	
khondok	
samun waeng	
bunnaak	flowers
bua luang	pollen
thong kham pleo	
chamot	
phimsen	

Equal parts, 14 items. Mix together, then add a decoction made from 1 *baht* of each of the following five ingredients:

chan thet	
krisanaa	
mali	flowers
phikun	flowers
yo thakaa	flowers

Prepare pills to be taken to treat *lom kumphan*, *lom baatthayak*, chest pain causing insomnia, agitation or hot fluid in the chest, mixed with aromatic water, *chan* seeds and *mahaa kaan* rhizome. This can be relied upon, without doubt.

Any doctor who is to treat [any of] the seven kinds of *lom* associated with *saang* should first examine the symptoms. If mild medicine is ineffective, then hot medicine will work. The doctor should increase [the dose of] the medicine to make it more effective, depending on the length of time the child has been ill. First, prepare these seven recipes: *Yaa hing*, *Yaa inthachak*, *Yaa mahaa chak*, *Yaa mahaa kaphrao*, *Yaa prasa nam khing*, *Yaa prasa dee plee* and *Yaa mahaa kaphrao yai*. These seven medicines are of medium strength. If ineffective, mix this:

[516] ***Waayo phinaat***

tree katuk		of each, 4 parts
kaan phluu		5 parts
hing yaang pho		
dong dueng		of each, 6 parts
phrik lon		
chetta muun phloeng	root	
kaarabuun		of each, 8 parts
bai naat		20 parts

10 items. Prepare pills, to be taken with *nam makruut*. This is a stomach mixture to get rid of all seven kinds of *lom* associated with *saang*.

[517] ***Mahaa chaiyawaat***

horaphaa	fruit	
krawaan		
kluea kratang		
kot so thet		
kaarabuun		
kluea sinthao		
marum	bark	
ching cho	root	
1 part of each		
krisanaa		
kralam phak		
phrik lon		
waan nam		
bai naat		
khing	dried	
2 parts of each		
yaa dam		
thian dam		
kaan phluu		
hatsakhun thet		
dong dueng		
chetta muun phloeng	root	
dee plee		
samo thet		
4 parts of each		
mahaa hing		8 parts

23 items. Pills to be taken with juice of *som saa*, ginger or *nam khaa*. This medicine can destroy all *lom* associated with the seven kinds of *saang*, easily overcoming them; and can cure *lom* of adults:

that is, *lom amphaat, lom raatthayak, lom thakkinnakhun, lom prawaattakhunna, lom san daan, lom klon, lom pattakhaat* and all kinds of *lom*.

[518] ***Hingkhaathichon***

lamphan thong		
sakhaan		
waan nam		
mahaa hing		
chaa phluu	root	
kluea sinthao		
khrai khruea		
phrik lon		
1 part of each		
thon dee	root	
krathiam		
thian khaao		
2 parts of each		
thian dam		3 parts
kot kraduuk		6 parts
khing	dried	
chetta phang khee		
8 parts of each		
dee plee		10 parts
samo Thai		11 parts

17 items. Prepare pills or a powder. The doctor should select the appropriate medicinal vehicle, in accordance with *Khamphee sapphakhun*, to treat *lom san daan, lom daan khun, lom chuk siat* and *lom* causing tightness in the chest and for *saang maa, saang wua* and *saang khwaai*, knotted and twisted muscles and tendons, internal disorders and *lom kumphan, lom baatthayak* and all the *lom* of the seven kinds of *saang*.

[519] ***Hingkhuwataa***

thian yaowa phaanee	
thian thang 5	
kot thang 5	
chan	seeds
krawaan	
kraai [plant]	fruit
kaan phluu	
son	flowers
samun waeng	
chetta muun	root
khon thee so	leaves
utta phit	

buk		
kloi		
kradaat thang 2		
chum het Thai	root	
plao thang 2		
khing	dried	
khee kaa thang 2	root	
ching cho yai	root	
samo Thai	fruit	
mahaa hing		
thon dee	root	
samae thang 2	heartwood	
1 part of each		
yaa dam		6 parts
nam prasaan thong		
sahatsakhun		
12 parts of each		
phrik Thai		14 parts
dee plee		24 parts

41 items. Prepare pills or a powder. To be taken mixed with juice of ginger root or *nam som saa* to treat *taan chon*, *khai charaa*,[28] *lom* which causes convulsions with spasms of the hands and feet, and all eighteen kinds of *lom*.

[520] ***Sawaang aarom***

teen pet ton	bark
teen pet khruea	bark
marum	bark
thong laang	bark
sakhaan	
chaa phluu	
khamin oi	
khamin khruea	
bencha raatcha phrik	
bencha khee lek	
kan krao	bark
maeng lak	leaves
rak khaao	leaves
salat dai	leaves
salot kin long	leaves
matuum	leaves
sawaat	leaves
saniat	leaves
khon thee so	leaves
ching cho thang 2	root

tree phalaa	
krameng	leaves
phinlangkaasaa	fruit
sahatsakhun thang 2	
mafai duean haa	
khaa taa daeng	
khing	dried
dee plee	
Equal parts, 40 items	
phrik Thai	an amount equal to the rest of the ingredients combined

Grind together. To be taken mixed with hot water, *nam som saa* or *nam makruut* to treat all seven major kinds of *lom*. The masters declare that this has been a very special remedy since former times.

The masters have described the symptoms of children born on Saturday. *Saang chon* is the predominant illness, *saang naangrin* is the minor *saang*, the *la* called *mahaaninlakaan* affects them in association with *saang chon*, the *la-ong phrabaat* is called *la-ong pleo fai faa* or *la-ong thap thim* and the *lom* which is a complication of *saang chon* is called *kumphan, baattayak* and *lom champraap*. It ends here.

NOTES

1 *saang chon* (จร): saang of a type said sometimes to occur during or following the course of birth *saang*, a complication of birth *saang*; translated here as 'minor *saang*'. This is to avoid confusion with the name of one of the birth *saang* called *saang chon* (โจร), transcribed identically. Similarly, *mae sue chon* (จร) and *sapphan chon* (จร) *Rāhū* are translated 'minor' *mae sue* and 'minor' *saphan Rāhū*.

2 Rāhū: an *asura* (demon) with half his body missing. The other half is called Phra Ket (Skt *Ketu*.) *PPPT*, p. 328. See also, Book I, note 42.

3 Misprint, correctly, pp. 106, 107.

4 Three months of age, or three months later, is debatable. The age of the child could not be known, as the minor *saang* sometimes starts during the course of birth *saang*, sometimes when it has finished. In this section, it is stated that the *saang kraai* follows *saang phloeng*, but, even so, the age of the child when the *saang phloeng* has finished cannot be known. What is important, is the approximate length of time between the development of subsequent symptoms.

5 *saang faai:* cotton *saang*, not to be confused with *saang fai*, fiery *saang*.

6 *la-ong kaeo witchian:* diamond *la-ong*; a form of follicular pharyngitis. *Mc*, p.130.

7 *la-ong phrabaat:* dust of the royal feet; dust of the Buddha's footprint.

8 There is a note included here: 'it says "*nam dee nguu tom*" at the beginning of this volume' ['*nam dee nguu tom*' meaning 'a decoction of snake's bile']. This explanation is, no doubt, to make it clear that *nam dee nguu ton*, juice from the plant '*ton*' called *dee nguu* is not intended. The transcriber of the text might, nevertheless, have been mistaken, since snake's bile is not usually boiled with water or alone in these prescriptions. It is usually used as a dry powder or the dried bile is mixed with (cold) water before adding to the other ingredients.

9 *klam:* a measure of volume equivalent to 2 *klom* or 8 grains of paddy.

10 This is very similar to the route of *pingkhalaa*, one of the ten major tendons or long, hollow, tubular organs of the body on which the Thai system of massage is based. See Mulholland, 'Traditional Medicine in Thailand', *Hemisphere*, Vol. 23, No. 4, July/August 1979, p.226.

11 Phrayaa Matchuraat: the god of death.

12 *chap:* malaria or chills and fever.

13 Omitted from the 1961 edition

14 See Book I, p.40; Book II, p.71.

15 *kaan:* probably bubonic plague.

16 See prescription no. 54.

17 *kaan singkhalee:* plague. *Mc*, p. 99.

18 *lom baatthayak:* tetanus.
lom kumphan; kumphan: a class of demons, giants or goblins;

kumphanthayak: an ancient name for a condition characterised by convulsions. *Mc*, p. 113.

19 *lakkapit; lakkapoet:* an oral disease characterised by periodic bleeding from the gums. *Mc*, p. 736.

20 Medicine called 'medicine to contract the nine orifices'.

21 *khuep:* a unit of linear measure from the end of the thumb to the tip of the middle finger when the hand is spread flat. *Mc*, p. 203.

22 Correctly, p. 151; prescription no. 398.

23 According to Thai traditional medicine, the therapeutic use of medicine is usually determined by taste.

24 These are possibly all names for tetanus.

25 108 times in the 1871 edition.

26 Massage is mentioned only twice in this text. (See Book V, Note 11, prescription no. 625.)

27 *puang nguu hao:* (lit.) cobra disease. The symptoms are like cholera, but milder. (PT)
puang: refers to a disease with symptoms of diarrhoea and vomiting. *PPPT*, p. 194.

28 *charaa:* debility consequent upon old age; senility. *Mc*, p. 280.
khai charaa: sickness or fever of old age, possibly refers to senility.

[Book IV]

Phrakhamphee prathom chindaa, Book IV, gives a summary of *apphayasantaa* and the seven major forms of *saang*,[1] *saang chon*, *saang phloeng*, *to* of *saang chon*, the fevers which occur with birth *saang* and the pustules of birth *saang* and of all the minor forms of *saang*, as follows.

Siddhikāriyaḥ We will begin by explaining next the supplementary texts which the masters took from *Phrakhamphee apphayasantaa* and included here in *Phrakhamphee prathom chindaa*, Book IV, in the hope that this will make it easy for inexperienced doctors, who have not got a complete grasp of the contents of the texts, to understand them.

Whether born at midday, during the early afternoon or at midnight, babies born on Sunday, Tuesday or Saturday will have *saang fai*, *saang daeng* and *saang chon* respectively, as their birth *saang*.[2] The doctor who treats these babies should be careful not to let the main *saang* of birth enter internally. Whenever it affects the liver or heart it is very difficult for the doctor to cure. If it affects the large intestine, it causes diarrhoea; if it affects the head, it causes swellings on the head; if it affects the eyes, they are damaged but the baby will not die. If it affects the liver or heart, it causes diarrhoea with fresh blood at first, then foul blood, and makes the face and body yellow and sallow and the mouth red. Whenever the eyes are yellow, it will make the baby pass mucus and blood, and the liver will hang down, and that will cause regular fever. Then it will affect the throat, so that the child cannot eat or drink and has a dry mouth and throat. If it affects the chest, it causes severe thirst, and having quenched its thirst, the baby's eyes are dry and it has no tears. If the wrong medicine is given, the infant will die [literally, reach its destiny (*karma*)].

About three months after leaving the fire of age, babies born on Monday or Wednesday in the morning or at midday will have *saang nam* or *saang sako* respectively. This starts in the throat and grows up over the palate and mouth, while another patch comes up to the base of the tongue from the outside of the intestines producing a scaly lesion resembling the [large] scales of the carp. Then it becomes inflamed, and sores develop at the rectum, after which the child has diarrhoea with red stained faeces, is thirsty and listless. If the doctor gives the appropriate medicine, the baby's life will be saved. To treat this:

[521]	*krabue* albino	horn
	benyakaanee	galls
	see siat thang 2	
	bunnaak	flowers
	bua luang	pollen
	nam prasaan thong	
	krathiam	

Equal parts, 8 items. Pills to be taken with *nam chan* for the diarrhoea of *saang nam*.

Medicine to treat the diarrhoea of *saang sako*:

[522]	*chan*	seeds
	khrang	
	see siat thet	
	bua luang	pollen
	bua khom	pollen
	nam prasaan thong	
	nguu lueam	bile

Equal parts, 7 items. Prepare pills using lime juice as excipient. To be taken mixed with alcohol for all diarrhoea whether continual or with mucus and blood.

Medicine for the diarrhoea of *saang nam* and *saang sako*:

[523]	*naam waai khom*	
	benyakaanee	galls
	nguu lueam	bile

Equal parts, 3 items. Pills to be taken mixed with *maphlap cheen* fruit juice, to counteract the diarrhoea of *saang nam* and *saang sako*, which looks like water used to wash meat and which causes unconsciousness.

Another:

[524]	*krathiam*	
	matuum	fruit
	chan daeng	
	mok man	bark
	benyakaanee	galls
	thap thim	under-ripe fruit
	nam taan	granulated

Equal parts, 7 items. Pills to be taken, mixed with hot water, to treat the diarrhoea of *saang nam* and *saang sako* which produces faeces like mucus, cotton or rotten eggs.

Saang faai comes up on the tongue and spreads out like a covering of white cotton. It causes diarrhoea, foul smelling, like rotten eggs. To treat this:

[525]	*nok yuung*	tail feathers scorched until brittle
	manaao	seeds
	bunnaak	flowers
	nguu lueam	bile
	nam taan	granulated
	nam phueng	

Grind together and give by mouth, mixed with lime juice.

One kind of *saang sako* causes a red mouth, severe diarrhoea and cold hands and feet. To treat this:

[526]	*khrang*	
	see siat thang 2	
	waan nam	
	cha-em	

krathue	
benyakaanee	galls
chan khaao	
ngaa chaang	
nam manaao	
nam taan	granulated

Equal parts, 11 items. Pills to be taken mixed with juice of wild ginger or garlic.

Saang kho and *saang chaang* are the birth *saang*, respectively, of infants born on Thursday or Friday. *Saang khaao plueak* is the minor *saang*. Whether the child is born at dawn or late in the evening, one month and fifteen days after the mother has left the fire, the major *saang* erupts at the throat and tongue, as white as tin. In two or three days time, it is as yellow as maize. If medicine is smeared on the throat with the finger, this will subside for a day or two, then it will start again around the eyes and on the backs of the thighs. It is flat and red or blue and causes severe diarrhoea. When the diarrhoea has ceased, spots erupt all over the body, making it as red as a ripe *tamlueng* fruit, like measles. But it is not measles, it is caused by a form of *saang*. Sometimes there are marks the size of *sabaa* seed or Chinese date leaves which spread out level with the flesh and are blue, black or red, as if the child has been beaten with a rattan or slapped with the hand. This kind of *saang* is very bad. It is as poisonous as typhoid fever. If an inexperienced doctor treats this condition, it is just the same as killing the baby. To treat this:

[527]	*mok man*	bark
	palong	bark
	haeo muu	
	kaang plaa daeng	root
	naam waai khom	
	faang sen	
	sakae	seeds
	nam taan tanot	

Equal parts, 8 items. Reduce to 1/3 volume by boiling. To be taken to counteract the internal poison which first causes diarrhoea. Follow this treatment with medicine called *Bencha taan* to clean out the abdomen. [See no. 92.]

Lotion:

[528]	*khanun lamut*	leaves
	sapparot	leaves
	yaa naang	leaves
	din prasiu khaao	
	din so phong	

Grind together and repeatedly spray the resulting liquid from the mouth on to the child's body.

Another:

[529]	*phak piang khaao*	leaves

plaai khaao saan
khamin oi
Grind together and apply likewise [as a spray from the mouth on to the child's body].

The female variety of *saang khaao plueak* starts with spots that look like sorghum or millet all over the body. The pustules are red. When they are ripe, they break, like *rok klaak* and *phanranai,*[3] causing a sore throat and the baby cannot eat or sleep and has flatulence. This *saang* starts in the large intestine, then appears at the root of the tongue and later erupts all over the body. To treat this:

[530] *chan daeng*
neraphuusee
waan keep raet
waan ron thong
saaraphat phit — fruit
Equal parts, 5 items. Pills to be taken mixed with *nam chan.*

The male variety of *saang phloeng* causes a red mouth, red palms of the hands and soles of the feet, diarrhoea with mucus and blood, a high temperature at regular times, and the baby is listless and stuporous. The doctor should examine the anus. If the area around the anus is as red as *sattabut* flowers,[4] this is a definite indication. If treatment is continued it will eventually be harmful and the child will die. To treat this:

[531] *yaa tak bai*
chan daeng
raet — molar tooth
chaang — molar tooth
Equal parts, 4 items. Pills. First give this medicine, mixed with alcohol or honey and *phimsen,* then prepare the following medicine to be taken.

Medicine to treat *saang phloeng*:

[532] *kot thang 5*
krisanaa
kralam phak
chaluut
khondok
phimsen
nam prasaan thong
khrai khruea — root
one part of each
thian thang 5
chan — seeds
chan — arils
krawaan
kaan phluu
waan keep raet
waan ron thong

	raatchadat	fruit
	saaraphat phit	fruit
	2 parts of each	

25 items. Pills to be taken mixed with *nam chan* to counteract the poisonous effects of *saang phloeng* and *saang haeng*.[5]

Decoction to treat the listlessness of *saang phloeng*:

[533]	*bunnaak*	flowers
	opchoei thet	
	kot kaan phraao	
	faek hom	root
	hua hom	
	matuum	under-ripe fruit
	krawaan	fruit
	phimsen	leaves

Equal parts. Reduce to 1/3 volume by boiling and give to counteract listlessness or stupor.

Application for the anus:

[534]	*song salueng*	leaves
	benyakaanee	galls
	neraphuusee	

To be applied mixed with sesame oil for redness and inflammation of the anus.

Medicine to expel the poison of *saang phloeng* in the chest or on the tongue:

[535]	*thalaai maak dip*	
	khamin oi	

[The remainder of this prescription is missing from the 1961 edition. The following items appear in the 1871 text:

	mayom tua phuu	leaves
	khaa kae	
	nguu lueam	bile

To be taken mixed with alcohol.]

Saang chon and *saang phloeng* are similar. Doctors should know this. They affect babies born on Saturday and Sunday. Sometimes an infant born on Sunday has *saang phloeng* as its birth *saang* and *saang chon* as its minor *saang*; sometimes a child born on Saturday has *saang chon* as birth *saang* and *saang phloeng* as minor *saang*. So both of these kinds of *saang* can be either birth *saang* or minor *saang*. When they occur together, the disease is called *saang chon saang phloeng*. It differs from *saang phloeng* in the following respects: the major pustules of *saang chon* erupt in the middle of the uvula, resembling rice flakes. It produces a dry throat, then the baby cannot eat, has blurred vision and the eyes become as yellow as candle smoke [? flame]. Subsequently, the child is listless and stuporous and the body is hot. If effective medicine is given, the symptoms will subside for four or five months, then they will recur and the child will have a craving for chillies and fishy and meaty food which favour the disease. When this exacerbation occurs, constant diarrhoea with blood and putrid mucus develops and the symptoms keep changing. The baby becomes so emaciated that the shinbones protrude and feel as rough and sharp as the skin of a stingray. The eyes develop *malet kadue*, then these become red and change to *to kon hoi*, [6]which break in four or five days. Then the baby dies. To treat this:

[536]	*som sieo*	root
	see siat thet	
	nam taan	granulated

Mix with milk and first paint the tongue four or five times, then treat as follows:

Medicine to treat the throat, cough, vomiting, and hiccoughs:

[537]	*tree phalaa*	
	kraphang hom	
	phak waan	
	kaphrao	leaves
	maklam khruea	leaves

Equal parts, 7 items. Mix with honey and paint the tongue. To treat *saang haeng*:

Medicine for painful diarrhoea, with mucus and blood in the stools:

[538]	*waan keep raet*	
	waan ron thong	
	chan thang 2	
	neraphuusee	
	prakham dee khwaai	fruit
	see siat thet	

Equal parts, 7 items. Pills to be taken mixed with alcohol to treat *saang chon saang phloeng*.

If this is ineffective:

[539]	*waan keep raet*	
	waan ron thong	
	chan daeng	
	benyakaanee	galls
	kathok rok	root
	phrik Thai	
	khing	dried
	hua hom	
	prakham dee khwaai	fruit roasted

9 items. Pills to be taken mixed with alcohol and python's bile.

Another:

[540]	*chaang*	tusk
	kwaang	horn
	thian thang 5	

Mix together and give for extreme distress.

Throat and mouth application for *saang chon saang phloeng*:

[541]	*phrik Thai*	
	khing	dried
	krathiam	bulb
	kaan phluu	
	khai fak	bark
	rong thong	

Equal parts, 6 items. Prepare a stick and use [mixed with a liquid] to paint the mouth.

Another:

[542]	*malaeng saap*	faecal matter
	kwaang	horn
	nok yuung	tail feathers, scorched brittle
	waai takhaa	
	phrik Thai	
	krathiam	bulb
	khaao mai	

Equal parts, 7 items. Prepare a powder or a stick to use to treat the child's tongue.

Medicine to treat internal heat:

[543]	*phung kho*	root
	nguan muu	root
	saniat	root
	khuun	root
	maduea	root
	salot nam	root

Equal parts, 7 items. Pills to be taken mixed with water used to wash rice to counteract heat, thirst and *saang chon saang phloeng.*

Medicine to treat *saang haeng*, that is *saang chon saang phloeng*[7] if it affects the eyes causing *klet kadee* [blepharitis], then pustules all over the body like a heat rash.

[544]	*hom daeng*	
	nom maeo	root
	khem lueang	root
	phrommi	
	kathue	
	phlai	
	krathiam	
	waan proh	
	thua phuu	root
	kwaang	horn
	raet	horn
	kui	horn
	suea	eye tooth
	chorakhe	eye tooth
	mee	eye tooth

muu	tusk
raet	eye tooth
kot thang 5	
thian thang 5	
kaarabuun	
nam prasaan thong	

Equal parts, 28 items. Prepare pills using aromatic water as excipient. To be taken mixed with cucumber juice to treat the four kinds of *to* and the *to* caused by *saang* in children.

Medicine to treat *to klet kadee*:

[545]	*bencha phak bung*	
	yaa chan kaat	root-stock
	taeng kwaa	flowers
	tamlueng	flowers
	banlangsinlaa	
	sang	
	din thanam	

Equal parts, 7 items. Prepare a stick, mix with cucumber juice and use as an eye lotion.

Medicine to treat blurred vision in children:

[546]	*bua luang*	pollen
	kradang ngaa	flowers
	salit	flowers
	saaraphee	flowers
	phimsen	

Equal parts, 5 items. Prepare a stick using dew drops, then mix with breast milk and a little *nam chai khrai* as excipient.

Medicine to treat *to kon hoi* [glaucoma]:

[547]	*sattabut*	flowers
	samo thet	
	thian dam	
	thian khaao	
	dee plee	
	din thanam	
	tuk tam nam thong	
	phut son	root
	anchan thang 2	root
	thong laang bai mon	root
	mafai	root

Equal parts, 12 items. Prepare a stick using lime juice as excipient, and mix with *nam tamlueng* to make an eye lotion to dissolve the film [on the eyes]. After 3 days, irrigate with half the lotion.

If it is necessary to remove more film:

[548] *kluea saek* [*thet*]

nam prasaan thong	
kaarabuun	
1 part of each	
krawaan	
chamot chiang	
nguu lueam	bile
chorakhe	bile
muu paa	bile
2 parts of each	
tuk tam nam thong	
dee plee	
kaan phluu	
chunsee	
thian dam	
thian khaao	
benyakaanee	galls
chan thang 2	
kot so	
kot hua bua	
kot chulaa lamphaa	
khondok	
chan	seeds
marum	bark
utta phit	rhizome
krachaai	
krathiam	
phrik Thai	
khing	dried
4 parts of each	
sang	
din thanam	
32 parts of each	

Mix together these 32 items, then prepare a stick using lime [juice] as excipient. Mix with *nam thao tamlueng* and use to irrigate the eyes. If something even stronger is required, add *lamut* seeds. This removes all *to.*

Medicine to dissolve *to kon hoi* [glaucoma] and *to lin maa* [pterygium]:

[549]	*maklam khaao*	fruit
	maklam dam	fruit
	chik	fruit
	yaang	fruit
	sabaa ling	seeds
	tamlueng laai	

khae daeng	seeds	
buk	tuber	
kloi	tuber	
utta phit	rhizome	
thao khan	rhizome	
khai fak	shell	
bia phuu		
sang		
tanot	rhizome	
(some editions say *khamot*) [sic]		
din thanam		
phimsen		

Equal parts, 17 items. Prepare a stick using *nam thao tamlueng* as excipient. Mix with water and irrigate the eyes to remove all *to*. Then prepare the following astringent eye lotion:

Astringent eye lotion for *to*:

[550]

samo thet		
fin		
maa mieo		
samo faai thet	under-ripe fruit	
nguu lueam	bile	

Equal parts, 5 items. Prepare a stick. Mix with milk or aromatic water and use as an astringent eye lotion to treat eye pain and irritation.

Medicine to treat *to lam yai* [cataract]:

[551]

hoi khong	shell	
sang		
bia phuu		
din thanam		

1 *baht* of each

Burn slowly with *mai sakae* then add

lin thale		1 *baht*
khaao saan dam		9 *grains*
phimsen		6 *klam*

Macerate in water, and express the liquid from

mafueng	leaves	1 *baht*
kaphrao	leaves	2 *baht*

Use as excipient to prepare a stick. Mix with breast milk or aromatic water and irrigate the eyes of the child.

Medicine to treat *saang chon* and *saang haeng*:

[552]

thian	leaves	
thap thim	leaves	
sawaat	leaves	
phimsen	leaves	

kraphrao thang 2	leaves
phrik Thai	
hua hom	
krachaai	
khamin oi	
plaa chon	burnt scales
waan keep raet	
waan ron thong	
khai fak	shell
nam prasaan thong	
lin thale	

Equal parts, 14 items. Pills to be taken mixed with alcohol to treat *saang chon* and *saang haeng* which cause craving for salt and pepper; thinness and yellowness; cough; breathlessness; and other symptoms.

Next is a summary of the *saang* of the seven days, from the supplementary texts. The masters have included it here so that doctors will know the origin of the pustules and fevers of *saang*.

If a child born on Sunday becomes ill, it is because of internal heat [one of the body elements]. The birth *saang* is *saang phloeng*, and this first occurs in the navel, then it spreads. Later, it returns to the navel again.

If a child born on Monday becomes ill, it is because of the element water. The birth *saang* is *saang nam*. If it comes up on the tongue, the baby cannot eat or drink and has diarrhoea and vomiting. The vomit is like rice water and mashed boiled eggs.

If a child born on Tuesday becomes ill, it is because of [the element] blood, and is very difficult to cure. The birth *saang* is *saang daeng*. This first develops around the navel and causes diarrhoea, cold hands and feet, listlessness and a stiff back.

If a child born on Wednesday becomes ill, they say it is because of eating the wrong food, and the illness is due to the element water. The birth *saang* is *saang sako*.

If a child born on Thursday becomes ill, it is because of [the element] internal heat. This causes headache, with a high temperature and cold hands and feet. The birth *saang* is *saang kho*, and if it affects the tongue, both tongue and chin stiffen and the baby cannot suck at the breast. Be very careful for three days and then it will be safe.

If a child born on Friday becomes ill, it is due to [the element] wind, which causes flatulence in the evening. The birth *saang* is *saang chaang*, which changes to *saang daeng* and is very difficult to cure. If the baby has this for a long time and does not die, [the disease] will gradually change to *taan chon*. The doctor will think that the child is better, but he should not rely on it.

If a child born on Saturday becomes ill, it is due to [the element] wind, which causes vomiting, difficulty in urinating, and constipation. The birth *saang* is *saang chon*. Doctors should understand this.

Next is a brief description of the minor forms of *saang*. Doctors should know the symptoms of *saang* which affects all children.

When it starts, pustules of *saang kraduuk* last for two days, then withdraw into the abdomen, causing diarrhoea and cold hands and feet. The major pustule then reappears at the root of the tongue. It is very hard, like a corn [on the foot, for example]. If the doctor recognizes this, he should break it first, before applying medicine and then it will go.

The pustules of *saang kranae* are small, black in the centres and red round the edges. When they subside, they enter the abdomen, causing the baby to pass mucus and blood. *Saang kranae* is a very bad type of *saang*.

The pustules of *saang naangrin* are white, like crystal clear water. When it enters the abdomen, it causes diarrhoea like water used to wash rice.

Saang prathommakan is caused by [the element] blood.[8] It makes the mouth red. When it enters the abdomen, it causes diarrhoea like spittle from a chewed quid of betel and areca nut.

The description of congenital *saang*,[9] both *saang* of birth and the minor *saang*, given here in *Prathom chindaa*, Book IV, explains only the appearance of the pustules. Their types and symptoms are explained in *Prathom chindaa*, Book III. Here the masters briefly discuss the pustules only.

If the doctor who intends looking after children does not study *Phrakhamphee prathom chindaa*, *Khampee apphayasantaaa* and this text, he is like a blind man who walks across a bridge without holding the railing. He will fall down. Those who just follow the prescriptions the masters have written, without learning, and use those prescriptions to treat patients just because they are greedy for profit, never know right from wrong. It is as is written in the Pāli texts: to give the wrong medicine once is like killing the patient with a spear; to give the wrong medicine twice is like killing the patient with fire; and to give the wrong medicine three times is like striking him with lightning. Without a doubt, the patient is sure to die.

If the doctor has studied *Khamphee prathom chindaa* and *Khamphee apphayasantaa* and becomes proficient in them, babies will be cool and happy, because they will be in no danger of dying.

NOTES

1 *apphayasantaa:* The name of a text on fevers, the various types of *saang* and diseases of the eye.

2 The reference to the time of day or night when the child is born may be a figure of speech, but its ambiguity may also provide a loophole should the predicted form of *saang* not eventuate. In the lunar system, the day starts at dark; in the solar system the day starts at dawn. The birth day might, thus, be different, depending on the system used in the calculation.

3 *rok klaak:* a kind of eczema.
phanranai: a skin condition which results in the outer skin flaking off.

4 *sattabut:* *Nymphaea lotus* L., Nymphaeaceae. The lotus - large white variety. (VJ) Clearly the name here refers to a red variety. The 1871 text is the same, but for the word '*rop*' rather than '*op*' following '*sattabut*' - a misprint in the 1961 edition.

5 *saang haeng:* coeliac disease, treated with bile salts. (DT)

6 *malet kadue* [*kadee*] and *to kon hoi:* types of glaucoma. There are many kinds of *to*, including *to hin, to klet kadee, to kon hoi* and *to klet hoi*, types of glaucoma; *to krachok* or *kachok* and *to lam yai*, cataract; also *to lin maa, to nuea* and *to saai lohit*, pterygium. (PT) See Book II, note 10.

7 See note 5.

8 See Book II, note 17.

9 *saang tae bandaa:* *saang* from or beginning with the parents.

[Book V]

Phrakhamphee prathom chindaa, Book V, gives a brief description of severe *taan chon*, birth *saang* and minor *saang*, severe illness of birth *saang*, and body parasites. It concludes with the effects of parasites after the time for birth *saang*, minor *saang* and *saang chon* has passed.

The culmination of a doctor's care for children is [the treatment of] *taan chon* which follows birth *saang* and minor *saang* when they have run their course.

In order to understand when birth *saang* and minor *saang* are finished, the inexperienced doctor should observe what the masters have explained, as follows.

A baby born on Sunday has *saang phloeng* as birth *saang*, *saang kraai* as minor *saang*. *Saang phloeng* affects the baby for 1 year and 11 months and *saang kraai* for 7 months; a total of 2 years, 6 months and 6 days. Then *saang phloeng* is finished.

A baby born on Monday has *saang nam* as birth *saang*, *saang faai* as minor *saang*. *Saang nam* affects the baby for 1 year and 6 months and *saang faai* for 6 months; a total of 2 years, 15 days. Then *saang nam* is finished.

A baby born on Tuesday has *saang daeng* as birth *saang*, *saang kranae* as minor *saang*. *Saang daeng* affects the baby for 3 years and 6 months and *saang kranae* for 1 year and 6 months; a total of 5 years and 8 days. Then *saang daeng* is finished.

A baby born on Wednesday has *saang sako* as birth *saang*, *saang kratang* as minor *saang*. *Saang sako* affects the baby for 1 year and 4 months and *saang kratang* for 1 year and 3 months; a total of 2 years, 7 months and 17 days. Then *saang sako* is finished.

A baby born on Thursday has *saang kho* as birth *saang*, *saang khaao plueak* as minor *saang*. *Saang kho* affects the baby for 2 years and 5 months and *saang khaao plueak* for 1 year and 6 months; a total of 3 years, 11 months and 19 days. Then *saang kho* is finished.

A baby born on Friday has *saang chaang* as birth *saang*, *saang kraduuk* as minor *saang*. *Saang chaang* affects the baby for 2 years and 9 months and *saang kraduuk* for 7 months; a total of 3 years, 4 months and 21 days. Then *saang chaang* is finished.

A baby born on Saturday has *saang chon* as birth *saang*, *saang naangrin* as minor *saang*. *Saang chon* affects the baby for 3 years and 8 months and *saang naangrin* for 1 year and 7 months; a total of 5 years, 3 months and 10 days. Then *saang chon* is finished.

These are the limitations of the seven kinds of birth *saang* and minor *saang*, showing the normal course of each disease from the onset to the time when it is finished, as stated previously.

Here, according to the masters, are set out the number of days the fever [*khai*] of each disease lasts and [the outcome]; whether a child will recover, get worse or die.

From its onset, the fever [*lom khai*] of *saang phloeng* lasts for eleven days, then it goes away.[1] If not, the baby will die.

From its onset, the fever of *saang nam* lasts for twelve days, then goes away. If not, the condition is grave.

The fever of *saang daeng* lasts for thirteen days, then it abates. Otherwise the child will die.

The fever of *saang sako* lasts for fourteen days before it subsides. If it does not go away by then, it gets worse.

The fever of *saang kho* lasts for fifteen days, then goes or else the baby dies.

The fever of *saang chaang* lasts for sixteen days before it abates or the baby dies.

The fever of *saang chon* lasts for seventeen days, and the baby will certainly die if it has not recovered by this time.

Here, the limitations of the course and severity of birth *saang* are given. If the normal time has passed and the disease has not yet abated, the child will fall into the hands of Phrayaa Matchuraat. When the birth *saang* and the minor *saang* are finished, then *taan chon* develops. There are seven kinds. This is an illness which is very tricky and, if the doctor does not know its origin and closes his eyes, it is just as if he has killed the baby with fire, because there is no doubt that the baby will die.

Intestinal Parasites and *Taan Chon*

Here we discuss children who have passed the age when birth *saang* [and minor *saang*] occur. They are then about five or six years old and might have *taan chon* because of eating things they are not used to. Just as when the brahmas came down to taste the sweetness of the earth. They developed physical abnormalities, because they were accustomed to being in the heavenly abode, and when they came down and tasted the sweetness of the earth their bodies changed to human form and they reproduced accordingly.[2] So the baby conceived in the mother's womb, having eaten strange food, get diseases and worms. There are 80 kinds of worms and they afflict all beings without exception. As explained here, unfamiliar food is the cause of the 80 kinds of worms that infest the bodies of living creatures.

Now, there are seven kinds of worms occurring in the digested food and the undigested food.[3] These are: *kata, otaka, khanthupaa* and *sukata*, making seven [sic] kinds.

There are two kinds of worms occurring in the bone marrow: *yaawa* and *sopphaa.*

There are two kinds of worms occurring in the spleen: *kata* and *raatawatthaa.*

There are four kinds of worms occurring in the heart: *thananta, mahaanantthata, lohita* and *mahaalohita.*

There are three kinds of worms occurring in the bile and mucus: *ninlaka, upawa* and *laamukkha.*

There are three kinds of worms occurring in the ocular cavities: *maana, takaa* and *nawa.*

There are three kinds of worms occurring in the pus: *manchu, mukkha* and *mikkhala.*

There are three kinds of worms occurring in the liver: *warana, tana* and *sawara.*

There are six kinds of worms occurring in the abdomen: *awitchaa, atthiwitchaa, watthaa, sitthaa, thatsaha* and *munnakkha.*

There are two kinds of worms occurring in the liquid fat: *phimanchaa* and *lemakkha.*

There are three kinds of worms occurring at the anus: *kitthaa, phaya* and *paalaata.*

There are four kinds of worms occurring in the middle of the body: *lohamukkha, mahaalohamukkha, munnachaa* and *mahaamunnachaa.*

There are six kinds of worms occurring in the lungs: *seta*, *lohita*, *chawakaan*, *siwaatchaa*, *akkha* and *mahaa-akkha*.

There are six kinds of worms occurring in the small and large intestines: *warasimahaa*, *waranataa*, *mahaawaranataa*, *sippapaa*, *mahasippapaa* and *santa-antaa*.

There are three kinds of worms occurring in solid fat: *sutthaacha*, *sinnehatchaa* and *mahaasinnehatchaa*.

There are five kinds of worms in the lower part of the body and down to the feet: *witsanhaa*, *siwaara*, *tetchanta*, *siwaraa* and *mahaasiwaraa*.

There are two kinds of worms occurring in the hair on the head: *phanlawaa* and *mahaaphanlawaa*.

There are three kinds of worms occurring in the nasal mucus: *nahaapattara*, *shanlamukkha* and *sattamukkha*.

There are three kinds of worms occurring on the tongue: *kaala*, *mukkhaa* and *mannapenla*.

There are three kinds of worms occurring in the finger and toe-nails: *leha*, *raakkha* and *awanna*.

There are three kinds of worms occurring in the flesh and along the tendons: *kanna*, *ratchaka* and *lohita*.

There are two kinds of worms occurring in the throat: *rammahaa* and *mahaarammahaa*.

Now, these 80 kinds of worms live inside the body of every human being and animal, without exception. When the worms mature they cause distress to animals and humans, resulting in various illnesses, as explained previously and to be continued below for the information of doctors, according to the masters, here in *Khamphee prathom chindaa*.

Here ends the description of 80 kinds of worms.

Finally, the masters give a brief description of *taan chon*, which is caused by eleven kinds of worms, to help doctors treating diseases in young children to identify and diagnose these eleven kinds of worms.

In other words, *taan chon* is associated with the four elements, as explained here, for the information of doctors.

Now, these eleven kinds of worms are: *purathaatubot*, *pattachiwahaa*, *santaa*, *uttharaa*, *phanlaphaha*, *khongsathaan fai*, *phrommakit*, *umuthaat*, *mutsakaayathaat*, *rattanapanlaathaat*. *Taan chon* embraces all these eleven kinds of worms.

Purathaatubot results from *saang phloeng*. At first it produces [rectal] bleeding, a yellow body, weakness and a craving for fresh meat and fish. Another called *patshannathaat* affects the child later. It develops in the nostrils and blocks the nose, like a bad cold with a foul smelling discharge. Then it passes down to the root of the tongue and all the way down to the feet. This causes incessant dribbling, a dry throat and the child cannot eat. As a result, various disorders develop which are very difficult to cure.

If a doctor wants to treat these two kinds of *taan chon*, he should first clear up the tongue and throat, then give medicine to stop the bleeding.

Medicine for *taan chon* of the tongue causing a dry throat and inability to eat or drink:

[553] *son thet* root

	see siat thet		
	cha-em		
	nam taan	granulated	

Equal parts, 4 items. Crush and apply to the tongue.

Medicine to treat excessive salivation [dribbling]:

[554]	*tree phalaa hom*		8 parts
	kraphang hom	root	1 part
	phak waan baan	root	1 part
	kraphrao	root	1 part
	maklam khruea	root	1 part

5 items. Prepare a stick. Mix with honey and paint the throat.

Another:

[555]	*yaa tai bai*	
	chan daeng	
	raet	molar tooth
	chaang	molar tooth

Equal parts, 4 items. Prepare a stick. Mix with alcohol and paint the tongue and mouth.

Medicine to cleanse the body of *taan chon:*

[556]	*chan*	seeds	
	chan	arils	
	krawaan		
	kaan phluu		
	tree katuk		
	thian thang 5		
	1 part of each		
	salot	fruit (purified)	2 parts

To reduce the toxicity of the *salot* [croton] fruit, soak in the liquor from fermented fish for one night in a narrow-mouthed jar. Then stuff the fruit inside *makruut* fruit and bake in a slow burning fire of paddy husks until well cooked. [Cf. nos.620,621,623.] Then combine all the ingredients, including the *makruut* fruit, and prepare pills the size of peppercorns. 5, 6 or 7 pills to be taken for a dose. If the child is from 3 to 6 years old, give 11 to 15 pills, depending on the elements and strength of the child.

Another:

[557]	*krathiam*	
	cheta muun phloeng	root
	makruut	skin
	kaarabuun	
	phrik Thai	
	dee plee	
	ching cho	root
	salot	leaves

matuum	leaves
sawaat	leaves

1 part of each. Steam the two [three] kinds of leaves before use, then measure out

rong thong	
yaa dam	
tong taek	root

2 parts of each. 12 items. Prepare pills, the size of cotton seeds, using *nam som saa* as excipient. From 1 to 9 pills to be taken, mixed with alcohol, the number of pills depending on the strength of the body elements of the child, whether heavy or light, to purge the body completely. **Then give the following medicine to stop the action of this medicine.**

[558]

waan keep raet	
waan ron thong	
chan daeng	
benyakaanee	
neraphuusee	
prakham dee khwaai	fruit
see siat thet	

Equal parts, 7 items. Prepare pills using *nam som saa* as excipient. To be taken mixed with alcohol to counteract the poisonous effects and diarrhoea of *saang chon.*

If that is ineffective, then prepare the following:

[559]

waan keep raet	
waan ron thong	
chan thang 2	
benyakaanee	
neraphuusee	
khan song	root
phrik Thai	
khing	dried
hom	
khamin oi	
prakham dee khwaai	fruit

Equal parts, 12 items. Prepare pills to be taken mixed with alcohol and a small quantity of python's bile.

If that is ineffective, then use the following prescription:

[560] ***Naatsaphit*** for the poison of *saang chon saang phloeng*

waan keep raet	
waan ron thong	
dee nguu thang 2 (dee nguu ton and khruea) [sic]	
krung khamao	
khrai khruea	root

neraphuusee	
raatchadat	fruit
rayom	root
prakham dee khwaai	fruit
phrakham kai	leaves
fin thang 2	
sang karanee	
chuk rohinee	
nguu lueam	bile
yaa fin	

Equal parts, 19 items. Python's bile, soaked in water, to be used as excipient to make pills. Mix with alcohol. To be given to counteract internal poisoning and the effects of any poison. Force open the child's mouth and pour the medicine in.

Medicine to treat *semha tee khuen:*

[561]

tree katuk	
kluea sinthao	
som kung	root
som poi	pods
muun kaa daeng	root

Equal parts, 7 items. Mix together, then combine

khanthatsakon	
nam taan	coarse
nam taan	granulated
nam manaao	
makhaam piak	fruit juice

and stir in with the rest of the ingredients. Paint the tongue frequently, until the child is able to swallow easily.

Medicine to treat inability to eat or drink, and weakness:

[562]

bua khom	tuber
khaao saan	

2 items. To be taken mixed with cow's milk or breast milk to strengthen the child, and increase the appetite.

Another:

[563]

krachap bok	
bua luang	pollen
lahung daeng	root

Equal parts, 3 items. To be taken mixed with water obtained when rice first boils.

Application to counteract the heat of *saang phloeng:*

[564]

mong	root
lamduan	root
yaa phraek	
din prasiu khaao	

Mix with water used to wash rice, and apply to overcome the high temperature of *saang phloeng.*

Medicine to treat thirst and the heat of *saang chon* and *saang phloeng:*

[565]	*khaao saan*	root
	bua luang	root
	thua phuu	root
	thong laang naam	root
	salot nam	root
	chan thang 2	
	salit	root
	thao yaai mom	root
	nam nong	root
	khaakrong	root
	puu chao loi thaa	
	phitsanaat	root
	see huat	root
	yaa naang	root
	san phraa naang ae	

Equal parts, 16 items. Prepare pills to be taken and applied mixed with water used to wash rice. For thirst and the temperature of *saang chon* and *saang phloeng.*

[566] **Yaa daeng** To treat *taan chon* affecting the stomach:

chan thang 2	
makluea lueat	bark
khee aai	bark
haang kraai	bark
neraphuusee	
sang karanee	
kaan phluu	
dee plee	
khing	dried
masaang	bark

Equal parts, 13 items. Use *marum* bark sap as excipient to prepare pills. To be taken mixed with *mamuang phruan* bark sap, *maduea* bark sap or *makok* bark sap for mucus and blood in the stools of *taan chon*, due to worms called *bunthaatubot.* If the child takes this medicine as set out here, he will survive.

Santaathaat results from *saang nam.* It makes the body cold and causes incessant flatulence. The child urinates and defecates with difficulty, it has gooseflesh while defecating, and rectal bleeding and the urine is as white as rice water because of milky coloured stones [urinary calculi].

Uttharaathaat occurs inside the navel within the abdomen. The child is listless, thin and breathless. The doctor can only give palliative treatment. If it continues for three to four months and the intestines swell and the abdomen grows larger, some say it is because the liver is enlarged and presses hard up against the rib-cage, the child will die.

Application for flatulence:

[567] *bai naat*

khon thee so	leaves
prakham kai	leaves
phak khet	leaves
phak sian phee	leaves
manaao	seeds
sabaa mon	seeds
mot yop	
kamyaan phee	
tree katuk	
saan som	
din prasiu khaao	
nam prasaan thong	
krachaai	
kathue	
phlai	
hom	
krathiam	
khamin oi	
nguu lueam	bones
nguu hao	bones
haan	bones
liang phaa	bones
mahaa hing	
yaa dam	
rong thong	

Equal parts, 26 items. Prepare pills or a stick, mix with *nam makruut* and apply to the abdomen. To treat flatulence, abdominal dropsy, *maan kasai lom*, swollen intestines, abdominal distension and flatulence, blue abdomen, inability to evacuate the bowels and bladder, convulsions with spasms of the hands and feet; convulsions with rigid back; *saphan*, *akkhamukkhee*, *lom baatthayak*, *lom kumphanthayak*, *lom thakkhinnakhun* and *lom prawaattakhun*. All will go.

[568] ***Prasa kaphrao*** *(noi)*

yaa dam
hing yaang pho
krathiam
phrik Thai
dee plee
waan nam

Equal parts, 6 items. Add an amount of *kraphrao* leaves equal to the rest of the ingredients. Pills to be taken mixed with *nam makruut* or alcohol to treat flatulence. Suitable as a stomach mixture for all children.

[569] ***Mongkhon rangap***

thian thang 5	
chan	seeds
chan	arils
krawaan	
kaan phluu	
sang karanee	
neraphuusee	
khrai khruea	
waan keep raet	
waan ron thong	
phan phak kaat	seeds
rangap	leaves
kameng	leaves
khee kaa daeng	leaves
nam tao	leaves
tree katuk	
khaa	
krachaai	
kathue	
phlai	
khamin oi	
hom daeng	
krathiam	

Equal parts, 27 items. Prepare pills using lime juice as excipient. To be taken mixed with alcohol to treat the flatulence and foul smelling faeces caused by *taan chon* and for the poison of all kinds of *taan* and *saang*.

[570] ***Mahaa kaphrao***

thian thang 5	of each, 1 part
tree katuk	of each, 4 parts
mahaa hing	
krathiam	

8 parts of each

kaphrao leaves, an amount equal to the rest

11 items. Prepare pills using alcohol as excipient. To be taken, mixed with alcohol, for mucus and blood in the stools, and pain.

[571] ***Hing*** (medicine to expel flatus)

phrik Thai	1 part
kaphrao	2 parts

dee plee		3 parts
mahaa hing		
kaarabuun		
makruut	skin	
waan nam		
phlai		

4 parts of each.

8 items. Prepare pills using alcohol as excipient. To be taken and applied to the stomach, mixed with *nam makruut* to treat stomach ache, flatulence and a cold body.

Laxative to treat *taan chon:*

[572]

makruut	skin
som saa	skin
marum baan	root
mawaeng ton	root
salot	purified fruit [see no. 556]

Equal parts, 5 items. Prepare pills the size of peppercorns, using leaf juice of *waan haang chaang* as excipient. Dose: one pill, depending on whether the elements are light or heavy. To expel all bad poison, and worms called *uttharaathaat.*

Also:

To treat swollen intestines, abdominal distension, and abdominal dropsy, causing swelling anywhere at all, in one place or the whole body, as a result of *taan chon*:

[573]

makhaam	leaves
som poi	leaves
som sieo	leaves
manaao	leaves
salot kin long	root

Equal parts, 5 items. Reduce to 1/3 volume by boiling. Decant the liquid then add

nam phueng	1 cupful
suraa	1 cupful
rong thong	
yaa dam	
din prasiu khaao	

1 part of each

dee kluea	2 parts

and mix together.

A child 5 or 6 years old should take an amount the size of the fruit of *bua kroh*, then the bowels will function properly and all illness will clear up.

Medicine to treat the *taan chon* called *sataothaat* (or *santaathaat*), which causes listlessness and stupor:

[574]	*chan daeng*	
	chan khaao	
	krisanaa	
	kralam phak	
	chaluut	
	khondok	
	bunnaak	flowers
	bua luang	pollen
	sattabut	flowers
	chaat cho sae	
	chamot	
	phimsen	

Equal parts, 12 items. Mix with dew then spread on a palmyra palm leaf to dry in the sun. Then mix again with aromatic water. Pills to be taken mixed with aromatic water to treat unconsciousness and restlessness. To treat weakness and exhaustion, mix with a decoction of *thua phuu* root. To treat diarrhoea, mix with a decoction of *samo Thai* fruit juice. For eye insensitivity, mix with lime juice and brain of the serpent-headed fish, and apply to the eyelids.

[575]	***Thip sawaang aarom***	
	thua phuu	seeds
	bua kroh	fruit
	thua phuu	root
	bua luang	root
	bua khom	tuber
	bua phuean	tuber
	bua phan	tuber
	haeo sot	
	krachap	raw
	yaa naang	root
	krisanaa	
	kralam phak	
	chaluut	
	khondok	
	chan chamot	
	cha-em thet	
	opchoei thang 2	
	kot hua bua	
	kot chiang	
	proh hom	
	bua luang	pollen
	bua phuean	pollen
	bua khom	pollen
	sattabut	pollen

sattabongkot	pollen
chong konlanee	pollen
saaraphee	pollen
phikun	flowers
bunnaak	flowers
mali son	flowers
mali laa	flowers
krung khamao	
chamot	
phimsen	
yaa faran	
amphan thong	

Equal parts, 37 items. Pills to be taken mixed with aromatic water to treat listlessness and stupor, and feebleness; to treat all *saang*; *saang* affecting the heart and in the chest, causing the child to be motionless and unable to open its eyes.

[576] ***Mahaa chaiyamongkhon* for breathlessness** (some editions call this *Mahaa chaiyaphak*') [sic]

krisanaa	
chan chamot	
san phraa naang ae	bark
yaa phan nguu daeng	
kammathan daeng	
malaeng saap	faecal matter
phak chee	fruit
raet	horn
chaang	tusk
kwaang	horn

Equal parts, 10 items. Pills to be taken mixed with lime juice, to treat breathlessness of *saang*. To treat *khai nuea*[4] make a decoction with sap of pomegranate leaves.

[577] ***Sukhum thaeng hom*** for breathlessness

nguu lueam	bones
nguu thap thaang	bones
nguu hao	bones
plaa chon	tail
krisanaa	
kralam phak	
son thet	
opchoei	
chan	seeds
chan	arils
chan thang 2	
chaluut	

	khondok	
	cha-em thet	
	yaa naang	root
	kot so	
	kot phung plaa	
	thian dam	
	thian khaao	
	bua luang	pollen
	bunnaak	flowers
	makruut	flowers
	manaao	flowers
	chaluut	flowers

Equal parts, 25 items. Add *kot hua bua*, an amount equal to the other ingredients combined. Prepare pills using aromatic water as excipient. To be taken mixed with aromatic water, together with a small amount of Borneo camphor and civet.

Decoction to treat *taan chon:*

[578]	*thap thim*	leaves	
	thian	leaves	
	boraphet		
	khamin oi		
	khon thee so	leaves	
	aai nieo	root	
	khai nao	bark	

Equal parts, 7 items. Add

makruut		1 fruit
som poi		7 pods

Reduce to 1/3 volume by boiling. To be taken to counteract the *taan chon* of *saang nam.*

Decoction to treat *taan chon:*

[579]	*krachap*	root
	sakae	root
	makluea	root
	lep mue naang	root
	fin ton	bark
	chum het thet	leaves

Equal parts, 6 items. Reduce to 1/3 volume by boiling. To be taken for abdominal pain and thirst.

Decoction to treat blood in the stools caused by *taan chon:*

[580]	*song maeo*	root
	to sai	root
	khamin oi	tuber

3 items. Take some of each and reduce to 1/3 volume by boiling. To be taken for swollen intestines and abdominal distension caused by the *taan chon* called *uttharathaat.*

Phalaphaha results from *saang daeng*, the birth *saang* of babies born on Tuesday. When the *saang daeng* is over, this might develop in the part of the intestines below the navel. The kidney on the left hand side is as large as a walnut. Then the child has abdominal colic, because it develops just like *saang daeng* and attacks the duct of the liver, as stated in *Phrakhamphee prathom chindaa*, Book III [II], Part 3 and set down here on page 109 of this volume of *Phaetthayasaat songkhroh.* Here we refer only to the effects of *taan chon.* Doctors should know, when it starts with a high temperature and regular fever, not to mistake it for hypertrophy of the spleen [*paang*] and enlarged spleen. It is the disease, *taan chon.* In which case the child has internal worms in the same way as some fish and lumps appear, covered in mucus. After three months, the faeces resemble water used to wash meat and contain mucus and blood. The child has severe abdominal pain and strains until it has a prolapse of the rectum; is thin and yellow, and craves hot-and-spicy and salty food, and fresh meat and fish. Then spots erupt all over the body. This should not be mistaken for *pradong*, it is the [*taan*] *chon* of *saang daeng*, and the main pustules of *saang* at the root of the tongue get worse and the child stops eating. Sometimes the tongue and chin stiffen and the main pustule of *saang* in the left ear causes earache and a discharge from the ear. The main pustules of *saang* in the eyes flare up, at first looking like *kradee* [fish] scales. If medicine is ineffective, *to kon hoi* [a type of glaucoma] develops, and after seven days the eye, or if both are affected, the eyes are damaged. Then the main pustules of *saang* on both shins erupt rough and sharp like the skin of a stingray, with roots like small blackheads. It can be cured if the doctor treats both the eyes and shins. Then the child will live.

Seven, eight or nine months later, another kind of worm called *phrommakit* develops in the intestines. It resembles black-mouthed scabies. It gives the child an insatiable appetite, and causes heavy bowel motions - white and smelly - blurred vision and a craving for prawns, fresh meat and fish. This results from *saang daeng* and the doctor will find it very difficult to cure and various conditions will develop, as described. If he treats it properly, it will clear up. Otherwise, it might move somewhere else. It will recur halfway through the child's lifetime, and again later, when tuberculosis will affect him. A doctor treating this should never give medicine to expel flatus, nor should he allow the patient to eat too much. This disease will change and cause difficulties in the end. To treat it, first prepare medicine to clean out the intestines, but do not give anything containing *salot* [croton]. The doctor should treat it as he would treat *sannibaat*, because this kind of *saang* results from [the elements] blood and internal heat and originates in the mother's womb at the time of conception. Whatever illness affected the mother was ultimately due to internal heat as has been stated in *Phrakhamphee prathom chindaa*, Book I, on pregnancy.

Decoction to clean out *taan chon* from the intestines:

[581]	*tree phalaa*		of each, 3 fruits
	makhaam	leaves	
	som poi	leaves	

khee kaa thang 2	root
hom	
tong taek	root

1 part of each

raatcha phrik pods, an amount equal to all the other ingredients

Reduce to 1/3 volume by boiling, and add *dee kluea* depending on whether the elements are light or heavy [perhaps, whether the patient is of light or heavy build]. To be given first to cleanse the intestines, then prepare a decoction to be taken for *chap* [possibly malaria].

Decoction for *chap* of *taan chon:*

[582]

khee lek	heartwood
sadao	heartwood
son	heartwood
chan thang 2	
yaa naang	root
makhaam pom	fruit
kradom	fruit
boraphet	
haeo muu	

Equal parts, 10 items. Mix with juice of *raatcha phrik* pods. Reduce to 1/3 volume by boiling. Dose to be taken depending on the strength of the child, to treat the *chap* resulting from *taan chon* due to internal heat and mucus.

[583] ***Chantharatsamee***

kum thang 2	
mayom tua phuu	leaves
phak khuang	leaves
phutsaa	leaves
phak bung khan	leaves
khee kaa daeng	leaves
prakham kai	leaves
makruut	leaves
manaao	leaves
mangua	leaves
som saa	leaves
khaa	
krachaai	
krathue	
phlai	
hom	
krathiam	
tree katuk	
khamin oi	
phan phak kaat	seeds

chan thang 2
waan keep raet
waan ron thong

Equal parts, 17 items. Add an amount of pepper equal to the rest of the ingredients combined. Prepare pills to be given according to the strength of the child. Add a small quantity of python's bile to treat *daan* [lumps], hypertrophy of the spleen and mucus, regular fever, abdominal worms, to contain the liver and to counteract the poison of *saang*. To treat any painful swelling, mix with alcohol and apply. For trembling, convulsions and delirium, give mixed with aromatic water. For epilepsy, give mixed with alcohol. For breathlessness, mix with *nam som saa*, aromatic water or syrup. To treat *taan saang* and mucus and blood in the stools, give mixed with alcohol. Mix with ginger root juice for *puang* [cholera] and mix with *nam khaa* for *lom*. To treat *sannibaat*, give with *nam som saa*, for asthma and coughs, mix with juice from *som poi* pods. For ear-ache, mix with *nam thalaai maak dip* and instill into the ear and apply externally. For insomnia, this mixture is to be given mixed with alcohol.

Medicine to expel worms from the abdomen:

[584] *khamin oi*

sakae	fruit	
maklam taa chaang	fruit	
makluea	fruit	
phalaan satruu	fruit	
nam prasaan thong		
lin thale		
samo thang 3		
one part of each		
maeng lak	leaves	
kaphrao	leaves	
salot	leaves	
salot kin long	root	
kaarabun		
2 parts of each		
kot nam tao		8 parts

16 items. Prepare pills the size of peppercorns, using alcohol as excipient. To be taken mixed with alcohol. Dose: Very young infants: 1 pill. Babies aged 4 to 5 months: 2 pills. Children aged 3 years: 3 pills. To expel worms, as explained under *saang daeng*; and also to expel *sai duean*.

Medicine to treat *la* in the throat and on the tongue:

[585] *nam prasaan thong*

plaa chon	burnt tail
hoi khong	calcined shell

chaang	tusk	
luuk on	excreta	
kaphrao	leaves	
khamao fai		
kon mo kaeng		
khamin oi		

Equal parts, 9 items. Prepare a stick. Mix with lime juice and paint the tongue.

Medicine to treat the primary pustule of *saang* at the base of the tongue:

[586]

chunsee sat		1 part
nam prasaan thong sat		2 parts
kluea	roasted	3 parts
dee plee	burnt	5 parts

4 items. Prepare a stick. Mix with lime juice and crocodile's bile and apply to *saang daeng pathommakan* which changes to *phayuha*.

Medicine to treat *to klet hoi:*

[587]

bencha phak bung Thai	
krachaai	rhizome
tamlueng	flowers
taeng kwaa	flowers
makhaam	flowers
yaa chan kaat	root-stock
plaa mo	roasted scales

Equal parts, 11 items. Mix together and add some Borneo camphor. Prepare a stick. Add cucumber juice and use as an eye lotion for *to klet hoi* and all forms of *to*; for pain and irritation, and to brighten the colour of the eyes.

Medicine to treat *to sai lohit:*

[588]

boraphet	
khamin oi	
baan mi ruu rooi khaao	root
yaa wong chaang	root
khulikaan [khunlikaa]	

Equal parts, 4 items. Soak in aromatic water and add a small quantity of crocodile's bile, to irrigate the eyes. For the treatment of *to sai lohit* in which there is a red film, like a flame, on the eye.

[589] ***Saawakalayaanee*** snuff

chamot
phimsen
kot hua bua
krisanaa
kralam phak
lin thale

	kaeo klaep	
	sang	
	som kung	root
	tuk tam nam thong	

Equal parts, 11 items. Powder finely, and blow into the child's nose to treat fainting, headache, red eyes and blurred vision.

Then prepare this plaster:

Plaster:

[590]	*mali*	flowers
	phikun	flowers
	kradang ngaa	flowers
	phutsaa	leaves
	phak pet	leaves
	khaao saan	root
	salit	root
	anchan	root
	muun kaa thang 2	root
	hua hom	
	din prasiu khaao	

Equal parts, 12 items. Grind together. Apply to the crown of the head as a plaster, from morning until midday, then remove it and prepare the following poultice to apply to the big toe.

Poultice for the big toe:

[591]	*yaa klet hoi yai*	
	bua bok (phak nok)	leaves
	saan nuu	

Use sufficient of these 3 ingredients to make a poultice for the big toe, then add

din prasiu khaao	2 *phai*
prot	1 *salueng*

Mix and apply as a poultice to the big toe to treat *to* in the eyes of both children and adults.

Irrigation to protect the eyes:

[592]	*raet*	horn
	suea	milk
	samo thet	fruit
	tamlueng tua phuu	

Equal parts, 4 items. Prepare a mass and mix with dew, to treat all *taan* and *saang* affecting the eyes.

Then prepare medicine called *Sapphakhunlikaa* to treat *taan chon.*

[593] ***Sapphakhunlikaa***

khing	dried	Crush on Sunday, and dry in the sun
haeo muu		Crush on Monday, and dry in the sun
phinlangkaasaa	fruit	Crush on Tuesday, and dry in the sun

khamin oi		Crush on Wednesday, and dry in the sun
phrik Thai		Crush on Thursday, and dry in the sun
dee plee		Crush on Friday, and dry in the sun
sadao	leaves	Crush on Saturday, and dry in the sun

Equal parts, 7 items. Soak in the urine of a Gaur ox. At the time of the next full moon, mix the medicine during the holy day.[5] Make an offering with lighted candles, flowers, rice,[6] and a tray containing curry and assorted condiments or sweetmeats to be eaten with the rice. Then success will be achieved. Also, the dispenser must undertake to observe 5 or 8 precepts.[7] From the commencement of the ceremony until the end of the ceremony to prepare the medicine, sanctify it by the repetition of this *gāthā:* '*Sabbarogavinimutto sabbasantāpavajjito sabbaveramatikkanto nibbuto ca tuvaṃ bhava. Sabbītiyo vivajjantu sabbarogo vinassatu mā te bhavatvantarāyo sukhī dīghāyuko bhava*, et cetera.'

When the medicine has been mixed and while it is being made into pills, repeat this magical formula 108 times: *Sabbāsī sabbāsī bra-itipiso bra-itipiso.*

Then it will work wonders. To treat mucus and blood in the faeces, pain and prolapse of the rectum resulting from *taan chon*, mix with a decoction made from the sap of *khae* bark; for scaliness, like the scales of the *kradee* fish, and roughness of the skin on the shins, like the skin of a stingray, it is to be taken [sic] mixed with lime water. If small pimples erupt, they will go completely. For thinness and dehydration, it is to be taken daily for the stomach, mixed with a decoction of the juice of *samo Thai* fruit. For painful swellings, apply mixed with lime water. For sprains and twisted tendons and broken bones mix with sesame oil and apply. And for flatulence, to be taken mixed with *makruut* juice.

Medicine to treat *to* of various kinds:

[594]	*phikun*	flowers	
	bunnaak	flowers	
	saaraphee	flowers	
	phuttha raksaa	flowers	
	bua luang	pollen	
	kot thang 5		
	phutsaa	bark	
	sahatsakhun thet		
	samun waeng		
	son	heartwood	
	sak khee		
	chan thang 2		
	1 part of each		
	yaa sapphakunlikaa		20 parts

Prepare pills using aromatic water as excipient. To treat insomnia, mix this with cold water and bathe the eyes. Do this for three days, and the child will sleep. To treat *to* of *taan chon*, mix with *nam tamlueng* and irrigate the eyes. To treat *thuuk horaa yaa phit* and arsenical poisoning, to be taken mixed with buttermilk diluted with 1/3 part of water. To treat running eyes, mix with dew and apply to the eyelids. To treat painful gum inflammation, mix with lime juice and apply. Also put some of the medicine in the child's mouth. To increase the child's strength, to be taken mixed with cow's milk or mother's milk. This medicine is useful for all the symptoms of *taan chon* described above.

Throat paint for *saang daeng:*

[595]	*sang*	
	chaat thang 3	
	banlangsinlaa	
	malaeng saap	faecal matter, roasted
	raet	molar tooth
	chaang	molar tooth
	suea	eye tooth
	chorakhe	eye tooth
	faan	horn
	yaa tai bai	
	bua luang	pollen
	phimsen	

Equal parts, 14 items. Prepare a stick, mix with *nam thalaai maak dip* and paint the mouth to treat putrid inflammation caused by *saang daeng.*

If *saang* occurs inside the ear canal causing putrid inflammation, with a foul odour and purulent exudate, they say that there is a creature like a *mareng rai* in the ear. [8] To treat this condition, the doctor should use this oil as ear drops and it will clear up.

Oily ear drops:

[596]	*lian*	leaf sap	1 cupful
	phak bung khan	leaf sap	1 cupful
	nam khamin oi		1 cupful
	maphraao	oil	1 cupful
	makhaam khop	bark sap	1 cupful
	din plak khwaai	moistened with water	1 cupful
	lamphong	fruit juice	1 cupful
	ngaa	oil	1 cupful

8 items. Boil until only oil remains, then mix together

benyakaanee	galls
see siat thang 2	
fin	
sinlaa yon	

Equal parts of these 5 ingredients. Combine with the oil and use as ear drops for boils and abscesses in the ears, *taan saang* and *to* in the eyes.

Oily application for the ears:

[597]	*faai thet*	juice of under-ripe fruit	1 cupful
	faai thet	sap of juvenile leaves	1 cupful
	muun kaa daeng	sap of juvenile leaves	1 cupful
	ching chaa chaalee	leaf sap	1 cupful
	boraphet	leaf sap	1 cupful
	ngaa	oil	1 cupful

6 items. Boil until only oil remains, then put in the inflamed and foul smelling ear.

If a child develops *saang* in the ears, and this becomes a boil or abscess or a growth, such as a chronic *fee mareng* of several months or years duration, prepare this oil to use as ear drops.

Oily ear drops:

[598]	*praduu*	bark sap	1 *thanaan*
	sadao	bark sap	1 *thanaan*
	mamuang khan	bark sap	1 *thanaan*
	waa	bark sap	1 *thanaan*
	phak bung khan	juice	1 *thanaan*
	lamphong	fruit juice	1 *thanaan*
	lian	bark sap	1 *thanaan*
	taa suea	bark sap	1 *thanaan*
	ngaa	oil	1 *thanaan*

9 items. Boil until only oil remains, then mix

nok yuung	bile	
mee	bile	
saan nuu		
4 parts of each		
rayom	root	8 parts
krabao	roasted seeds	1
lamphong	seeds	1
see siat		
takhian	resin	1

8 items. Combine with the oil, to use as ear drops for inflamed and foul smelling ears.

Oily ear drops:

[599]	*lamphong*	fruit juice	1 cupful
	manaao	seed oil	1 cupful
	prakham dee khwaai	fruit juice	1 cupful
	nam yaa fin		1 cupful
	nam het muun kho		1 cupful
	nam neraphuusee		1 cupful
	nguu lueam	liquid bile	1 cupful
	ngaa	oil	1 cupful

8 items. Boil until only oil remains, and use as ear drops for boils, abscesses and growths in the ear. If the disease spreads to the external ear, this can be cleared up by applying this oil. If there is a discharge from the ear, moisten a small roll of Chinese straw fibre paper with the oil, gently insert this into the ear and leave it there for half an hour.

Medicine for diarrhoea with mucus and blood in the stools, caused by *taan chon:*

[600]	*phimsen*		
	thian thang 5		
	chan	seeds	
	chan	arils	
	krawaan		
	kaan phluu		
	chan thang 2		
	krisanaa		
	kralam phak		
	cha-em thet		
	opchoei thet		
	proh hom		
	kaarabuun		
	waan keep raet		
	waan ron thong		
	dee plee		
	lin thale		
	kanchaa		
	phan phak kaat	seeds	
	bua luang	pollen	
	mali son	flowers	
	mali laa	flowers	
	phikun	flowers	
	3 parts of each		
	yaa fin		1 part

Mix together these 29 items and add python's bile. Prepare pills using water as excipient. To be taken mixed with aromatic water to treat painful diarrhoea with mucus and blood caused by *taan chon.*

[601] ***Maha songkhroh***

thao yaa naang	both roots and aerial parts
thap thim	both roots and aerial parts
makluea	both roots and aerial parts
sakae	both leaves and roots
phung do	both leaves and roots
chan	seeds
chan	arils

krawaan	
kaan phluu	
phrik Thai	
khing	dried
dee plee	
khamin oi	
nam prasaan thong	
raatcha phrik	pods
boraphet	wrap around patient's head
ching chaa chaalee	stem, wrap around patient's head
muun kaa thang 2	

Equal parts, 19 items. Boil with a mixture of equal parts of water and alcohol over a slow fire of paddy husks. To be taken to counteract the mucus and blood in the faeces resulting from *taan chon.*

Decoction to stop the vomiting of *taan chon:*

[602]	*kot thang 5*	
	thian thang 5	
	chan	seeds
	chan	arils
	krawaan	
	kaan phluu	
	sang karanee	
	neraphuusee	
	chan thang 2	
	waan keep raet	
	waan ron thong	
	benyakaanee	galls
	kammathan daeng	
	yaa dam	
	1 part of each	
	taan thang 5	
	chetta phang khee	root
	kaphrao	root
	khai nao	root
	makluea	root
	phayaa muun lek	root
	phung do	root
	mawaeng thang 2	root
	makhuea thang 2	root
	thap thim	root
	lep mue naang	root
	sakae	root
	kraphang hom	root
	chaa phluu	root

salot nam	root	
chetta muun phloeng	root	
maklam thang 2	root	
kaang plaa daeng	root	
to sai	root	
krot	root	
phak khraat	root	
khon thee so	root	
boraphet		
ching chaa chaalee	stem	
haeo muu		
sakhaan	stem	
khaa		
phlai		
som poi	pods	
yaa tai bai		
krathuep yop		
khop chanaang thang 2		
4 parts of each		
muun kaa daeng		3 fruits
muun kaa khaao		3 fruits
khamin oi		3 rhizomes
makruut		3 fruits

68 items. Boil with a mixture of equal parts of water and alcohol. To be taken to treat mucus and blood in the faeces and as medicine to eliminate *taan chon* and all *taan saang* from the abdomen.

[603] ***Thong naep nuea (yai)***

yo	fruit pulp
samo thet	fruit pulp
din thanam	
thian yaowa phaanee	
kot so	
khrai khruea	root
kamlang wua thaloeng	
kaarabuun	
cha-em thet	
nam prasaan thong	
phimsen	

Equal parts, 11 items. Boil with fruit juice of *samo Thai.* To be taken to build up the body and to improve the appetite.

[604] ***Thong nuea ngaam***

thian thang 5
1 part of each
phlai

kaarabuun	
2 parts of each	
samo Thai	fruit pulp
samo phiphek	fruit pulp
yaa dam	
mahaa hing	
khamin oi	
kluea sinthao	
makruut	skin
waan nam	
4 parts of each	

Add an equivalent amount of samo thale leaves. 16 items. Prepare pills using alcohol as excipient. To be taken mixed with *nam makruut* or lime juice to build up the body and improve the appetite. To use to expel flatus, mix with a triturate of ripe tamarind fruit pulp in water, sodium sulphate and python's bile.

Amunlathaat occur when *saang* starts in the part of the intestines below the navel, and they are the size of maize kernels. After nine or ten days, they disperse and cause incessant diarrhoea which looks like fish water, then clots of blood are passed for three or four days, then blood with purulent mucus, causing thirst, listlessness, a high temperature, revulsion to food and emaciation. The doctor should first treat it as for dysentery with acute pain, mucus and blood. If the child does not respond, prepare a cleansing decoction to be taken.

Medicine to clean up the damage caused by *taan chon:*

[605]	*kaphrao thang* 5		
	kraphang hom thang 5		
	khee kaa		2 1/4 fruits
	makruut		2 1/4 fruits
	boraphet	a piece the length of the sole of the patient's foot	
	khamin oi		7 pieces
	som poi		7 pods
	samo thang 3		of each, 3 fruits
	yaa dam		1 *baht*
	raatcha phrik	pods	1 *baht*

12 items. Reduce to 1/3 volume by boiling, and add sodium sulphate. Dose to be taken according to the strength of the elements of the patient, to completely clean out all the badness, as explained. Then prepare the following protective medicine to be taken.

Medicine to treat mucus and blood in the stools, resulting from *taan chon:*

[606]	*thian*	leaves
	thap thim	leaves

	phak khuang	leaves	
	khamin oi		

Equal parts, 4 items. Mix together, prepare a stick and boil with bark sap of *khae*. To be taken.

If that is ineffective, prepare this decoction:

[607]	*mamuang kalon*		3 seeds
	chan thang 2		1
	krisanaa		1
	sak khee		1
	chan	seeds	1
	benyakaanee	galls	1
	palong	bark	1
	fin thang 2	bark	1

10 items. Mix together. Reduce to 1/3 volume by boiling and give to the child by mouth.

[608]	***Mahaa ut***	
	khrang	
	chan	seeds
	benyakaanee	galls
	see siat thet	
	takhian	resin
	khamin oi	

Equal parts, 6 items. Mix together and stuff in under-ripe pomegranates. Cover with layers of cow manure and heat on a slow fire of paddy husks until well cooked. Then mix all together, including the pomegranates, and prepare pills. 5 pills to be taken mixed with lime water. Then give mixed with medicine called *Tree phalaa hom* and some shallot and Borneo camphor. Then treat with medicine called *Bencha taan* [no.92], as described at the beginning, and following this, to treat *taan chon*, and listlessness:

[609]	*khat mon*	leaves
	chan	seed juice
	saniat	decoction of fruit juice

Add some Borneo camphor. To be taken for mucus and blood in the stools.

[610]	***Thong phan chang***	
	taan thang 5	root
	mawaeng thang 2	root
	ching cho	root
	makluea	root
	makhuea khuen	root
	lep mue naang	root
	khaa	
	khing	

khamin oi		
tree phalaa saam		
muun kaa thang 2	fruit	
horaphaa	fruit	
thian yaowa phaanee		
haeo muu		
boraphet		
1 *baht of each*		
yaa dam		3 *baht*

24 items. Reduce to 1/3 volume by boiling. To be taken to treat *taan saang* and *taan chon*, as medicine to clean out the abdomen and for mucus and blood in the stools. For all seven types of *saang* for children from 3 months to 12 years of age, by which time *saang* ceases. After giving the medicine to clean out the abdomen, then give medicine called *Thong nuea ngaam*, mixed with *som saa* juice to be taken for the stomach and to improve the appetite, build up the body and improve the complexion.

Mutsakaayathaat results from *saang kho.* At first the baby has itchy spots, resembling measles, all over the body. But the spots are white and contain no fluid. After eight or nine days, it goes inside and upsets the stomach and causes diarrhoea looking like water used to wash meat, and the baby craves something fresh or fishy or meaty. After two or three months, the eyes are red and the baby is listless, and the primary pustule of *saang* has appeared on the side of the tongue, as big as a seed of Job's tears, and as hard as a corn [*taa plaa*]. If the doctor applies the medicine inside the mouth with the finger and the disease doesn't clear up, it will remain for six months from the time it started, and the *saang* which was on the body and withdrew internally will come up again as red spots like *khai rabutchaat*, and it will appear regularly, causing a high temperature, but the hands and feet will always be cold. The baby will also be thirsty, and pant and have a stiff tongue and lockjaw.

Any child with these symptoms is said to be in the hands of [the god of death] Phrayaa Matchuraat. If a doctor wants to treat it, he should start when it begins, when the spots first come up. First apply the lotion called *Phrasuriyachanthanang* to the body, then treat with other remedies as follows.

Treatment for itching:

[611]	*phraamon*	leaves
	phut son	leaves
	ching chaa chaalee	leaves
	boraphet	leaves
	khamin oi	
	krabue chet tua	leaves

Equal parts, 6 items. Mix and add a little camphor. Prepare a stick, mix with river water and apply to the body to stop itching.

[612] ***Yaa daeng*** **to treat diarrhoea:**

chan thang 2	
son	
sak	
krak khee	
sang karanee	
neraphuusee	
waan keep raet	
waan ron thong	
reesee prasom laeo	
rangap	leaves
phak khuang	leaves
chan	seeds
chan	arils
benyakaanee	galls
see siat thang 2	

Equal parts, 17 items. Prepare pills using alcohol as excipient. To be taken mixed with bark sap of the red corkwood tree for diarrhoea. If this does not stop it, then prepare *Yaa prasa daeng yai.*

Throat paint to reduce the temperature:

[613]	*makruut*	fruit	
	tree katuk saam		
	krathiam		
	mawaeng khruea	fruit	
	phlai		
	suphannathan daeng		

Equal parts, 8 items. Mix and add an amount of borax equal to the rest combined. Prepare pills. Mix with lime juice and paint the throat. If this is ineffective, then add

chunsee sat		1 *klam*
kapee dee	partially burnt	2 *klam*

Mix 1 pill with *salot nam* juice and apply to the throat. Then the temperature will fall.

Throat paint to treat coughs and vomiting:

[614]	*waeo nok yung*	eyes of tail feathers, scorched brittle
	maeng daa	calcined shell
	plaa chon	burnt tail
	nam prasaan thong sat	
	krathiam	
	hua hom	
	khrai hom	
	phak khraat	flowers

Equal parts, 8 items. Prepare a stick, mix with lime juice and apply to the throat to treat cough. To treat vomiting, mix with a decoction of *yo* fruit. If it fails to respond to any medicine, sharpen a piece of sappan wood to a point, and break it. If this is not clean, cut with the finger nail, so that it breaks, then prepare the prescription called *Sapphakhunlikaa.* Mix with zedoary juice and apply to the throat 3 or 4 times a day, then prepare this astringent medicine and apply it.

[615] ***Fai chit mahaa wong*** astringent paint:

makhaam pom	root
maklam thang 2	root
chan thang 2	
nam prasaan thong sat	
benyakaanee	galls
see siat thet	
kui	horn
kwaang	horn
chaang	tusk
raet	horn

Equal parts, 12 items. Prepare a stick. Mix with river water, add some Borneo camphor, opium, honey and rock salt, and paint the mouth, to treat a stiff tongue and lock-jaw and bleeding from the mouth.

[616] ***Saeng kabinlaphat***

sappha dee thang 8	
thian thang 5	
1 part of each	
kot thang 5	
2 parts of each	
raatchadat	fruit
saaraphat phit	fruit
waan keep raet	
waan ron thong	
sang karanee	
neraphuusee	
krachao thang 2	
akkhanee chawaa	
suraamrit	
cha-em thang 2	
chan	seeds
chan	arils
yaa raak khaao	
yaa raak dam	
khrai khruea	root
khem daeng	root
taeng nuu	root
rangap	leaves
sawaat	leaves

sadao	leaves
kaphrao	leaves
phrakham dee khwaai	leaves

4 parts of each

42 items. Prepare pills using a decoction of *marum* bark sap as excipient. To be taken mixed with alcohol for delirium and unconsciousness. To use as a throat paint for *saang*, mix with lime juice and add borax and alum and apply to the throat. To treat delirium, mix with burnt bones of a vulture and burnt rhinoceros skin, and give by mouth. To treat the poison of boils, abscesses and snake-bite, this mixture is to be taken mixed with alcohol. To treat the poison of *saang*, *taan chon* and fever,[9] to be taken mixed with aromatic water and *Borneo camphor*. This is effective against all forms of *saang* poisoning resulting from *mutsakaayathaat*.

[617] ***Prasa kaarabuun*** stomach mixture

tree katuk	2 parts
kaan phluu	5 parts
mahaa hing	6 parts
phrik Thai lon	8 parts
chetta muun	8 parts
kaarabuun	8 parts

8 parts of each

bai naat	
dong dueng	tuber

20 parts of each

Prepare pills to be taken mixed with *nam makruut* or *som saa* juice for all the *lom* of *saang*. The mixture is called *Waayo phinaat* if 8 parts of each of the following are added:

phlai	
waan nam	
makruut	skin
krathiam	

and this may be used in the treatment of adults.

Sutchimukkhakaanlahira results from *saang chang* and can turn into *saang chon*. This worm arises spontaneously in the ileum and colon. It looks like a small, white snake, about the size of a *mai muan*.[10] It could be described as *sai duean* [an earthworm]. It has life and consciousness, and nests in the large intestine. When mature, they start to irritate beings, making them emaciated, causing distension of the abdomen, insatiable appetite, sometimes abdominal colic, sometimes vomiting. After a month, when they are more mature, they cause restlessness, because they group together and roll about in a ball, and create noises in the stomach. Sometimes they crawl out through the mouth, sometimes through the anus, causing the child severe pain, and a regular fever, with high temperature. Sometimes they affect the eyes, making them red. To treat this, the doctor should give an anthelmintic, but be careful. If the worms are not expelled, they might become stuck in the throat and anus and die, and this is very difficult. These worms come with every kind of *saang* of the seven days of the week. They occur because unfamiliar food disagrees with the elements. To get rid of them, the doctor should first give the medicine called *Sapphakhunlikaa* mixed with fresh fruit juice of *makluea*, and then treat with the other medicines as follows.

Medicine to expel *sai duean:*

[618]	*suphannathan daeng*		1 part
	sakae	seeds	
	salot	fruit	
	makluea	seeds	
	4 parts of each		

Take 2 *phai* of the powdered mixture and stir in with an egg and fry it. The whole to be taken to expel *sai duean.* If this causes restlessness and distress, mix with coarse sugar, lime juice and Borneo camphor. Then give the following aromatic medicine.

Decoction to expel *sai duean*, and to act as an astringent on the intestines:

[619]	*lep mue naang*	root	1 part
	raatchadat	fruit	
	phalaan satruu	fruit	
	kraai [plant]	fruit	
	2 parts of each		
	kot kakkraa		4 parts
	yaa dam		8 parts
	prik	root	
	thap thim	root	
	18 parts of each		
	muun kaa		3 fruits
	som poi		7 pods
	makruut		3 fruits
	khamin oi	a rhizome	1 *khuep* long
	boraphet	wrap around the patient's head	

14 items. Boil with a mixture of water and alcohol in equal parts and give to the child. To expel *sai duean* from the intestines and reduce abdominal distension.

Worms resulting from *saang chon* come from the spine up to the brain, spreading through all the tendons. They cause wind in the large intestine to move up and down, then they get into the bladder causing retention of urine and bladder stones, and abdominal distension, and the intestines become swollen. They also cause blurred vision, and painful defecation with mucus and blood, and the child is emaciated, because these worms are in the flesh and tendons. There are three kinds in the tendons - *kanna*, *ratchaka* and *awanna*. They all look like fleas, and crawl in the flesh, causing emaciation, as described. To expel them, the doctor should first prepare medicine to cleanse the body, then they will disappear. Doctors should understand this.

Medicine to expel the mucus of *taan chon:*

[620]	*chan*	seeds	
	chan	arils	
	krawaan		
	kaan phluu		
	phrik Thai		
	khing	dried	
	dee plee		
	1 part of each		
	salot	purified	2 parts

Mix together these 8 items. To purify the *salot*, remove all traces of skin, soak in salt water for two nights, then stuff inside *makruut* fruit and cook in the fire until shrivelled. [Cf. nos.556,621,623.] Then mix all the ingredients together, including the *makruut* fruit, and prepare pills. To be taken mixed with alcohol. Dose: 7 pills. For children aged 3 to 4 years, 9 pills. This will get rid of the mucus of *taan chon.*

Medicine to expel the worms of *taan chon:*

[621]	*phimsen*	
	kaarabuun	
	chan	seeds
	chan	arils
	kaan phluu	
	kaphrao	leaves
	sawaat	leaves

2 parts of each. Mix together these 7 items, then prepare *salot* fruit, 14 parts, as follows. Remove and discard the skin, wash thoroughly in water, wrap in a cloth and put in a pot with rice until dry, and stir 3 times. Then roast with fish sauce until crisp, express the oil, then mix with the rest of the ingredients. Prepare pills the size of mung beans, and give to the child to take by mouth to treat emaciation and yellowness and mucus and blood in the faeces.

Dose:	1 year	7 pills
	2 years	9 pills
	3 years	11 pills

To be taken according to the strength of the child. This may be taken by adults also. To treat constipation, add *chan hom* and apply to the body. If the result is excessive, mix with *mataat* fruit, stir with raw sugar-cane juice and boil. If this is taken, the looseness will cease.

Medicine to expel the worms of *taan chon:*

[622]	*dee plee*	
	krawaan	
	chan	seeds
	chan	arils
	phak chee	fruit

samo Thai	fruit
samo thet	fruit
kluea sinthao	
chaat kon	
1 part of each	
salot	fruit with black skin, 2 parts

Do not purify the *salot*, use it all, including the skin.

kaan phluu 4 parts

10 items. Prepare pills the size of peppercorns, using honey as excipient. 3 pills to be taken if the elements are [the build is] heavy, 1 if light. This is very beneficial and completely successful in cleaning out the worms of *taan chon.*

Laxative for young children from 1 month to 3 years old:

[623]	*kaan phluu*	
	khamin oi	
	phlai	
	khaao	cooked
	salot	fruit

Equal part, 5 items. Purify the *salot* [croton] by boiling with one handful each of *makhaam* leaves, *som poi* leaves and salt until cooked. Spread out to dry in the sun, keeping only the *salot* pulp. Mix with the rest of the ingredients. Prepare pills the size of cotton seeds. Feed the child this medicine mixed with rice by placing it in the child's mouth.

Now it does not matter whether this laxative is for *saang* or not, but a skilled doctor should determine the strength of the disease whether it is severe or mild. It has been explained that a child cannot escape birth *saang* and minor *saang* whatever day it is born. They say absolutely not to administer a laxative and medicine containing *salot* to a very young child who still has little strength. Only give it to those aged 5 years or more. They advise absolutely against giving medicine containing *salot* to people over 60 because old age weakens and debilitates them. The masters say *salot* is an extremely valuable and excellent [drug]. If you understand the administration of medicine, it is the easiest of all to use.

In addition, the external parasites which infest the skin and the flesh producing the symptoms previously described are treated by applying a body lotion which makes them drop off.

Body lotion for parasites:

[624]	*plaa lai phueak*	root
	ueang phet maa	
	manaao	seeds
	chum het thet	seeds
	muun lek	fruit
	krabao	bark
	krabian	bark

lian	bark
thong laang naam	root
thong phan chang	root
mawaeng khruea	fruit
makhuea khuen	fruit
banlangsinlaa	
horadaan thong	
yaa fin	
phimsen	

Equal parts, 20 items. Prepare pills using lime juice as excipient. Mix with *nam chan daeng* and apply to the body to dislodge parasites, whether raised or flat [on the skin].

These external parasites which infest the skin, flesh and spine cause the child to become emaciated and dehydrated. To treat this, prepare this oily application.

Oily application to treat external parasites and the tendons and muscles:

[625]	*buk*	juice	1 *thanaan*
	kloi	juice	1 *thanaan*
	ngaa	oil	1 *thanaan*
	kho	urine	4 *thanaan*

Boil until only oil remains, then combine with

salot	seeds	1 *baht*
khing	dried	1 *baht*
dee plee		2 *baht*

Mix together and add to the oil, then apply to the parasites. Then massage the weak, aching, withered and palsied muscles, tendons and bones. [11] Then prepare medicine called *Phitsadaan* to be taken mixed with alcohol. The parasites will go.

Decoction to expel worms:

[626]	*lan thom*	root
	lep mue naang	root
	sakae	root
	khamin oi	
	chueak thao khan	
	bencha madan	

Equal parts, 10 items. Mix and reduce to 1/3 volume by boiling. To be taken to expel parasites and *sai duean.*

When the child is completely purged of all poison, the wind which rises and descends and rumbles in the stomach such that there is enlargement of the spleen and waves of nausea, will disappear. If not, prepare medicine called *Inthachak* to be given next. If the child does not respond to any treatment, then prepare the medicine called *Fai aawut* to be taken next.

[627] ***Fai aawut***

chan	seeds

chan	arils	
kaan phluu		
kot thang 5		
thian thang 5		
cha-em thet		
kanchaa		
samae thale	heartwood	
1 part of each		
utta phit		
samun waeng	bark	
dee plee		
phimsen	leaves	
2 parts of each		
ching cho	root	
som kung	root	
plao noi	root	
plao yai	root	
sakhaan	root	
phaat shon	root	
3 parts of each		
sahatsakhun thet		4 parts
buk ro		9 parts
phrik Thai		
khing	dried	
chetta muun	root	

16 parts of each. 32 items. Prepare pills using lime juice as excipient. To be taken to treat the seven kinds of *saang* and twelve kinds of *taan chon*; for the seven kinds of *huet nam nom* [? asthma]; for cough with thinness and yellowness; and for intestinal swelling and abdominal distension; for pot-belly and colic; hypertrophy and enlargement of the spleen; for the piercing pain of a mass of mucus in the abdomen; for mucus and blood in the faeces after which the child becomes unconscious and haemorrhages from the bowel; and for fevers resulting from the elements mucus and wind.

[628] ***Tree phalaa thulao***

phimsen		
samo Thai		
samo phiphek		
thian dam		
thian daeng		
thian yaowa phaanee		
horaphaa	fruit	
2 parts of each		
phlai		4 parts

makham pom	12 parts
raatcha phrik	flesh of the pods only, an amount equal to the rest of the ingredients

10 items. Prepare pills the size of peppercorns. Dose: 1 pill at a time, to be taken mixed with alcohol, as a laxative for young children.

[629] ***Plaap phranakkhon***

bencha mafai	
taan mon	root
taan sian	root
to sai	root
takhop	root
kaang plaa daeng	root
tako	root
sakae	root
yaa tai bai	

Equal parts, 13 items. Reduce to 1/3 volume by boiling. To be taken for mucus and blood in the stools and when the child either goes to sleep while sitting or bites its nails.

Decoction to treat *taan chon* affecting the eyes and causing blurred vision:

[630]

bencha kaphrao		
kraphang hom thang 2		
phlai		
khamin oi		
boraphet		
bencha yaa nguang chaang		
bencha thop thaep		
som poi	pods	
anchan khaao	root	
yaa chan kaat	root-stock	
tree katuk		
hua hom		5 bulbs
khee kaa		3 fruits
makruut		3 fruits

17 items. Prepare a decoction to be taken for *taan chon* affecting the eyes or *to* causing blurred vision. This medicine eliminates internal worms.

Eye lotion to treat *taan chon* affecting the eyes:

[631] *bencha phak bung*

sang

din thanam

Equal parts, 3 items. Prepare a stick; mix with *nam thao tamlueng* and irrigate the eyes.

Snuff to treat *taan chon:*

[632]	*thep thaaro*		
	waan nam		
	chan thang 2		
	krisanaa		
	cha-em thet		
	lin thale		
	chamot		
	phimsen		

Equal parts, 9 items. Powder and blow into the nostrils to treat a child whose vision is obscured or blurred.

Poultice to apply to the abdomen to treat *to* resulting from *taan chon:*

[633]	*phikun*	flowers	
	kradang ngaa	flowers	
	hua hom		
	din prasiu khaao		
	song baadaan	leaves	

Equal parts, 5 items. Prepare a poultice to apply to the abdomen of a child with *to* in the eyes, blindness or blurred vision.

Decoction to treat [bladder] stones of *taan chon:*

[634]	*yaa chan kaat*		
	haeo muu		
	phlai		4 parts
	khrai haang naat		
	yaa khaao yen		
	krathung maa baa	root	
	thao wan priang		
	yaa naang	root	

Equal parts, 8 items. Reduce to 1/3 volume by boiling and give by mouth.

Poultice to apply to the supra-pubic area to treat bladder obstruction or inability to urinate:

[635]	*nam tao*	leaves	
	sawaat	fruit	

Mix with water used to wash rice and apply as a poultice to the supra-pubic area, then the urine will flow.

Another:

[636]	*plaa thuu*	dried head	

Powder and mix with lime juice, then apply as a poultice to the supra-pubic area and urine will flow similarly.

Decoction to treat blood in the urine resulting from *taan chon:*

[637]	*khon thaa*	leaves	
	nom tamria		

	kamchaai	root
	mai daeng	bark

Equal parts, 4 items. Reduce to 1/3 volume by boiling and give to the child.

Another:

[638]	*saan som*	
	son	heartwood

Reduce to 1/3 volume by boiling and give to the child.

Another:

[639]	*bia phuu*	3 shells
	sang	4 *baht*

Soak overnight in lime juice, then add

khee lek	7 leafy tips of new shoots, steamed over a fire until cooked
phrik Thai	8 peppercorns
khing	7 pieces
krathiam	7 cloves

To be taken mixed with lime juice.

Decoction to treat *taan chon:*

[640]	*khee lek*	leafy tips of new shoots
	oi daeng	root
	yaa khaa	root
	nam klaep	

Boil together and add *krathue*, spread out and expose to the sun and dew for a day and a night. To be taken mixed with proof spirit.

Decoction to treat bladder stones resulting from *taan chon* in children who have reached 10 years of age:

[641]	*lamut seedaa*	7 leafy tips of new shoots
	lam chiak	7 leafy tips of new shoots

Reduce to 1/3 volume by boiling. To be taken.

To treat bladder stones in children who have reached 12 years of age:

[642]	*sakae*	ash
	taeng kwaa	juice
	khanthatsakon	
	din prasiu khaao	

Mix together. To be taken.

The masters have explained birth *saang* and minor *saang*, the actions of the seven kinds of fever and the 80 kinds of worms which follow birth *saang* and minor *saang*; also the *taan chon* resulting from sixteen kinds of worms. It ends here.

NOTES

1 *lom khai:* in this context, could refer to the *lom* diseases such as tetanus which are associated with birth *saang*. However, the term used in the introductory statement to this passage is simply *khai*, not *lom khai*, leaving the matter open to question, since each of these terms *lom* and *khai* can mean simply 'disease'.

2 Cf. p.15.

3 The digested food and the undigested food are two of the 20 earth elements, that is, parts of the body having the quality of solidity or hardness. (See Mulholland, *JSS*, 1979.)

4 *khai nuea* or *khai paa:* a form of malaria occurring in Northern Thailand; jungle fever. *Mc*, p.172.

5 *ubosot:* the Buddhist holy day or fast day, occurring on the days of the new and full moon. *Mc*, p.1006.

6 *baai see:* (lit.) 'propitious or auspicious rice', that is, rice offered to the mysterious psyche hoping to bring good fortune. *Mc*, p.481.

7 *seen:* a system of moral rules laid down by the Lord Buddha. *Mc*, p.799.

8 *mareng rai kin yuu nai huu:* (lit.) cancer mite destroying the inside of the ear.

9 *phit khai:* a very high temperature resulting in delirium but not loss of consciousness; *khai phit* is toxic fever. (VJ)

10 *mai muan:* the vowel mark 'ใ' in Thai script.

11 Massage is mentioned as treatment only twice in this text. (See Book III, Note 26, prescription no. 512.)

[Book VI]

Summary of the characteristics of *taan chon* complete with a description of the birth elements, the combination of the elements, abnormal elements, disintegration of the elements and moribund elements.

(Ayaṃ kāyo dhātuhetuko ayaṃ kāyo dhātunihāno ayaṃ kāyo āhārahetuko ayaṃ kāyo dhātunidāno tiṇṇaṃ utūnaṃ davādasākāraṃ asi.)

Description of another seven kinds of *taan chon* which develop in association with the four elements, according to the Pāli text, as follows. When a life has been conceived in the mother's womb, the element appropriate to the season of conception is the birth element.

If a woman becomes pregnant in the fifth, sixth or seventh month, [the baby] has the characteristics of the element, fire. When the foetus has developed the five branches and the 32 parts complete, the element fire is the birth element with which the other elements combine.

If a woman becomes pregnant in the eight, ninth or tenth month, [the baby] has the characteristics of the element, wind. When the foetus has developed the 32 parts complete, the element wind is the birth element which combines with the mother's elements.

If a woman becomes pregnant in the eleventh, twelfth or first month, [the baby] has the characteristics of the element, water. When the foetus has developed the 32 parts complete, the element water is the birth element which combines with the mother's elements.

If a woman becomes pregnant in the second, third or fourth month, [the baby] has the characteristics of the element, earth. When the foetus has developed the 32 parts complete, the element earth is the birth element which combines with the mother's elements.

Finally, whichever season it is and whichever element is the birth element, that season and that element will be the primary causes of disease in that child up to the time of birth and from birth up to 5 or 6 years of age. Then, at 5 or 6 years, when *taan saang* has run its course, *taan chon* develops. If the doctor prepares medicine which is not effective, he is advised to consult *Phrakhamphee thaatbanchop* and treat according to the birth element. The masters have simplified it by explaining in four parts. A wise doctor will give it his consideration.

To treat the birth element, fire:

[643] *dee plee*
phrik Thai
khing dried
waan proh
haeo muu

Equal parts, 5 items. First prepare pills to be taken mixed with hot water, then treat with all the following medicines.

To treat the birth element, wind:

[644]	*phrik Thai*	
	thian yaowa phaanee	
	phak chee	fruit
	mok man	bark

Equal parts, 4 items. Pills to be taken mixed with hot water. Then each of the other medicines is to be taken.

To treat the birth element, water:

[645]	*chetta muun phloeng*	root
	thian yaowa phaanee	
	phak chee	fruit
	mok man	bark

Equal parts, 4 items. Pills to be taken mixed with hot water. Then each of the other medicines is to be taken.

To treat the birth element, earth:

[646]	*krathiam*	
	sadao	leaves
	khon thee so	leaves
	son	heartwood

Equal parts, 4 items. Pills to be taken mixed with hot water. Then each of other medicines.

The fire element, when abnormal, causes flatulence, distension of the abdomen, nausea, difficulty in breathing, constriction in the chest, swollen hands and feet, and constant coughing. When it has these symptoms, if it does not respond to treatment the baby will die in eight days.

Medicine to treat abnormalities of the fire element:

[647]	*chetta muun phloeng*	root
	mawaeng thang 2	root
	phak khuang	root
	boraphet	
	sadao	leaf stalks
	chaa phluu	root

Equal parts, 7 items. Reduce to 1/3 volume by boiling and give by mouth. If this is ineffective, augment it by combining it with medicine to treat the fire element of the mother.

[648]	*phak phaeo daeng*	
	kot khamao	
	opchoei thet	
	makhaam pom	fruit
	khrai ton	
	waan proh	
	sawaat	root
	yaa rang kaa	

Equal parts, 8 items. Combine with the previous prescription to make one mixture. Reduce to 1/3 volume by boiling. If pills are made, hot water should be used as excipient. These pills are to be taken mixed with cow's milk or mother's milk. If no milk is available, use hot water.

The wind element, when abnormal, causes deafness, an offensive discharge from the ears and blurred vision. When pressure is applied to the inner corner of the eye, the patient cannot see any light. It also causes muscular pain in the hands, feet and both legs, as occurs in adults, causing cramps, backache and bruises all over the body, giving the appearance of abscesses in the tendons; also vomiting and sometimes dry retching, but the baby still has abdominal pain due to wind, flatulence, belching and so on, even though it does not eat. This is because the element wind is abnormal, as explained.

Medicine to treat abnormalities of the wind element:

[649]	*kot kaan phraao*	
	sakhaan	stem
	khat mon	root
	kathok rok	
	haeo muu	
	son thet	heartwood
	sak khee	
	khing	dried
	makruut	leaves
	manaao	leaves

Equal parts, 10 items. Reduce to 1/3 volume by boiling. First give this and observe the results. If it is ineffective, augment it by combining it with medicine to treat the wind element of the mother.

[650]	*mok man*	bark
	mok luang	bark
	phrik Thai	
	khing	dried
	salot nam	root
	amphan	
	haeo muu	
	yaa rang kaa	
	phak phaeo daeng	
	samo Thai	fruit
	khrai khruea	root

Equal parts, 10 items. Combine with the previous mixture to make a single preparation. Prepare pills to be taken mixed with urine of a Gaur ox or with alcohol.

If that is still ineffective, then combine the previous mixture for the wind element with the following:

[651]	*mahaa hing*	
	waan nam	
	dee plee	
	sabaa mon	seeds

	raatchadat	fruit
	cha-em thet	
	kot khamao	
	yaang saai	leaves
	krung khamao	

Equal parts, 9 items. Combine with the previous mixture and prepare pills to be taken mixed with hot water.

If that is still ineffective, combine the previous mixture with the following:

[652]	*chetta muun phloeng*	root
	cha-em thet	root
	ching cho	root
	tong taek	root
	phrik Thai lon	
	khing	dried
	dee plee	
	amphan	
	bai naat	
	salot	leaves

Equal parts. Boil together with salt water and dry in the sun. Then add an equivalent amount of camphor. Mix all together with the previous medicine, and make pills to be taken mixed with hot water, cow's milk or urine, or urine of a young boy.

If that is still not effective, then discard all but the previous prescription for the wind element [no.649], then add this:

[653]	*phak sian phee*	
	phak pet daeng	leaves
	phak khraat	leaves
	hua waen	
	yaa rang kaa	
	phak chee thang 2	fruit
	phan phak kaat	seeds
	chong konlanee	flowers
	sakhaan	stem
	taeng mo	seeds

Equal parts, 10 items. To be mixed with the previous compound, made into pills and taken with alcohol. To treat abnormalities or disorders of the wind element, as explained previously.

The water element, when abnormal, causes diarrhoea, epigastric pain, cold hands and feet, and the intestines coil up tightly into a lump in the abdomen. Sometimes it causes constipation, retention of urine, discomfort in the supra-pubic region, sometimes mucus and blood in the stools, and colic or stabbing pain around the sides. This occurs on the left side in a female and on the right side in a male. If the child has these symptoms, it is very difficult to cure.

Medicine to treat abnormalities of the water element:

[654]	*waan nam*	
	plao thang 2	
	peep	root
	khrai nam	root
	phluu kin kap maak	root
	ching cho yai	root
	khrop chakrawaan	root

Equal parts, 8 items. Reduce to 1/3 volume by boiling. Give this to the child first. If it is ineffective, combine it with the following mixture:

[655]	*phak chee lom [lon]*	fruit
	amphan	
	mok luang	bark
	nam tao khom	
	kradom	fruit

Equal parts, 5 items. Add to the previous preparation, reduce to 1/3 volume by boiling and give to the child.

If that is ineffective, combine the previous medicine with this prescription to treat the water element in the mother.

[656]	*ching cho luang*	root
	tree katuk saam	
	raatchadat	fruit
	khamin oi	
	kraphang hom thang 2	
	khaao khaa	root-stock

Equal parts, 9 items. Mix with the previous compound and prepare pills to be taken mixed with *chueak thao [khao] muak.*

If this last is still not effective, combine it with the following:

[657]	*makhaam pom*	fruit
	tree katuk saam	
	tree phalaa saam	
	chaa phluu	root
	sakhaan	stem
	khaa	dried
	chan	seeds

Equal parts, 11 items. Combine with the previous preparation and make pills to be taken mixed with *nam kluai teep*, to treat abnormalities of the water element.

The earth element, when abnormal, causes severe abdominal pain, inability to eat, distension of the abdomen, like an adult with *ritseeduang*, thinness, jaundice and backache. It may change to gonorrhoea, causing rectal and urethral haemorrhage with pus. If it does not respond to treatment in five days, the baby will die.

Medicine to treat abnormalities of the earth element:

[658] *dee plee*

	thian dam	
	sang karanee	
	san phraa naang ae	bark
	kradom	fruit
	yaa chan kaat	root-stock
	yaa dam	
	samee	root
	manaao	33 leaves

Equal parts, 9 items. Reduce to 1/3 volume by boiling and give to the child by mouth.

If this is ineffective, augment the previous prescription by combining it with medicine to treat the earth element in the mother.

[659]	*yaang saai*	root
	krathiam	
	dee plee	
	matuum	under-ripe fruit
	mawaeng thang 2	root
	sakhaan	stem
	phak phaeo daeng	
	amphan	
	thian sattabut	
	samo Thai	
	khing	dried

Equal parts, 12 items. Combine with the previous mixture and reduce to 1/3 volume by boiling. To be taken.

If that is ineffective, combine it with the following:

[660]	*mahaa hing*	
	waan nam	
	tree katuk saam	
	tree phalaa saam	
	nguan muu	root
	kot chadaa mangsee	
	phlai	
	khat mon	root

Equal parts, 12 items. Combine with the previous prescription and prepare pills to be taken mixed with cow's milk or mother's milk.

If the last compound is ineffective, then mix it with this:

[661]	*kraphang hom thang 2*	
	boraphet	
	mawaeng thang 2	root
	muun kaa daeng	root
	khat mon thang 2	root
	chueak thao pharuan	

Equal parts, 9 items. Combine with the previous mixture. Prepare pills to be taken mixed with *nam chan* or *nam cha-em*, for the abnormal earth element.

This summary of the characteristics of the four elements, has been taken from *Phrakhamphee thaatbanchop*, and included here in *Phrakhamphee prathom chindaa* by the masters, so that doctors will know which of the four elements is the cause of any symptoms which may arise. For example, *taan chon* results from birth *saang* because the doctor has been unable to get rid of the birth *saang* before the child reached the age when it ceases, then it changes to *taan chon*, as already explained. If a doctor has not become proficient in his understanding of *Phrakhamphee prathom chindaa*, and *Phrakhamphee apphayasantaa*, and cannot get rid of the *taan chon*, then it will remain until the age of 30 or 40 years, then it will turn to a form of *ritseeduang*, depending on the kind of birth *saang* and minor *saang*, as explained in *Phrakhamphee apphayasantaa*.

The question may be asked, however, why is it called *taan chon*? The answer is, there are sixteen kinds of *taan chon*. In the main body of the text, it says about the child born on Sunday, that *saang phloeng* is the birth *saang*, *saang krai* is the minor *saang* and *la utthayakaan* is the *la*. Here, despite what is said at the beginning of the text, we say of *taan chon* that *saang phloeng* is the birth *saang* of Sunday; sometimes *saang kranae chon* occurs, sometimes *saang kratang chon*; that not only *la utthayakaan* occurs with *saang phloeng*, but that *la ninlakaan*, *la saeng phloeng* and *la ninlaphloeng chon* sometimes accompany it. Similarly, not only is *la-ong pleo fai faa* the *la-ong phrabaat* associated with *saang phloeng*, but also *la-ong kaeo morakot*, *la-ong phloeng* and *la-ong thap thim* sometimes occur with it. This is the way these diseases are manifested.

If the doctor is not fully aware of what is stated here in *Khamphee prathom chindaa*, many people will be killed. That is why the masters call this disease *taan chon*, because this *saang* changes its form. It is so strange that it is beyond description. Here, we have explained only one kind of *saang*, but doctors should realize that all seven kinds of [birth] *saang* behave similarly.

Puna ca paraṃ Next, we discuss *taan chon* resulting from *atisaan*. (*Ācāriyena*) 'The masters' (ābhataṃ) 'have taken '(atisāraṃ) 'from *Phrakhamphee atisaan'* (*abhāsi*) '[this knowledge which] should be explained' (*antevāsikaṃ*) 'for the information of medical students.' (*Maraṇaṃ*) 'Death' (*dārakānaṃ*) 'in children' (*tividhaṃ*) 'has three signs' (*soviggahaṃ*) 'which indicate deterioration' (*atisāraṃvā*) 'for example, the ill effects of *atisaan'* (*maranaṃ*) 'indicate death' (*dārakānaṃ*) 'in children.' (*Visucikā*) 'That is, abnormalities of the urine and faeces' (*bhaveyya hemāḥa bhave*) 'such as affect all creatures in this world' (*iti hemāḥa imināpakārena*) 'as follows:'

There are eleven impurities and each has three forms, making 33 altogether. For example, *atisaan* and similarly, the *tridoṣa*. They are *butsathaat*, *patshannathaat*, *rattannathaat*, *patsathaat*, *mutsakaayathaat*, *kaanlathaat*, *patthaweethaat*, *aapothaat*, *waayothaat*, *techothaat*, *aakaasathaat*. So they are called *thaat banchop* [the combined elements], in this way.

The masters explained at the beginning that *amutsakaayathaat* (sometimes called *amuunlathaat*) has three symptoms. In *Phrakhamphee saarasongkhro* they say that the element of fire called *parinaamakkhee*, which digests the food, causes nausea and incessant diarrhoea. When all the food has been excreted, the faeces resemble water which has been used to wash meat and which has a very offensive, fishy odour, like the snapping turtle, and the child has abdominal pain, extreme thirst, dry throat and chest, and dry mouth and teeth, because the element fire is in great disorder and rises fiercely to the palate. The saliva is the liquid which comes from the food. It rises up to the palate like liquor being distilled. The juices from the food filter out to the tip of the tongue and the teeth, and become saliva.

If a person is going to die, the fire element will leave his body. It can be compared to someone cooking rice, using too much fire, so that the water boils over and extinguishes the fire itself. The digestive juices dry up in a similar manner. This is why the patient has a dry throat and dry mouth. If this happens, you should put your hand in the patient's throat. If the throat is extremely cold, it is hopeless. He will definitely die that same day. Doctors should be in not doubt about this.

Description of the element of fire called *atsittaatchiwachaawak*. It causes swelling (some editions say weakness and exhaustion) [sic] of the whole body, then the faeces become green and black. In three days the patient will die.

Description of *patshannathaat*. Anyone affected by this will have liquid faeces as red as the juice of a chewed quid of betel, and watermelon juice. They will die in seven days.

Description of the *lom* called *kutshisayaawaataa*, the wind which blows in the intestines. Whenever this wind comes out of the body, it makes the person ill. This kind of wind element will cause incessant diarrhoea, but it cannot be allowed to go unchecked. If it is, the patient will suffer colicky pain, and will have a feeling of constriction in the throat, so that he cannot eat, drink or take medicine, because it makes him vomit all the time and the saliva becomes very viscous. Whenever the saliva becomes sticky, the patient is sure to die.

Description of the earth element leaving the body, as explained in *Phrakhamphee saarasongkhro*, which discusses the 20 elements of earth - the hair on the head, body hair, nails, teeth, skin, flesh, tendons, bones, bone marrow, spleen, heart, liver, connective tissue, abdomen, lungs, small intestine, large intestine, digested food, undigested food and the brain. These are all the parts which are of the earth element. If you wish to know which earth [element] came out of the body, it says in this text that it is usual for four kinds of elements to leave the body - the tendons, the undigested food and the digested food, bone and flesh. If anyone becomes ill, no matter how severely, the digested food will never all go completely. But when that person is going to die, he will have continuous diarrhoea, until all the digested food and undigested food is gone. The faeces will be abnormal is some way. Sometimes they contain putrid mucus and blood, sometimes they look like rat droppings, because the disease prevents medicine from being absorbed, then the wind and mucus combine, to [produce faeces] resembling rat droppings, sometimes covered in mucus and sometimes the faeces are as green as a leaf.

They say it is because the bile overflows. When all the digested food has gone from the stomach, it comes out as yellow as fresh turmeric water or as green as a leaf. It is called *muun thao.* [1] If anyone is as sick as this, they need Indra to bring them back to life.

If the doctor wants to know whether the gall bladder has overflowed or burst, when the gall bladder has overflowed, the faeces are yellow, like fresh turmeric, the face, eyes and hair are yellow. The doctor who is ignorant of this might think it is *kaan singkhalee.* He should attach importance to the faeces and whether the patient is delirious or possessed by a spirit, and whether people think it is a *krasue.*[2] To treat it, the doctor is advised to give the right medicine, then the patient will live. But some die and some are cured. If the gall bladder bursts it is incurable. So the question arises, What injures the gall bladder, and what makes it overflow? The masters are positive in their reply that there are four reasons: *kaan* [3]develops in the gall bladder; the patient has a toxic fever; the patient has a fever resulting from *saang*; or the patient has been struck a blow by someone or has had a fall from a high place. The liver and gall bladder consequently rupture.

The gall bladder overflowing results from a disorder of the fire element or everything being poisoned and excessively hot. Then the bile spills out from the gall bladder. Just as when rice is being cooked, if the fire is too hot, the water boils over and the fire then extinguishes itself, so the person destroys himself. Such a person will certainly die. '*Semhakiṃakāraṇāti.*' Then the question is asked '*Bho ācāriya.*' 'Why, venerable masters, and what is the cause, and why do they die?' The masters, who know precisely, reply, 'Verily now, mucus is the cause.' In other words, the water element, of which there are twelve kinds, and altogether there are 108 elements derived from the element water. Mucus is an example. Mucus can cause twelve kinds of illness. We will give you three illustrations - mucus in the throat, mucus in the chest and mucus in the rectum.

The mucus in the throat can move up and down. Whenever someone has an illness with coughing and vomiting, mucus will come out. The mucus in the throat is about seven *niu* [inches] thick and covers the throat. This is normal for all beings. When food is swallowed, the mucus opens out and makes way for the food to slide down. After the food is swallowed, the mucus comes together again. Just as when a stone is thrown into stagnant water covered with green scum, the scum moves apart, then comes together as before, for example.

Mucus in the chest. Whenever someone has an illness caused by the fire and wind elements being stronger than the water element, the mucus becomes viscous and hard for two to five inches below the upper chest, causing a regular fever. Just as when someone has enlargement of the spleen, it makes the complexion, body, faeces and urine yellow, like *khai kaan singkhalee.* If the treatment is ineffective, the condition changes to *maan kasai*, which results in blood and purulent mucus in the faeces, and causes distension of the abdomen, like someone with dropsy. It is very difficult to cure. If you give the appropriate medicine, you might win or you might lose. If you give the wrong medicine you will lose.

Mucus in the rectum; that is, blood and pus. When someone is ill, blood and pus come from the rectum. It looks like water used to wash meat, and the spittle from a quid of betel and areca nut. It is foul smelling, like the smell of a corpse. It is very painful, the patient feels faint, has flatulence, with a feeling of fullness right up to the chest, dry retching, no desire to eat. He finds everything smells fishy, whenever he stands up he faints, has blurred vision, convulsions, his eyes roll back, and he has spasms of the hands and feet. If these symptoms occur together it is his *karma* [his time has come].

So the question is asked 'Venerable masters, what is the appearance of urine and faeces which indicate *atisaan*?' The masters reply 'There are eleven indications that people with *atisaan* will die. It has been explained in *Khamphee atisaan.* Here we will describe them briefly for the information of the doctors. There are eleven kinds of *atisaan*, which are divided into two categories - deeds performed during the present life and deeds performed during the past. There are six kinds of *atisaan* resulting from deeds performed during the present life, which can be treated successfully, and five kinds which are incurable. Here we summarise for doctors the five kinds of incurable *atisaan.* These five kinds of *atisaan* are associated with the four elements. If anyone has one of the five kinds of *kaan* affecting the chest - be it *kaan fee mee phit, kaan phit, kaan singkhalee mee phit, kaan suut* or *kaan mut* - it seems that Phrayaa Matchuraat [the god of death] has reached that person. His life cannot be prolonged.

Kaan fee mee phit starts at the liver and makes the liver hang down. If it affects the edge of the liver, the patient will first pass blood in the faeces. When he takes medicine, this will stop for four or five days, then he will pass mucus stained with blood for two or three days and it will become purulent mucus and blood, causing pain, and the poison will come up to the chest, causing dry retching two or three times, then hiccoughs. When the hiccoughs stop, the patient will have diarrhoea, and when that stops, the hiccoughs will return. Then red and black spots like birthmarks will appear all over the body, and the patient will have a high temperature, and be restless. When he is about to die, he will pass fresh blood for one day and one night, then die.

Kaan phit symptoms: diarrhoea like water used to wash meat and purulent serum with an offensive odour like a rotting corpse; panting, severe thirst, irritability and confusion like an insane person, because *kaan phit* affects the heart and the liver. Only one in 100 of such cases can be saved. Even to save one is difficult.

Kaan singkhalee affects the gall bladder, injuring it and causing the bile to overflow. Then the face, eyes, body, hands and feet become yellow, also the faeces, urine and bones are yellow, and changes occur all the time. Anyone with these symptoms will die in three days and when the patient is about to die, he will suddenly start and jerk upright, then die.

Kaan suut. There are three kinds of symptoms. The bile causes first diarrhoea, like filthy water, which smells like gunpowder, then severe thirst. Food acts as a laxative, causing diarrhoea. Then there is vertigo involving the whole body, heavy perspiration with drops the size of maize kernels, and constant severe vomiting. Treatment is ineffective, because the patient cannot take medicine, as it will pass straight through, and *lom sunthonwaat* blows up strongly, causing epigastric pain, and the patient cannot expel it, so he has flatulence. Death will come when the diarrhoea ceases.

Kaan mut affects the heart. It causes diarrhoea four, five, nine or eleven times a day. At first fresh blood is passed, then it affects the liver, breaking it away as a black mass like a piece of charcoal. The faeces are like *muun thao* [those of a foetus] and the patient is restless, sometimes listless and stuporous, has cold hands and feet, and is absent-minded and delirious. People think it is because the patient has been possessed by a spirit, but that is not so, it is just this group of fevers which gives the appearance of being possessed by a greedy spirit, because *kaan mut* affects the heart, then the liver. It causes the patient to pass blood, and then the liver breaks up. If it affects the lungs, it causes severe panting; if it affects the edge of the spleen, it causes regular fever and thirst; if it affects the upper chest, *lom sunthonwaat* will also arise. When the end of the patient's days has come, that *lom* will blow strongly, causing hiccoughs and sobbing breath. The film of mucus which has been in the upper chest since seven days after birth increases and becomes thick in the throat, causing dim vision and dull eyes, and the patient cannot sleep, and he sits down with his head bowed and does not want to see anybody.

The doctor might think that a demon or spirit has possessed this person, but that is not so, it is the severity of the disease itself. *Khai kaan mut* devours the heart and the liver, just like a greedy spirit, sending the patient out of his mind and causing other symptoms. These five kinds of *kaan atisaan* can happen to anybody when they are dying. Doctors should understand that any doctor who is to treat children or adults, who has not learnt the three texts, *Phrakhamphee atisaan, morannayaansuut* and *thaatbanchop*, is like a blind man, who is unable to see a being dying, he closes his eyes to treat the patient, not knowing whether he will win or lose. Even if he knows the texts *Khamphee roknithaan, prathom chindaa* and *apphayasantaa*, he will not know whether his treatment will succeed or not - he will be like a blind man.

Puna ca paraṃ. Here we discuss the urine and faeces of children from seven years of age down to three months. Regardless of the day of birth or the *saang* which affects a child, the main thing is to examine the faeces. If they are abnormal in any way and cause any illness, the doctor should understand it, as summarized here.

If a child has yellow faeces, not in lumps, it has enlargement of the spleen or a mass in the abdomen. Anyone seeing only the faeces and not the child would predict that the child had a high temperature and regular fever. If left a long time, the child will have convulsions, with the feet arched, hands clenched and the eyes rolling up. If it continues for three months, it is very difficult to cure. If a child has white faeces, the colour of rice water, it has worms called *sai duean* in the large intestine, and they say it is normal for everyone to have *sai duean* in their intestines. Even if they do not become ill, they will have them all their lives, as explained here.

One type of *taan chon*[4] is called ***kara***. It causes diarrhoea with white faeces like *din so phong* [soft chalk]. If the right medicine is given, it will stop, but there will be spots all over the body, like a heat rash, then blurred vision, and *klet kadee* [blepharitis]. The patient craves salt and shrimp paste. These *sai duean* worms are self-producing. They move about the body and the intestines become swollen and the abdomen distended, so that the chest and heart are constricted for about seven days. Then they mature, some crawl out through the anus, some through the throat and they make the patient vomit, and cause abdominal pain, and they bite the inside of the abdomen, making it so painful the patient thinks he is going to die. He feels hot and restless, and looks pale and anaemic. After about eight days he will die. From the onset of the disease until death is a total of fifteen days. This disease is incurable.

Taan chon called *santukkamit* is caused by *khai phikkhaat.* When the baby starts to walk and run, and falls down, hitting the ground or a piece of wood with its face, nose and chest, and getting bruised, this can be the cause of *khai phikkhaat.* It causes a high temperature, cold hands and feet, writhing of the body, small pustules over the body. It looks like measles. When it goes inside, it gives the child incessant diarrhoea, with blood and mucus, pain and thirst, and makes him stuporous. The child has a cough, and cannot eat or drink. Doctors are warned to be careful in treating it. For every one saved, two are lost.

Taan chon saaraphakara makes all the hairs stand up and pustules develop in the ears and nose. When the pustules break, they bleed, become swollen, and discharge foul smelling pus. It keeps recurring for years. If it occurs in the nose, it is very serious, because it goes to the brain, then the abdomen, causing diarrhoea, like pus and brains, and the child cannot eat. When the child dies, blood comes out of his ears and nose, rectum and urethra. If the symptoms are like this, it is not treated. The child cannot live.

Taan chon phrommakit starts in the navel. It looks like an abscess called *akkhaneesan.* After three days, the child passes fresh blood, then it goes inside and affects the gall bladder, liver, heart and intestines, then the patient becomes confused and delirious, hot and cold alternately, and sometimes passes blood and putrid mucus. If the symptoms are like this, a good doctor can cure it in fifteen days to one month. If the symptoms are intractable, the child will certainly die. When death approaches, blood will come out through every pore. If the child does not die, both eyes will be damaged, because there will be *to kon hoi* in the eyes.

Here the masters end the summary of the characteristics of the five kinds of *taan chon* which can be fatal.

(Ācāriyena) In *Phrakhamphee apphayasantaa* the teachers discuss (*sabbesattā āhāraṭṭhitikā*) all the unusual food which has come into existence since the recreation of the earth. When sixteen brahmas came down and tasted the sweetness of the earth, and their bodies changed to the forms of women and men, and they threw off their lower and upper garments, and had intercourse, and took pleasure in the five senses, and then indulged together in the pastimes of the earth. Then maize and wheat grew, and they derived sustenance from that wheat from that day to this.

Now, for millions and millions of cycles of years all beings which came to be born in *Jambū Dvīpa* ate wheat, whether they came from gods, from humans, from beasts or from hell; whether from ghosts or apparitions or self producing. When, in time, they all came to eat things like prawns and fish and all sorts of food in its crude, natural state, all of which can be impure or unclean, various diseases were produced.

Then the god Phakaaphrom, who is the head of all the brahmas, caused four trees to grow - one in each *dvīpa.* In Udon kaaro, he planted the *kanlappa phrik.* Three of the trees are quite divine, but not the one he gave us in Jambū Dvīpa. As all beings used to eat bad food and become ill, he gave us the *raatcha phrik,* because he hoped that it would cure all diseases of mankind. And these four trees are the lords of trees, because they originated before all other plants, and they are the important trees of the *dvīpa.* Then millions and millions of trees and plants and grasses grew in the soil of the earth. After that, he decreed that all plants would be medicinal. Not only that, the god Phakaaphrom bid a brahma of great intelligence to be reborn in the world of human beings who could care for all creatures affected by disease. And that brahma said 'I would like to ask four blessings.' And the god Phakaaphrom said 'May your every wish be fulfilled.'

The brahma then asked 'When I am born in the world of human beings in Jambū Dvīpa, let me be like all medicines so that I will know the symptoms of diseases by myself. And my second blessing: let all medicinal plants be able to speak, so that they can tell me the diseases they can cure. And the third blessing is: when any [one who is] ill and has come to the end of his life comes to me to ask to be cured, please don't let him find me. The fourth blessing: let me have whatever I desire.'

End of *Phrakhamphee prathom chindaa.*

NOTES

1 *muun thao:* early evacuated faecal matter of a foetus.

2 *krasue:* a group of female evil spirits or demons, reputed to feed on putrid meat and to inhabit women. *Mc*, p.46.

3 *kaan:* in this sense possibly refers to bubonic plague. It could mean that the bile is black.

4 *taan chon* (ตาน จร): the term '*chon*' (จร) translated previously as 'minor', to differentiate it from 'chon' (โจร) meaning 'robber'. This is probably a misprint.

Appendix I

Medicinal Substances: Animal, Mineral and Plant

Arranged in Roman alphabetical order

Note: Items marked with an asterisk* are mentioned in the text but not included as ingredients in prescriptions for medicine.

The code set out below is used for the description of the medicinal substances which follow:

Thai name transcribed	Thai name Thai script	Thai classification according to taste	Parts thus classified by *PP*
Thai synonyms			
Scientific name			
Genus species author(s)			
Scientific synonyms			Family
English name(s)			
Other names			Source(s)

Parts used in *KPC* prescriptions (not always the same as the parts to which the taste is attributed).
Other comments

Animals and Animal Products

amphan khee plaa อำพันขี้ปลา
Ambergris (PT)

bia chan เบี้ยจั่น
Cypraea moneta (L.) Cypraeidae
Monetary cowrie
calcined shell

bia tua phuu เบี้ยตัวผู้
bia phuu เบี้ยผู้
Cypraea eglantina (Duclos.) Cypraeidae
Eglantine cowrie
calcined shell
This shell measures 60-70mm x 35-40mm
There are eight types of monetary cowrie (VJ)

chaang ช้าง
Elephas maximus (L.) Elephantidae
Elephant see *kraam chaang* (plant)
tusk (*ngaa chaang*); molar tooth (*kraam chaang*)
A triturate of powdered elephant molar tooth in water is obtained by rubbing the tooth in water on a rough surface (VJ)

chamot ชะมด cool and fragrant
1. *chamot chet* ชะมดเช็ด
2. *chamot chiang* ชะมดเชียง
1. *Viverra zibetha* (Schneider) Viverridae (VJ)
   Asian civet
   Viverra megaspila Bluth.
   Burmese civet (VJ); *CS*, p.578
   Viverricula malaccensis thai (Kloss)
   Thai civet (VJ); *CS*, p.581
2. *Moschus moschiferus* (L.) Moschidae
   Musk deer
the secretion of the odoriferous gland of
1. both sexes of the civet cat
2. the male musk deer (VJ)

*cho** จอ
Dog

*chok** จอก
Monkey

chorakhe จระเข้ bitter bile

Crocodylus siamensis (Schneider) Crocodylidae *CS*, p.464
Crocodile, usually the above fresh water crocodile (VJ)
bile, teeth

*chuat** ชวด
Rat

chum phaa ชุมพา, ชุมภา
Llama
horn

dee mee ดีหมี
1. Plant
2. Animal:
Bile of a bear
see *mee* (animal) and *dee mee ton* (plant)

dee nguu ดีงู
1. Plant
2. Animal: see *nguu lueam*
Dried bile of a snake, usually the reticulated python (VJ)

duang ด้วง
Worm, grub of the beetle (VJ)

faan ฟาน
keng เก้ง
Muntiacus feae (Thomas et Doria) Cervidae
Barking deer (VJ); *CS*, p.593
horn

fong kai ฟองไก่
Hen's egg see *kai*

haan ห่าน
Goose
bone

hin kaa rang (daeng) หินการัง(แดง) see *sinlaayon*

hoi eerom หอยอีรม

naang rom นางรม
Ostrea edulis Ostridae Mc, p.928
Oyster shell

hoi khom หอยขม salty shell
Vivipara spp. Viviparidae *CS*, p.52
Freshwater snail (VJ)
calcined shell

hoi khong หอยโข่ง salty
Pachylabra celebensis (Quoy et Gaimard) Ampullaridae
(*Ampullaria celebensis* (Fischer et Dautzenberg)) (VJ); *CS*, p.54
burnt operculum of the shell; fresh shellfish, including the shell

hoi khraeng หอยแครง salty shell
Arca granosa (VJ)

*hoi maeng phuu** หอยแมงภู่ salty shell
Mytilus smaragdinus Mytilidae Mc, p.928
Sea mussel (PT)

hoi phimphakaarang หอยพิมพะการัง
Pholas orientalis Gmelin Pholadidae
Piddock (VJ)
shell

hoi sang หอยสังข์ see *sang*

kaa กา
Corvus coronoides andamanensis (Beavan) Corvidae
Crow (VJ); *CS*, p.647
feathers, bone, head

*kadee** กะดี่ see *kradee*

kae แกะ
Ovis aries (L.) Bovidae
Sheep
horn

kai ไก่
Gallus domesticus (VJ)

Chicken

kapi กะปิ
Acetes spp. Sergestidae
Caridina spp. Atyidae
Shrimp paste made from partially fermented tiny shrimps (VJ)

kapi dee กะปิดี
Mesopodopsis orientalis (Tattersall) Mysidae
Shrimp paste made from partially fermented, tiny shrimps (VJ)

katang muut กะตังมูตร
kluea kratang เกลือกระตัง
Concrete deposit from collected, kept human urine (VJ).
Uric acid salts *Mc*, p.122.

keng เก้ง see *faan*

*khaan** ขาล
Tiger

khai fak (plueak) เปลือกไข่ฟัก
Shell of hatched hen's egg (VJ)

khanom nom noei ขนมนมเนย
Sweet biscuits made from milk and butter (VJ)

khao nuea เขาเนื้อ
Deer horn see *kwaang*

khee ขี้
Excreta

khee kho sot ขี้โคสด
khee wua sot ขี้วัวสด
Fresh cow dung see *kho*

khee malaeng saap ขี้แมลงสาบ
khee maeng saap ขี้แมงสาบ see *muun malaeng saap*

khee thao luuk kho ขี้เทาลูกโค

khee thao luuk wua ขี้เทาลูกวัว
Faeces of a newborn calf

khee thao luuk kho nai thong ขี้เทาลูกโคในท้อง
Early evacuated faecal material of the foetus calf (VJ)

kheio เขี้ยว
Eye tooth; canine tooth

khieo chorakhe เขี้ยวยวจรเข
Eye tooth of a crocodile see *chorakhe*

khieo mee เขี้ยวหมี
Eye tooth of a bear see *mee*

khieo ngaa เขี้ยวงา
Eye teeth and tusks

*saaraphat khieo ngaa*สารพัดเขี้ยวงา
Probably a variety of eye teeth and tusks

khieo raet เขี้ยวแรด
Eye tooth of a rhinoceros see *raet*

khieo suea เขี้ยวเสือ
Eye tooth of a tiger see *suea*

kho โค oily milk
wua วัว salty urine
Bos taurus (L.) Bovidae
Cow
Roast beef; pure, fresh cow's milk; fresh cow dung; urine; early evacuated faecal matter of the foetus calf; faeces of a newborn calf

kho dam โคดำ see *krathing*

khon คน
Homo sapiens
Human being
breast milk, roasted hair from the head, urine

see also *katang muut, nam muut dek*

khon men ขนเม่น see *men*

khon nok ขนนก
Bird's feathers

khrang ครั่ง
Laccifer chinensis (Mahdihassan) astringent
Laccifer lacca (Ker.) Coccidae
(*Tachardia lacca* (R. Blanchard))
(*Lakshadia indica* Mahdihassan)
Lacs; Stick-lac insects; Coccus. *L. chinensis* is Siam lacs (VJ)
solution (*nam khrang*) similar to cochineal. A red coloured solution made by steeping powdered stick-lacs in water (VJ) See also *Mc*, p.179.

khunlikaa คุลิกา see *sappha khunlikaa*

khwaai ควาย see *krabue*

kluea kratang เกลือกระตัง see *katang muut*

*kraai** กราย
1. Plant
2. Fish: Notopteridae
Notopterus chitala (Buchanan) *CS*, p.202, (VJ)
A species of featherback with 7 or 9 black spots along the sides of the body. (Dept. Agri. & Fishersies). *Mc*, p.51. A large fish with silvery scales which glitters; looks and moves very smoothly. Becomes fierce when protecting young, and bites. Has a row of black spots at the lower part of the body on both sides. (VJ)

kraam chaang กรามช้าง see *chaang*
1. Molar tooth of an elephant
2. Plant: *kraam chaang (kluai)* a species of banana *Mc*, p.51

kraam raet กรามแรด see *raet*
Molar tooth of a rhinoceros

kraben กระเบน toxic
kaben กะเบน
kraben thale กระเบนทะเล

Dasyatis bleekeri (Blyth.) Dasyatidae
Dasyatis spp.
Ray; Stingray (VJ); *CS*, p.135

krabue กระบือ
khwaai ควาย
Bos bubalis (L.) Bovidae
Water buffalo (VJ); *Mc*, p.38
horn, burnt horn from an albino buffalo, water squeezed from the dung of a water buffalo

*kradee (plaa)** ปลากระดี่
kadee กัดี่
malet kadue เมล็ดกะดี [misprint *klet kadee* เกล็ดกะดี่]
Trichogaster trichopterus (Pallas) Osphronemidae
Trichopodus trichopterus
Trichopodus maculatus
A species of fresh-water fish (VJ); *CS*, p.339
scales (*klet* เกล็ด

krasuu กระซู่
kasuu กะซู่ see *raet*

*krataai** กระต่าย oily liver
Lepus peguensis siamensis (Bonhote) Leporidae
Rabbit; Siamese hare (VJ)

krathing กระทิง
1. Plant
2. Animal
3. Fish

2. *krathing* กระทิง
kho dam โคดำ
wua dam วัวดำ
Bos gaurus (Ham-Smith) Bovidae
Gaur ox (VJ)
Indian bison, known in Malaysia as *seladang* *Mc*, p.35
urine

3. *krathing (plaa)* ปลากระทิง
kathing กะทิง Mastacembelidae

Mastacembelus armatus (Fowler) (VJ); *CS*, p.205;
Spiny eel - a flat, long fish, with a pattern of yellow and brown patches and marks

*krot** กรอด
1. Plant กรด
2. Bird กรอด see *nok krot*

kui กุย
Nemorhaedus crispus (Temm.) Bovidae
horn (VJ)

*kun** กุน
Swine

kwaang กวาง
nuea เนื้อ
Cervus spp. Cervidae
Deer (VJ); *CS*, p.591
horn, newly grown horn

liang phaa เลียงผา
Nemorhaedus sp. *Mc*, p.754
Goat antelope; Serow (VJ)
horn, bone

lin thale ลิ้นทะเล
Os sepiae (Latin name)
Sepia esculenta (Hoyle)
Sepia officinalis (L.)
Sepia spp. common to Thai waters
Sepiidea (Zoological name)
Bone of the cuttle-fish, mainly crude calcium carbonate (VJ)

lueat raet เลือดแรด
lueat daeng เลือดแดง[misprint]
1. Plant
2. Rhinoceros blood see *raet*

maa mieo ม่าเหมี่ยว
1. Plant
2. Insect of the Scaraboeidae (VJ)

maaraa (*rang*) รังหมาร่า
Ishnemon
Hornet (nest)
The Thais use earth or mud from seven places for medicine. For example, a graveyard, river bank, etc. In this case, it might be the earth or mud used to make the nest, which is useful. The earthen nest is burnt, thus producing a mineral or mineral compound and at the same time, sterilizing it and killing microorganisms. (VJ)

maeng daa แมงดา
Lethocerus indicus
The giant water-bug or the giant electric-light bug, an insect of blue and green colouring found in the fields during the rainy season *Mc*, p.324
shell

maeo dam แมวดำ
Felis
Black cat
roasted head

malaeng mum taai saak แมลงมุมตายซาก
Carcass of a spider (VJ)

malaeng saap แมลงสาบ
maeng saap แมงสาบ
Pariplaneta australasie (Fabricus)
Common cockroach
faecal matter (*muun* มูล; *khee* ขี้)

*mamae** มะแม
Goat

*mamia** มะเมีย
Horse

*marong** มะโรง
Naga

*maseng** มะเส็ง
Snake

mee หมี	toxic	bile
1. *mee khon* หมีคน		
mee khwaai หมีควาย		
mee dam หมีดำ		
2. *mee maa* หมีหมา		
mee muu หมีหมู		
1. *Arcticonus thibetanus* Cuver		
2. *Helarctos malayanus* Raffles		Ursidae
1. Himalayan black bear		
2. Malay bear		(VJ)
eye tooth		

men (*khon*) ขนเม่น		
khon men		
Porcupine quills		(VJ)

men (phung) พุงเม่น
Viscera of the porcupine

muk มุก
Pearl

muu หมู	oily	liver
Sus scrofa (L.) var. *domesticus* (Gray)		Suidae
Pig		(VJ)
tusks		

muu thuean หมูเถื่อน		
muu paa หมูป่า		
Sus spp.		(VJ)
Sus cristatus (Wagner)		Suidae *CS*, p.588
Wild boar		
bile		

muun มูล
Excreta

muun kho มูลโค		
muun wua มูลวัว		
Cow dung	see *kho*	

muun kho tok mai มูลโคตกใหม่
Fresh cow dung see *kho*

muun luuk on มูลลูกอ่อน
Faeces of a nursing baby (VJ)

muun malaeng saap มูลแมลงสาบ
khee malaeng saap ขี้แมลงสาบ
muun maeng saap มูลแมงสาบ
khee maeng saap ขี้แมงสาบ see *malaeng saap*
Faecal matter of the cockroach (VJ)

muun wua khaang phom มูลวัวข้างพ้อม
Cow dung taken from the outer wall of a granary. The granary is made from woven bamboo sealed with cow dung. see *kho* (VJ)

muut kho dam มูตรโคดำ
Urine of a Gaur ox see *krathing*

muut maa มูตรม้า
Urine of a horse

nam khee khwaa น้ำขี้ควาย see *krabue*
Liquid squeezed from the dung of water buffalo (VJ)

*nam khrang** น้ำครั่ง see *khrang*
nam khrueng น้ำครึ่ง[misprint]
A red coloured solution made by steeping powdered stick-lacs in water (VJ)

nam kraam chaang น้ำกรามช้าง see *chaang*
A triturate of powdered elephant molar tooth in water

nam muek น้ำหมึก see *plaa muek*
Ink

nam muut dek น้ำมูตรเด็ก salty
Urine of a child

nam muut dek chaai น้ำมูตรเด็กชาย salty
Urine of a male child

nam nom kho น้ำนมโค
Cow's milk — see *kho*

nam nom khon น้ำนมคน — see *khon*
Human breast milk

nam phueng น้ำผึ้ง — sweet
nam phueng ruang น้ำผึ้รวง
Honey

nam plaa น้ำปลา
Fish sauce

nam plaa raa น้ำปลาร้า
The supernatant liquid from the juices of decomposed fish to which have been added salt and roasted paddy rice grains (VJ)

nam saaraphaat khieo ngaa น้ำสารพัดเขี้ยวงา see *khieo ngaa*

ngaa chaang งาช้าง
Elephant tusk — see *chaang*

ngaa chaang dee งาช้างดี
Undamaged elephant tusk, as opposed to *ngaa chaang kamchat* (VJ)

ngaa chaang kamchaai งาช้างกำจาย
An elephant's tooth that has been broken — *Mc*, p.102

ngaa chaang kamchat งาช้างกำจัด
When an elephant attacks a tree with its tusks, sometimes a tusk breaks and the broken end remains embedded in the tree. This is *ngaa chaang kamchat*. (VJ)

nguu hao งูเห่า
Naja naja (L.) — Colubridae
Cobra — (VJ)
Cast off skin, bile, head, bones, scales

*nguu khieo** งูเขียว
Green snake

nguu lueam งูเหลือม | bitter | bile
| toxic | bones
Python reticulatus (Schneider) | Boidae
Reticulated python | (VJ); *CS*, p.493
dried bile, kept as the whole gall bladder; grease
The reticulated python, *nguu lueam*, is very close to *nguu laam*, but they are not identical. It is usually *nguu lueam* which is used in medicine. (VJ)

nguu tabong phalam งูตะบองพะลำ
A species of snake
bile

nguu thap thaang งูทับทาง
Bungarus multicintus (Bluth.) | Elapidae
Many banded *krait*
bones
There are three or more such snakes. This is a deadly poisonous snake. It is said that if it bites, the victim will drop dead on the path, as the name implies. (VJ)

no raet นอแรด
Rhinoceros horn | see *raet*

noei (nam man) น้ำมันเนย
Ghee

nok นก
Bird
feathers

*nok krot** นกกรอด
nok prot นกปรอด
Pycnonotus blanfordi conradi (Fensch) | Pycnonotidae
Bulbul; Indochinese streaked-eared bulbul | (VJ); *Mc*, p.496
The eggs are very pale turquoise colour and speckled | (VJ)

nok yuung นกยูง
Pavo muticus (L.) | Phasianidae
Peacock; The common peafowl | (VJ); *CS*, p.614
bile, tail feathers, 'eyes' of feathers (the distinctive circular pattern near the tips of the tail feathers) scorched brittle

The peacock feather, in its natural state contains a toxic irritant. Peacock's bile contains a deadly poison at all times. In Thailand, in the mating season, it is forbidden to eat the peafowl's meat because it is very poisonous then. (VJ)

nom kho khon นมโคข้น
nom wua khon นมวัวข้น
cream see *kho*

nuea เนื้อ see *kwaang*

nuea kho yaang เนื้อโคย่าง
Roast beef see *kho*

nuu ring หนูหริ่ง
Crocidura murina *Mc*, p.917
Rattus spp. Muridae
Species of rat (VJ)
droppings

nuu thuean หนูเถื่อน
Rattus spp. Muridae
Wild rat (VJ)
droppings

phae แพะ
Goat
milk, horns

phom khon phao ผมคนเผา see *khon*
human hair from the head, roasted or burnt

phung men พุงเม่น
The viscera of the porcupine

plaa ปลา
Fish

plaa chon ปลาช่อน
Channa striatus (Bloch.) Channidae *CS*, p.336
(Ophiocephalus striatus Bleeker)
Serpent-headed fish; Snake-head fish (VJ)

scales

plaa mo ปลาหมอ
Pristolepis fasciata Nandidae *CS*, p.139

*plaa muek** ปลาหมึก salty bone
Squid; Cuttle fish *Mc*, p.912

plaa phayuun ปลาพะยูน, ดูหยง (มลายู)
Halicore dugong (Erxleben)
Sea cow; Dugong Manatidae (VJ)
tusk

plaa taphian ปลาตะเพียน
Puntius gonionotus (Bleeker) Cyprinidae
A kind of carp (VJ)

plaa thuu ปลาทู
Rastrelliger chrysozonus Scombridae *Mc*, p.420
dried fish

*pluak** ปลวก
Termite; white ant (of which more than 30 species in Thailand) (VJ)

priang phrakho เปรียงพระโค
priang เปรียง
nam priang phrakho น้ำเปรียงพระโค
tak ตักร
Buttermilk mixed with a third part of water *Mc*, pp.532, 358

*prot** ปรอด see *nok krot*

puu naa ปูนา
Paratelphus sexpunctatum (Lanchester) Gecarcinucinae *CS*, p.170
A very small crab; Field crab (PT)
carapace or shell

puu thale ปูทะเล salty claws; carapace
Scylla serrata (Forskal) Portunidae
Sea-crab; Blue crab *CS*, p.173
claws, carapace

raak din รากดิน
sai duan ไส้เดือน
Earthworm (VJ)

raeng แร้ง
1. *Sarcogyps calvus* (Scopoli) Accipitridae
2. *Pseudogyps bengalensis* (Gmelin)
1. Black vulture
2. Indian white backed vulture; Brown, white backed vulture (VJ); *CS*, p.611
skull, bones

raet แรด
krasuu กระซู่
kasuu กะซู่
see also *lueat raet* (*ton*) เลือดแรดต้น, a plant called rhinoceros' blood
1. *Rhinoceros sondaicus* (Desmarest) Rhinocerotidae
2. *Didermoceros sumatrensis*
(*Rhinoceros sumatrensis* Gairdner))
1. One-horned rhinoceros
2. Asiatic two-horned rhinoceros (VJ); *CS*, p.587
molar teeth, eye teeth, horn, blood, burnt hide

*rai** ไร
rai nam ไรน้ำ
Moina macrocopa (Strauss) (VJ); *CS*, p.127
Daphnia
A very small, reddish brown, transparent fresh water animal about the size of a pinpoint

*rakaa** ระกา
Cock

rang maaraa รังหมารา see *maaraa*

saai ทราย
Cervus porcinus annamiticus (Hende) (VJ)
Hog deer

saaraphat khieo ngaa สารพัดเขี้ยวงา
Canine teeth, tusks of a variety of animals (VJ)

sai duan ไส้เดือน — see *raak din*

sang สังข์ — salty — calcined shell
hoi sang หอยสังข์
sang naam สังข์หนาม
Strombus canarium (L.) — Strombidae
Conch shell. There are many kinds. — (VJ); *CS*, p.63
calcined shell

sappha dee thang 8 สรรพดีทั้ง๘, สารพัดดีทั้ง๘
saaraphat dee สารพัดดี
8 kinds of bile
moistened with water

sapphakhunlikaa (yaa) ยาสรรพคุณลิกา
khunlikaa , *khulikaa* คุลิกา
khulikaan คุลิการ [misprint]
An ancient remedy made from enlarged glands of monkeys or baboons *Mc*, p.206

*shalu** ฉลู
Ox

sing สิงห์
Unicorn (mythical) — (PT)
Lion — *Mc*, p.864
horn

sinlaayon ศิลายอน
hin kaa rang daeng หินการังแดง
pravala Skt
Corallium rubrum
Os corallii
obtained from
Corallium elatius Ridl. — Gorgonidae
C. konojoi Kishin
C. japonicum Kishin
Composition: $CaCO_3$ 83%, $MgCO_3$ 3.5%,
Iron oxide 4.5%, organic compounds 8%
Red coral — (VJ)
Flint or very hard rock — *Mc*, p.667

suea เสือ
Felis tigris (L.) Felidae
Tiger (VJ); *Mc*, p.889
teeth, bones, milk

taen (rang) รังแตน
Wasp (nest)

tao lueang เต่าเหลือง
Testudo elongata (Blyth.) Testudinidae
Tortoise (VJ)
carapace

taphaap nam ตะพาบน้ำ
Trionyx cartilagineus (Bodd.) Trionychidae (VJ)
Soft-shelled turtle
bile, carapace

thoh เถาะ
Hare

tuk kae ตุ๊กแก
Gecko (PT); *CS*, p.471
faeces

*ueng yaang** อึ่งยาง [?misprint for *ueng aang* อึ่งอ่าง]
ueng aang อึ่งอ่าง
P.kaloula mediolineata (Smith)
Bull frog (VJ)

waeo nok yuung แววนกยูง see *nok yuung*
The eyes of the feathers of a peacock's tail, usually scorched brittle

wua วัว see *kho*

wua dam วัวดำว see *krathing*

Minerals and Mineral Products

amphan อำพัน
Amber; a fossil resin *Mc*, p.997

banlangsinlaa บัลลังศิลา,บัลลังก์ศิลา
Red coral (VJ)

chaat ชาด
1. Plant: *Bixa orellana*
2. Mineral:
chaat kon ชาดก้อน
chaat cho sae ชาดจอแส
chaat chu sae ชาดจุแส [misprint]
chaat horakhun cheen ชาดหรคุณจีน
Red mercuric sulphide
Cinnibar; Chinese red; Vermilion

chaat (nam) น้ำชาด
Vermilion-coloured paint

chaat horakhun ชาดหรคุณ
chaat sakhun ชาดทรคุณ[misprint]
chaat horakhun Thai ชาดหรคุณไทย
Iron pyrites

chaat horakhun thet ชาดหรคุณเทศ
?

chaat phong ชาดผง
Chinese *ngîng čhū* จิ่งจู
A red pigment (VJ)

chaat thang 3 ชาดทั้ง๓
1. *chaat kon* ชาดก้อน
2. *chaat cho sae* *chuusaa* (Chinese)ชาดจอแส,จูซา(จีน)
3. *chaat horakhun cheen* ชาดหรคุณจีน
Three different grades of the same drug
Mercuric sulphide

Cinnibar; Chinese red; Vermilion

chunsee จุนสี
Copper sulphate
Verdigris (VJ); *Mc*, p.254

chunsee sat จุนสีสตุ
Anhydrous copper sulphate (VJ)

*dee buk** ดีบุก
Tin

dee kluea ดีเกลือ
Sodium sulphate (PT)
Epsom salts, Magnesium sulphate *Mc*, p.339

dee kluea farang ดีเกลือฝรั่ง
Magnesium sulphate (PT)

din kin ดินกิน
?

din ping ดินปิ้ง
Baked clay (PT)

din plak khwaai ดินปลักควาย
Mud; soil from a swamp (PT)

din prasiu ดินประสิว
Potassium nitrate
Nitre; Salt petre (VJ)

din prasiu khaao ดินประสิวขาว
Potassium nitrate, purified
Purified nitre; Salt petre (VJ); *Mc*, p.329

din so phong ดินสอพอง bland
din see phong ดินสีพอง
A soft prepared chalk *Mc*, p.329
Marl (Soil consisting of clay and carbonate of lime) (VJ)

din thanam ดินถนำ

din thanam tham ดินถนำถ้ำ (VJ)

1. Plant
2. A golden-coloured clay It is reported to fall from heaven or to be of meteoric origin and is believed to endow all who partake of it with miraculous virtues.

Mc, p.329

fun ฝุ่น

fun cheen ฝุ่นจีน

Talcum powder, Chinese (PT)

hin fan maa หินฟันม้า

Feldspar (VJ)

horadaan หรดาล

horidaan หริดาล

horadaan thong หรดาลทอง

horadaan kleep thong หรดาลกลีบทอง

Arsenic trisulphide As_2S_3

Yellow orpiment; Auripigment; Orpiment; Yellow arsenic; King's gold; King's yellow, *Haratala* (Hindi) (VJ)

kabang กะบัง see *krabang*

kammathan กำมะถัน

kammathan lueang กำมะถันเหลือง

maat lueang มาศเหลือง

suphan than สุพรรณถัน

Sulphur

Brimstone (VJ)

kammathan daeng กำมะถันแดง(กำมะดันแดง)

horadaan daeng หรดาลแดง

suphan dan daeng [suphan than daeng] สุพรรณดันแดง(สุพรรณถันแดง)

Arsenic disulphide As_2S_2

Red orpiment; Realgar (VJ)

kammathan thang 2 กำมะถันทั้ง๒

1. *kammathan* กำมะถัน
2. *kammathan daeng* กำมะถันแดง

1. Sulphur
2. Arsenic disulphide; Red orpiment (VJ)

kham คำ
Mineral: Gold see Plants: *kham foi*
khamao fai เขม่าไฟ
Carbon black; Soot (VJ)

khamao lek เขม่าเหล็ก
1. Mineral: Iron oxide
2. Plant: *Desmodium cephalotoides* Craib Papilionaceae (VJ)

khee takran lek ขี้ตะกรันเหล็ก
The scum precipitated in the bottom of an iron boiler, (usually resulting from hard water) (VJ)

kluea เกลือ
Sodium chloride
Common salt

kluea khua เกลือคั่ว
Common salt, baked or dry roasted by tossing in a pan over a fire to purify it (in the sense of to 'cleanse' it); Table salt (VJ)

kluea sinthao เกลือสินเธาว์ salty
Crude sodium chloride (VJ)
A form of medicinal salt found in salt-licks
Rock salt crystals *Mc*, p.123

kon mo kaeng ก้นหม้อแกง
khamao mo kaeng เขม่าหม้อแกง
The bottom of an earthenware cooking pot heated with wooden fuel. It might, therefore, mean 'soot', that is, very fine particles of carbon. (VJ)

krabang กระบัง
kabang กะบัง
Kaolinite (in very fine purified powder form) (VJ)

maat lueang มาศเหลือง see *kammathan*

muek hom หมึกหอม

A superior variety of Chinese ink block. Carbon particles, with the addition of some aroma and glue; Indian ink. The bark of the coconut fruit, i.e. coir, is burnt, and the resulting soot is held together with glue to form a block. Since the glue will ferment in plain water, liquor is added to prevent this, and some fragrance is added - the more the better, and the more expensive. Indian ink is Chinese. The Chinese knew that carbon absorbs toxins, they may not have known that it also absorbs colours. (VJ)

naam chaat น้ำชาด see *chaat*

nam khaang น้ำค้าง
nam raem khuen น้ำแรมคืน
dew drops

nam khram น้ำครำ
Polluted water from under a native kitchen platform (VJ)

nam kluea น้ำเกลือ
Salt water; Saline water (VJ)

nam man din น้ำมันดิน
Coal tar *Mc*, p.455

nam prasaan thong น้ำประสานทอง
Borax; Sodium borate

nam prasaan thong sat น้ำประสานทงสตุ
Anhydrous sodium borate (VJ)

nam puun sai น้ำปูนใส
Lime water see *puun*

nam raem khuen น้ำแรมคืน see *nam khaang*

nam thaa น้ำท่า
River water (VJ)

ngoen เงิน
Silver

nom phaa นมผา
Stalactite or stalagmite

phluang พลวง
1. Plant
2. Metal:
Antimony

prot ปรอท
Mercury; Quicksilver; Hg

puun ปูน
puun khaao ปูนขาว
Calcium hydroxide; Slaked lime; Calx

puun daeng ปูนแดง
Calcium hydroxide tinted with a minute amount of turmeric; Red calx;
Pink calcium hydrate
The Indians use a paste of slaked lime with no turmeric in betel leaf and areca nut chewing (VJ)

saan nuu สารหนู toxic
saan yuak สารหยวก
Arsenic trioxide (PT)

saan som สารส้ม
Alum; Common potash alum *Mc*, p.858

saan som sat สารส้มสตุ
Anhydrous alum

sinlaayon ศิลายอน see Animals

suphan than สุพรรณถัน see *kammathan*

suphan than daeng สุพรรณถันแดง see *kammathan daeng*

thaan fai paa chaa ถ่านไฟป่าช้า
Glowing charcoal from a cremation

thong kham pleo ทองคำเปลว
Gold leaf (VJ)

thong ngoen ทองเงิน
Gold and Silver (VJ)

tuk tam nam thong ตุ๊กต่ำน้ำทอง
Golden coloured Biotite; $K.(Mg,Fe)_3.AlSi_3O_{16}(OH)_2$
Used to treat inflammation of the inner membrane lining the mouth (VJ)

yaa khieo khee thong ยาเขียวขี้ทอง
Medicine containing the green oxide of brass (Copper oxide)
Used externally (VJ)

yaa yong fai หญ้ายองไฟ
khamao fai เขม่าไฟ *PP*, p.185
A soot coated kitchen cobweb. Cobweb-like filaments of soot or carbon found above a wood burning stove. (VJ)

Plants and Plant Products

aai nieo อ้ายเหนียว
ai nieo ไอ้เหนียว
ee nieo อีเหนียว
Desmodium gangeticum DC. Papilionaceae
root (PT); (VJ)
Both male (*ai nieo*) and female (*ee nieo*) forms can occur on the same tree (VJ)

akkhanee chawaa อัฆนีชวาอัคนีชวา
akkhee thawaan อัคคีทวาร
Clerodendron serratum Spreng. *FT*, p.1063; *WW*, p.818

amphan dok mai อำพันดอกไม้
amphan thong อำพันทอง
lamphan thong ลำพันทอง [misprint]
Amber from pine; Pine amber; Yellow amber (PT)
This is used as an expectorant

anchan อัญชัน
anchan khaao อัญชันขาว
Clitorea ternata L. Leguminosae (VJ)

White flowered variety (Papilionaceae)
leaves

anchan thang 2 อัญชันทั้ง๒
1. *anchan khaao* อัญชันขาว
2. *anchan khieo* อัญชันเขียว
Clitorea ternata L. Leguminosae (VJ)
Both white and blue varieties (Papilionaceae) (PT)

angkaap อังกาบ
Barleria cristata L. Acanthaceae (PT)
leaves, root

baan mi ruu rooi khaao บานมิรู้โรยขาว
Gomphrena globosa L. Amaranthaceae (PT)
White flowered variety
Globe amaranth
root

bai ใบ
leaves

bai bua thee taai klaang sa ใบบัวที่ตายกลางสระ see *bua luang*
Lotus or water lily leaves which have died in the pond or because of disease or drought. They die because of lack of nutrients in the water. (PT)

bai mai thang 5 ใบไม้ทั้ง๕
Five kinds of leaves; which kinds depend on the recipe

bai naat ใบหนาด see *naat*

bai ngoen bai thong ใบเงินใบทอง bland leaf
bai ngoen ใบเงิน
bai thong ใบทอง
bai naak ใบนาก
The name given to the plant varies depending on the colour of the leaves - silver, gold or red. There are two kinds of flowers. The red one is Acanthaceae
Graptophyllum pictum Griff. (VJ); *TS*, p.168
When the flower is a five pointed star, it is Acanthaceae
Pseuderanthemum atropurpureum Radlk. (VJ); *TS*, p.275

which is one plant called *bai naak*. One plant produces one or two of the three colours of the leaves, but all are the same species. This is used by the Indonesians for haemorrhoids - it is a mild laxative. Caricature plant is the English name given to these two species of the two genera. *bai thong* is also the name of another plant.
leaves, young leafy shoots

bai thong ใบทอง
B. monosperma Ktze. — Leguminosae
(Butea frondosa) Roxb. — (Papilionaceae) (VJ)
leaves, young twigs

bencha เบญจ
Prefix meaning 'the five', here usually five parts of a plant: the whole plant; stem, root, leaves, flowers and fruit

bencha khee lek เบญจขี้เหล็ก — see *khee lek*

bencha kradom เบญจกระดอม — see *kradom*
kradom thang 5 กระดอมทั้ง๕
Gymnopetalum cochinchinense Kurz — Cucurbitaceae (VJ)
whole plant, i.e. stem, root, leaves, flowers and fruit

benyakaanee (phon) ผลเบญกานี
Quercus infectoria Olivier — Fagaceae
Aleppo gall; Nutgall — (VJ); *FT*, p.472
'*phon*' here means gall, not fruit

bit ปิด
1. *kabit* กะปิด
1. *Zingiber* sp. — Zingiberaceae (PT)
2. *mabit* มะปิด
2. *Helicteres isora* L. — Sterculiaceae
fruit

bong (mai) ไม้บง — see *mai bong*

boraphet บอระเพ็ด — bitter — stem
boraphet daeng บอระเพ็ดแดง
Tinospora tuberculata Baumé — Menispermaceae (VJ)
(*T. crispa* Miers. ex Hook. f. Thoms.) — *WW*, p.432
(*T. rumphii* Boerl.)

stem, leaves, leaf sap

bua bok บัวบก	cool and fragrant	
a. *phak nok* ผักหนอก		
b. *waan phrachan* ว่านพระจันทร์		
a. *Centella asiatica* (L.) Urb.		Umbelliferae
(*Hydrocotyle asiatica L.*)		(VJ); *HE*, p.5
b. *Stephania erecta* Craib		Menispermaceae
a. Asiatic pennywort		(VJ); *HE*, p.17

A herb of the genus *Hydrocotyle*, allied to the Marsh pennywort (Sek)
The whole plant of *Centella asiatica* is used as an alterative and to treat diarrhoea *HE*
C. asiatica is a small creeping plant. The *bua bok* mentioned here (in the text, *KPC* p.221, but not necessarily in the prescriptions), being an auspicious plant, should not be too small - not as low as *Centella asiatica* - and is therefore *Stephania erecta* Craib. (VJ)
b. The corm is used as a stomachic, anodyne, antimicrobial and to treat arthritis.

bua khom บัวขม		bitter
Nymphaea lotus L.		Nymphaeaceae (VJ)
Bitter variety, with a small white flower		

bua kroh บัวเกราะ		
Nelumbo nucifera Gaertn.		Nelumbonaceae (VJ)
fruit	see *bua luang* below	

bua luang บัวหลวง	astringent	flowers
Nelumbo nucifera Gaertn.	cool and fragrant	pollen
Sacred lotus	oily	root,seeds
rootstock, pollen, flowers,		Nelumbonaceae
juvenile leaves, seed husks *(plueak)*		(VJ); *HE*, p.13

The receptacle and leaves are used for checking haemorrhage; the embryo is used as a coronary vessel dilator; and the seeds and rhizome as a nutrient *HE*

bua phan บัวผัน	oily	rootstock
bua ninlubon บัวนิลุบ		(VJ)
Nymphaea cyanea Roxb.		Nymphaeaceae (VJ) (PT)
Blue water lily or lotus		
rootstock		

bua phuean ดอกบัวเผื่อน		
Nymphaea stellata Willd.		Nymphaeaceae
Water lily		(VJ)
flowers, root, pollen, rootstock		

bua thang 5 บัวทั้ง๕
bua nam thang 5 บัวน้ำทั้ง๕
1. *bua chong konlanee* บัวจงกลนี
2. *bua sattabut* บัวสัตตบุษย์
3. *bua sattaban* บัวสัตตบรรณ
4. *bua lin chong* บัวสินจง
5. *bua phan* บัวผัน
Nymphaea lotus Nymphaeaceae
Flowers of five kinds of water lilies (VJ)
flowers, pollen

buk บุก
Amophophallus campanulatus Bl. ex Decn. Araceae
Elephant yam; Stanley's water-tub (PT); *LP*, p.158
tuber

buk ro บุกรอ
Amophophallus saraburiensis Gagnep. *Araceae TS, p.20*

bunnaak บุญาค,บุนนาค cool and fragrant flowers
Mesua ferrea L. Guttiferae
Indian rose chestnut (VJ); *HE*, p.12
flowers
The flowers are used as a stimulant, and in making aromatic powder; the root is used as a carminative *HE*

chaa phluu ช้าพลู
Piper rostratum Roxb. Piperaceae
root, fruit
The fruits are used as an ingredient in an asthma remedy *HE*, p.14

chaak จาก
nam luuk chaak น้ำลูกจาก
Nypa fruticans Wurmb.
Nipa palm; Atap palm (VJ)
kernel sap (*nam luuk chaak*)

chaat ชาด
1. Mineral: Mercuric sulphide
2. Plant: *Bixa orellana* *Bixaceae Mc*, p.291

Annato or Arnatto — see *kham Thai*

chabaa ชะบา
Hibiscus rosa-sinensis L. — Malvaceae
Common red hibiscus; Shoe flower; China rose — (PT)
leaves

cha-em ชะเอม
cha-em Thai ชะเอมไทย — sweet — root and fruit
Acacia pennata subsp. *insuavis* Nielsen — Leguminosae *TS*, p.14
Albizia myriophylla Benth. — (Mimosaceae) *TS*, p.2

cha-em thang 2 ชะเอมทั้ง๒
possibly
1. *cha-em Thai*
2. *cha-em thet*

cha-em thet ชะเอมเทศ
1. *Glycyrrhiza glabra* L. — Leguminosae
2. *G. uralensis* Fisch. — (Papilionaceae)
(also called *cha-em khaa kai* ชะเอมขาไก่)
3. *Abrus praecatorius* L.
Liquorice — (VJ); (PT)
root

chaluut ชลูด
chaluut khaao ชลูดขาว
Alyxia reinwardtii Bl. — Apocynaceae
Alyxia reinwardtii Bl. var. *lucida* Marlegr. — *TS*, p.18

chamot ton ชะมดต้น
faai phee ฝ้ายผี
Abelmoschus moschatus Medic. — Malvaceae
(*Hibiscus abelmoschus* L.) — *HE*
root, seeds (*thian chamot*)
The seeds are used as a carminative, stomachic and antispasmodic *HE*

champaa จำปา — cool and fragrant — flowers
Michelia champaca L. — Magnoliaceae (VJ)
flowers, petals

chan จันทน์
Myristica fragrans Houtt Myristicaceae
Nutmeg
seeds (*luuk* ลูก), seed + aril (*luuk* + *dok* ดอก), i.e. nutmeg and mace, roasted seeds.
The use of the word '*phon*' ผล in this context is an error, as *phon* can only mean 'fruit', while '*luuk*' can mean 'fruit' or 'seeds', or anything round. On the other hand, '*dok*' here means the 'aril', not 'flower', although '*dok*' usually means 'flower'. The kernel of nutmeg contains an amphetamine derivative. It also contains a volatile oil which irritates the kidneys, and in this way could be considered to be an aphrodisiac. The seed, with the seedcoat removed, is used for curry. (VJ)

chan chamot จันทน์ชะมด
chan hom จันทน์หอม
Mansonia gagei Drummond Sterculiaceae
wood
Used as a cardiac stimulant. (VJ)

chan daeng จันทน์แดง bitter wood
chan phaa จันทน์ผา
Dracaena lourieri Gagnep. Agavaceae
Dracaena (VJ); *HE*, p.8
wood (the infested medulla is used, but this is always referred to as wood) (VJ)
The infested medulla, which becomes hard and red, is used as an aromatic powder and colouring agent *HE*

chan hom จันทน์หอม see *chan chamot*

chan khaao จันทน์ขาว cool and fragrant wood
chan thanaa จันทน์ทนา
Tarrena hoanensis Pitard Rubiaceae (VJ)
wood

chan koh [kroh] จันทน์เกาะ (เกราะ)
Myristica see *chan* above
There are two species of *Myristica* used in Thailand. Mostly *M. fragrans* Houtt., the longer one, is used; sometimes *M. argentenea* Warb., the rounder one. '*Kroh*' means 'armour', and this name refers to nutmeg with its hard seed coat. The other form, *chan*, which is used for curry, has the seed coat removed. (VJ)
seed

chan phaa จันทน์ผา see *chan daeng*

chan takhian ชันตะเคียน
chan mai takhian ชันไม้ตะเคียน   astringent   bark, resin
takhian ตะเคียน
Hopea odorata Roxb.   Dipterocarpaceae (PT)
bark, resin

chan thanaa จันทน์ทนา   see *chan khaao*

chan thang 2 จันทน์ทั้ง๒
1. *chan thet* จันทน์เทศ
2. *chan daeng* จันทน์แดง
wood   see *nam chan thang* 2

chan thet จันทน์เทศ   bitter   heartwood
chan himalaya จันทน์หิมาลัย   hot-and-spicy   fruit
Santalum album L.   Santalaceae
Sandalwood; White sandalwood
Chan thet in the old medical texts is *S. album*; it now means *Myristica fragrans.* (VJ)
Other sources give *M. fragrans* for *chan thet*, and *S. album* for *chan khaao.* In prescription No. 246, there is fruit of *chan thet*, which can only mean nutmeg, *M. fragrans*, in this context. The part used is always called 'wood'; this is actually the heartwood.   (VJ)

chetta muun เจตมูล
Erythroxylum cuneatum Kurz   Labiatae
A tree with red heartwood   (Erythroxylaceae) (VJ)

chetta muun phloeng เจตมูลเพลิง   hot-and-spicy   root, leaf
1. *Plumbago indica* L.
(*Plumbago rosea* L.)
2. *Plumbago zeylanica* L.   Plumbaginaceae
1. Rose coloured leadwort   (VJ); WW, p.234
2. White leadwort; Ceylon leadwort   (PT)
root, leaves

chetta phangkhee เจตพังคี   hot-and-spicy   root
Adenochlaena siamensis Ridl.
(*Cladogynos orientalis* Zipp. ex Span.)   Euphorbiaceae

chik จิก

chik naa จิกนา — *HE*, p.3
Barringtonia acutangula Gaertn. — Barringtoniaceae
B. racemosa Roxb. — (VJ); *TS*, p.43
root
Twigs of *chik naa* are used as an antiscorbutic, expectorant and for headache *HE*

ching chaa chaalee ชิงชาชาลี — bitter — stem
Tinospora cordifolia Miers. — Menispermaceae
stem, leaves, fruit — (VJ); *HE*, p.18; *WW*, p.256
The whole plant is used as a bitter tonic, febrifuge and stomachic

ching chee ชิงชี่ — bitter — root
Capparis micracantha DC. — Capparidaceae (Capparaceae)
root — (PT); *LB*, p.23; *WW*, p.256

ching cho จิงจ้อ
1. *ching cho luang* จิงจอ้อหลวง
   ching cho yai จิงจ้อใหญ่
2. *ching cho liam* จิงจ้อเหลี่ยม — sweet — root
1. *Ipomoea vitifolia* Sweet. — Convolvulaceae (VJ)
2. *Operculina turpethum* S. Manso — *TS*, p.190; (PT)
   (*Ipomoea turpethum* R.Br.) — Convolvulaceae (VJ)
leaves, root

ching cho thang 2 จิงจ้อทั้ง๒
1. *ching cho luang*
2. *ching cho liam*
1. *Ipomoea vitifolia* Sweet. — Convolvulaceae (VJ)
2. *Operculina turpethum* S. Manso. — *TS*, p.190; (PT)
   (*Ipomoea turpethum* R.Br.) — (VJ)
root

ching cho yai จิงจ้อใหญ่ — see *ching cho luang*

chok ช้อก — see *mamuang* — *Mc*, pp.227, 234

*champhuu** ชมพู่ — Myrtaceae
Rose apple — *FT*, p.949

champhuu saarek ชมพู่สาแหรก

Eugenia malaccensis L. — Myrtaceae *FT*, p.950
A species of rose-apple tree

Eugenia Jambos L.
chong kho ชงโค
Bauhinia purpurea L. — Leguminosae (PT)
root

chong konlanee จงกลนี
Nymphaea lotus L. var. *pubescens* Hk.f. et Th. — Nymphaeaceae (VJ)
Water lily - pink, double, with frilled petals
flowers, pollen

chueak khao fai เชือกเขาไฟ
sueak khao fai เซือกเขาไฟ[misprint]
Bauhinia integrifolia Roxb. — *Leguminosae (VJ)*
(*B. flammifera* Ridl.)

chueak khao muak เชือกเขามวก
chueak khao muak khaao เชือกเขามวกขาว
chueak thao muak เชือกเถามวก [misprint]
Parameria barbata Schum. — Apocynaceae (PT)

chueak khao muak daeng เชือกเขามวกแดง
Xylinabaria minutiflora Pierre — Apocynaceae (PT)

chueak khao muak thang 2 เชือกเขามวกทั้ง๒
1. *chueak khao muak khao* (white)
2. *chueak khao muak daeng* (red)

chueak thao khan เชือกเถาคัน
Collumella trifolia Merr.
Cissus carnosa Roxb. — Vitidaceae
Cissus trifolia L. — (Ampelidaceae) (VJ)

chueak thao muak เชือกเถามวก[misprint] see *chueak khao muak*

chueak thao phruan เชือกเถาพรวน
A big strong rope, usually made from a bunch of rattans stranded together (VJ)

chuk rohinee จุกโรหินี

thao phung plaa เถาพุงปลา
Dischidia rafflesiana Wall. Asclepiadaceae
(PT); *TS*, p.128

chum het ชุมเห็ด
chub het ชุบเห็ด [misprint] Leguminosae
chum het Thai ชุมเห็ดไทย (Caesalpiniaceae)
Cassia tora L. (VJ); *HE*, p.5; *WW*, p.260
Foetid cassia; Sickle senna; Toradhal (India) (VJ)
leaves, root
The leaves are used as a purgative; an infusion of roasted seeds is used as a diuretic and to treat insomnia *HE*

chum het thet ชุมเห็ดเทศ exotic toxic leaves
chub het thet ชุบเห็ดเทศ [misprint] Leguminosae
het thet เห็ดเทศ (Caesalpiniaceae)
Cassia alata L. . (VJ); *HE*,p.5; *WW*, p.260
Candelabra bush, Seven-golden-candlesticks (VJ)
leaves, flowers, root, water (probably flower water), seeds

daang sakae ด่างสะแก see *sakae* salty ash
Wood ash from *Combretum quadrangularis Kurz* Combretaceae
Ash in water produces an alkaline solution used in washing (PT)

daeng (mai) แดงไม้
Xylia kerrii Craib-Hutch. Leguminosae (PT)
bark

dee mee (ton) ดีหมีต้น bitter wood
Cleidon javanicum Blume Euphorbiaceae
(*C. spiciflorum* Merr.) *PB*, p.68; *LB*, p.45

dee nguu ดีงู
1. Snake's bile
2. Plant

dee nguu ton ดีงูต้น bitter
kom khom กอมขม *LB*; *PP*, p.167; Mc, p.68
Picrasma javanica Bl. Simaroubaceae

(VJ); *LB*, p.49

dee nguu khruea ดีงูเครือ
Heterostemma wallichii Wight — Asclepiadaceae (VJ)

dee nguu thang 2 ดีงูทั้ง๒
1. *dee nguu ton*
2. *dee nguu khruea*

dee plee ดีปลี — hot-and-spicy — flowers, stem
1. Piper longum L. — Piperaceae (VJ); (PT
(P. longum C.DC.) — (VJ); (PT); *WW*, p.294
2. Piper retrofractrum Vahl. — *HE*, p.14; (PT)
(*P. officinarum* C.DC.)
Piper chaba Hunter
(*P. longum* Bl.(non L.)) — (VJ)
Long pepper
flowers, baked (this is done to kill fungi etc.) — (VJ)
The fruit are used as a carminative, stomachic and tonic, also to treat haemorrhoids
HE, p.14

din thanam ดินถนำ
1. A golden-coloured clay (see Minerals)
2. A plant: *Lycopodium fernallies* — Lycopodiaceae *Mc*, p.329

dong dueng ดองดึง — hot-and-spicy — tuber
dong dueng hua khwaan ดองดึงหัวขวาน
phan mahaa พันมหา
Gloriosa superba L. — Liliaceae
Glory lily; Superb lily; Climbing lily — (VJ); *HE*, p.10
tuber
The tuber is used to prepare a poultice for application to ulcers *HE*

duei เดือย
Coix lachryma-jobi L.
(*C. lachryma* L.)
(*C. agrestis* Lour)
(*C. chinensis* Tod.) — Gramineae
Job's tears; Adlay — (VJ)
kernel

en เอ็น

thao en เถาเอ็น
Cryptolepsis buchanani Roem.et Schult. — Asclepiadaceae
fruit
The stem and milky sap are used to strengthen muscle tone — *HE,* p.8

faai ฝ้าย
Gossypium spp. — (PT)
seeds

faai daeng ฝ้ายแดง
Gossypium arboreum L. — Malvaceae
Red flowered cotton tree; Tree cotton — (VJ); *HE* 10
young twigs, leaves, roots
This has a red flower and green seed; the other kind has black seed (VJ)
The leaves are used as an antipyretic and diaphoretic — *HE*

faai thet ฝ้ายเทศ
Gossypium barbadense L. — Malvaceae
(*G. brasiliense* MacFar.) — (PT); *TS*, p.167
Cotton plant; Sea island cotton; Pernambuco cotton
leaves, juice of juvenile leaves, fruit (*samo* สมอ)

(samo) faai thet สมอฝ้ายเทศ
fruit of *Gossypium*
('*samo*' here means fruit; this term is never used for any other fruit, in much the same way as the term 'hip' is used in 'rose hip') — (VJ)

faang ฝาง
faang sen ฝางเสน
Caesalpinia sappan L. — Caesalpiniaceae
Sappan — (VJ); (PT); *HE*, p.7
bark, root, wood
The wood is used as an alterative, and as a colouring agent

faeng แฟง
Wax gourd; White gourd — see *fak* ฟัก

faek hom แฝกหอม — cool and fragrant — root
Vetiveria zizanioides Stapf. — Gramineae (VJ)
(*V. odorata* Vivey)
Vetiveria zizanioides Nash — *HE*, p.18
Vetiver

The rhizome is used as a carminative and as a heart stimulant *HE*

fak ฟัก
Benincasa hispida
(*B. cerifera*) Cucurbitaceae (PT)
This gourd, when young, is called *fak* or *fak khieo* (Green gourd), while the rind is hispid. When the gourd is older, the hispid hairs vanish and the rind becomes waxy. This stage is called *faeng* (Wax gourd or White gourd). (VJ)
Wax gourd; White gourd; Chinese preserving melon; Chinese water melon
fruit, tendrils (*mue* มือ)

fak khaao ฟักข้าว
Momordica cochinchinensis Spreng. Cucurbitaceae (VJ)
leaves, root

fak khieo ฟักเขียว see *fak*
Green (young) gourd

fin ฝิ่น exotic toxic
yaa fin ยาฝิ่น
Papaver somniferum L. Papaveraceae
Medicinal opium (VJ); *WW*, p.521
dried or partly dried latex obtained from the opium poppy capsule

(nam yaa) fin น้ำยาฝิ่น
1. A residual deposit in the opium pipe after smoking. This is scraped out and put in water to wash it and make an aqueous extract for use as a very potent method of stopping the diarrhoea of cholera
2. Raw opium boiled with water to improve the otherwise foetid odour of the crude opium (VJ)

fin ton ฝิ่นต้น toxic leaves
kradong daeng กระโดงแดง astringent bark
Linociera microstigma Gagnep.
Linociera sangda Gagnep. Oleaceae (VJ)
Tree opium [which contains no opium]
bark
The leaves used to be chewed to avoid craving for opium, but nothing of significance has been found in them

A comparatively recently introduced ornamental plant is also known as *fin ton*. This is:
fin ton ฝิ่นต้น

malako farang มะละกอฝรั่ง
Jatropha multifida L. Euphorbiaceae
This is not the *fin ton* of the ancient prescriptions. (VJ)
Jatropha multifida L., recently introduced to Thailand, is named *malako farang* (exotic Papaya) because of the resemblance of the leaf blade to Papaya leaves. (VJ)
There is some disagreement about the identity of *fin ton*, and the inclusion of opium as one of the two *fin* (see below) might also be questioned since one prescription includes both *fin thang* 2 and *yaa fin*, the last being a synonym for *fin* (opium).

fin thang 2 ฝิ่นทั้ง๒
1. *fin*
2. *fin ton*
The two *fin*.

haang chaang หางช้าง
Sorghum vulgare Pers. Gramineae (VJ)
Sorghum see *khaao faang*

haang maa หางหมา
Setaria italica L. Gramineae (VJ)
Foxtail millet see *khaao faang*

haang chorakhe หางจรเข้ see *waan haang chorake*

haang kraai หางกราย
hom kraai หอมกราย
possibly *haam kraai* หามกราย
Terminalia triptera Stapf. Combretaceae (VJ)
bark

haang krarok หางกระรอก
Justicia bentonica L. Acanthaceae *FT*, p.116
root

haeo แห้ว exotic oily tuber
haeo cheen แห้วจีน
Eleocharis tuberosa Schultes. Cyperaceae *PB*, p.10
Chinese water chestnut (VJ)
tuber (a raw truffle)

haeo muu แห้วหมู

Cyperus rotundus L. Cyperaceae
Nutgrass (VJ); *HE*, p.8;
rhizome *WW*, p.812
The rhizome and root is a diuretic, febrifuge and stomachic

haeo sot แห้วสด sweet flesh
Cyperus esculentus L. Cyperaceae (VJ)
Raw truffle of Chufa (VJ)
Water chestnut (PT)
A truffle can be a mushroom or it can be a fungal infestation of a plant, e.g. Chufa is a mushroom type truffle
Zizania latifolia Turez. (Gramineae) grows in water. If it is not infested with fungus it cannot be eaten. The fungus makes it large and soft like canned asparagus. (PT)
This is called *no mai nam* q.v. (VJ)
cf. *krachap*

hatsakhun หัสคุณ see *salot*

hatsakhun Thai หัสคุณไทย
Micromilum minutum Wight et Arn. Rutaceae
This is a carminative and expectorant (PT)

hatsakhun thang 2 หัสคุณทั้ง๒ hot-and-spicy root
sahatsakhun thang 2 สหัสคุณทั้ง๒
1. *hatsakhun Thai*
2. *hatsakhun thet*
1. *Micromilum minutum* Wight et Arn. Rutaceae
2. *Croton* sp. Sterculiaceae

hatsakhun thet หัสคุณเทศ
sahatsakhun thet สหัสคุณเทศ[incorrect]
Croton sp. (VJ)
Hatsakhun thet is very close to *salot*, *Croton tiglium*, but whereas the leaves of *C. tiglium* are glabrous, the leaves of *hatsakhun thet* have an irritant surface covered with fine hairs (VJ)

het thet เห็ดเทศ see *chum het thet*

het muun kho (nam) น้ำเห็ดมูลโค
Juice from a mushroom which grows in a cow pat (PT). That is, juice from the Magic mushroom; an hallucinogenic mushroom.
Psilocybe cubensis (Earle) Sing Agaricaceae (VJ)

hing หิงค์ — see *mahaa hing*

hing haai หิงหาย
Crotalaria bracteata Roxb.
root
Leguminosae (Papilionaceae) (VJ)

hing yaang pho หิงค์ยางโพ
A kind of asafoetida which looks like the latex of the Bo tree. *KPC* B.E. 2495 (AD 1952) edn. uses *mahaa hing* for *hing yaang pho*. (VJ)

hom หอม — salty — leaf
hot-and-spicy — bulb
Allium ascalonium L. — Alliaceae
Shallot — (VJ)

hom daeng หอมแดง
Eleutherine palmaefolia — Iridaceae *HE*, p.9

hora duei kai โหราเดือยไก่
Aconitum carmichaeli Debx., and *Aconitum* spp. — Ranunculaceae (VJ)

horaphaa โหระพา
Ocimum basilicum L. — Labiatae
fruit — (PT)
Basil; Sweet basil

horaphaa thet โหระพาเทศ
possibly *Ocimum* sp. — (VJ)
seeds (*phon*)

horaa ammarit โหราอำฤตย์
Phyllanthus emblica L. — Euphorbiaceae (VJ)
Emblic myrobalan

horaa thao sunak โหราเท้าสุนัข
horaa teen maa โหราตีนหมา
Balanophorn abbreviata Bl. — Balanophoraceae (VJ)
(*B. polyandra* Griff.)

hua waen หัวแหวน
waen แหวน — see *phak khraat*

inthanin อินทนิล
Lagerstroemia flos-reginae Retz. — Lythraceae (VJ) *HE*, p.11
(*L. speciosa* (L.) Pers.)
Queen of flowers
heartwood
The leaves are used in an infusion as a diuretic and anti-diabetic; the seeds are used as an anti-diabetic and narcotic — *HE*

kaa kathing กากะทิง — see *krathing ton*

kaa ron การ่อน
kaare kaa ron กาเรการ่อน
Cymbidium aloifolium SW. — Orchidaceae
C. findlaysonianum Lindl., and
C. simulans Rolfe
leaves — (VJ)

kaan phluu กานพลู
Eugenia caryophyllata Thunb. — Myrtaceae
(*E. aromatica* Kuntze) — (VJ); *LB*, p.62
Eugenia caryophyllus Bullock et Harrison — *HE*, p.9
Clove tree
flower buds
The flower buds are used as a stimulant, aromatic and carminative; the oil is used as a local anaesthetic and antiseptic — *HE*

kaang plaa ก้างปลา
Bridelia monoica Merr. — (VJ); *HE*
Fluggea microcarpa Bl.
F. virosa Baill. — Euphorbiaceae
root — (VJ); *LB*, p.287
The root is used as a febrifuge and antibiotic — *HE*

kaang plaa daeng ก้างปลาแดง — bland — root
Phyllanthus reticulatus Poir. — Euphorbiaceae
root — (VJ); *WW*, p.49

kaarabuun การบูร — hot and spicy
Cinnamomum camphora (L.) Nees et Ebermaier — Lauraceae

Gum camphor; Laurel camphor; 2-Camphanone (VJ); *LB*, p.21
obtained from wood
There are other kinds of camphor, see *naat* and *phimsen*

*kaaraket** การะเกด
Pandanus distans Craib Pandanaceae
A kind of screw pine (VJ)

kabao กะเบา see *krabao*

kaeo kaa long แก้วกาหลง see *krabao*

kaeo klaep แก้วแกลบ salty powder
Silica, SiO
Obtained by burning paddy husks (VJ)
powder
(nam) klaep น้ำแกลบ
Perhaps the tarry, pyroligneous product obtained from burning (i.e. dry distilled) paddy husks, if for application. In this context it is for worms. (VJ)

kamchaai กำจาย
1. *Caesalpinia digyna* Rottler Leguminosae
2. C. decapetala (Roth) Alston (Caesalpiniaceae)
(*C. sepiara* Roxb.)
Teri-pod plant (VJ), *LB*, pp.116
1. pod
2. bark, root, seeds

kamlang wua thaloeng กำลังวัวเถลิง
Anaxagorea luzonensis Gray Annonaceae
(VJ)

kamphaeng chet chan กำแพงเจ็ดชั้น see *khamin khruea*

kamyaan กำยาน
Styrax tonkinensis (Pierre) Craib et Hartwick Styracaceae
Siam benzoin (VJ)

kamyaan phee กำยานผี
possibly *Styrax* sp.

kan krao กันเกรา

Fagraea cochinchinensis A. Chev. — Loganiaceae
(*F. fragrans* Roxb.) — (VJ)
bark

kanchaa กัญชา — exotic — toxic
Cannabis sativa L. — Cannabidaceae
Indian hemp; Marihuana; Marijuana — *HE*, p.4; *WW*, p.35
The flowering tops of the female plant are used as a bitter tonic, and as an hallucinogenic — *HE*

kanchaa thet กัญชาเทศ — exotic
kanchaa cheen กัญชาจีน
chaa kanchaa ช้ากัญชา (pseudo or fake *kanchaa*)
Leonurus sibiricus L. — Labiatae
Siberian motherwort — *LB*, p.80; *WW*, p.35
seeds, root, leaves, stalk

kanlappa phrik กัลปพฤกษ์ — exotic
1. *Cassia grandis* L. — Leguminosae (VJ); *WW*, p.36
2. *Cassia bakeriana* Craib — (Caesalpiniaceae) *WW*, p.36
1. Horse cassia
2. Pink shower
secondary meaning, wishing tree — (VJ)

kannikaa กรรณิกา
Nyctanthes arbor-tristis L. — Verbenaceae (VJ); *WW*, p.5
root

kaphang hom กะพังโหม — see *kraphang hom*

kaphrao กะเพรา — see *kraphrao*

kathee * กะที — exotic (Karen)
Saccharum officiniarum L. — *WW*, p.32

kathi กะทิ
Cocos nucifera L. — Palmae
The cream squeezed from shredded coconut meat, which is oilier than ordinary coconut meat; coconut cream — (VJ)

kathing ton กะทิงต้น

kaa kathing กากะทิง
Calophyllum inophyllum L. Guttiferae *WW*, p.37

kathok rok กะทกรก
khuea eethok เครืออีทก
tee mia buea yaang ตีเมียเบื่อย่าง
Olax scandens Roxb.
root Olacaceae (VJ)
The stem is used as an antidote for poison, and as a stomachic; the root is used as a febrifuge *HE*, p.13

kathue กะทือ see *krathue*

khaa ข่า
Alpinia galanga Swartz Zingiberaceae (VJ); (PT); *LB*, p.59
Alpinia galanga Willd. *HE*, p.2
Greater galangal; Fake galangal; Galangal
rhizome, dried rhizome, young rhizome, mature rhizome, juice from the rhizome
Used as stomachic, carminative and food seasoning *HE*

khaa hom ข่าหอม
khaa luang ข่าหลวง
possibly *Alpinia* sp.

khaa ling ข่าลิง
1. *Globba schomburgkii* Hook. f. Zingiberaceae
2. *Alpinia conchigera* Griff. Zingiberaceae (VJ)

khaa taa daeng ข่าตาแดง
Alpinia sp. Zingiberaceae (PT)
Alpinia galanga Swartz (perhaps)
Red budded galangal

khaai khaao plueak คายข้าวเปลือก see *khaao plueak (khaai)*

khaakrong คากรอง
Imperata cylindrica Beauv. Gramineae (VJ)
root

khaan hua duan คานหัวด้วน

A shoulder pole for carrying any weight, with the end(s), the useful parts, cut or bored by the carpenter bee (*Xylocopa*) and so rendered useless (VJ)

khaao ข้าว
Oryza sativa L. Gramineae (VJ)
Paddy plant; Cooked rice
grain

khaao faang ข้าวฟ่าง
1. *khaao faang haang maa* ข้าวฟ่างหางหมา
2. *khaao faang haang chaang* ข้าวฟ่างหางช้าง
1. *Setaria italica* Beauv. Gramineae
2. *Sorghum vulgare* Pers. Gramineae (VJ)
1. Foxtail millet
2. Sorghum, Korean corn
root

khaao kanyaa ข้าวกัญญา,ข้าวกันยา
Oryza sativa L. var. Gramineae (VJ)
Dark purple, glutinous rice
grain

khaao khaa ข้าวข้า
Euphorbia sessiliflora Roxb. Euphorbiaceae (VJ)
rootstock

khaao khua ข้าวคั่ว
khaao mai ข้าวไหม้
Oryza sativa L. Gramineae
Desmodium thorelli Gagnep. Leguminosae (Papilionaceae)
Diospyros wallichii King et Gamble Ebenaceae (VJ)
Burnt rice, i.e. charred starch (C) and yellow (rice) dextrin made by roasting rice grains (VJ)

khaao mao เมล็ดข้าวเม่า
Ordinary white rice, i.e. husked rice, flattened, then roasted or popped to make rice flakes
malet khaao mao might be the seed of *Antidesma* sp. such as
A. ghaesembilla Gaertn. Stilaginaceae(VJ)

khaao nieo ข้าวเหนียว
Orzya sativa L. var. *glutinosa* Gramineae

White gluten rice

khaao nieo kanyaa ข้าวเหนียวกัญญา(กันยา)
khaao tok kanyaa ข้าวตอกกัญญา
A black variety of gluten rice (VJ)
grain

khaao on (ram) รำข้าวอ่อน (VJ)
Fine rice bran; Rice polishings

khaao phot ข้าวโพด
Zea mays L. Gramineae
Maize; Corn; Indian corn (VJ); *LB*, p.15
kernels, style and stigma

khaao plueak (khaai) คายข้าวเปลือก
Whole grain rice; Rice husks; Paddy; Unmilled rice; Rice still in the husks
(VJ)

*khaao saalee** ข้าวสาลี
Triticum aestivum Lam. Gramineae Wallis, p.8
Wheat

khaao saan ข้าวสาร
Rice; dehusked, uncooked rice; glutinous or non-glutinous (long grain) (VJ)
Rice which has been hulled and cleaned; Milled rice; White rice *Mc*, p.156

khaao saan (ton) ข้าวสารต้น
Raphistemma hooperianum Decn. Asclepiadaceae
R. pulchellum Wall. (VJ)
root

khaao saan dam ข้าวสารดำ
Uncooked, dehusked rice, black in colour, perhaps soiled or stained (VJ)

khaao saan khaang khrok ข้าวสารข้างครก
Uncooked, dehusked white rice which is close to the inner wall of the wooden mortar (VJ)

khaao suk ข้าวสุก
Cooked rice (VJ)

khaao tit naa taphon ข้าวติดหน้าตะโพน
Pounded, sticky cooked rice put at the centre of the skin piece of a drum (*taphon*) and mixed with powdered rice husk charcoal and ash (that is, burnt rice husks) (VJ)

khaao tok ข้าวตอก (VJ)
Popped rice, (that is, white dextrin)

khaao tok kanyaa ข้าวตอกกัญญา see *khaao nieo kanyaa*

khae แค astringent bark
Sesbania grandiflora L. Leguminosae
Cork wood tree (Papilionaceae)
bark (decoction)
The leaves and flowers are used as a mild febrifuge; the bark, as an astringent, and to counteract bacillary dystentery and diarrhoea *HE*, p.16

khae daeng แคแดง astringent bark
Sesbania grandiflora Pers.
Agati; Cork wood tree
There are two varieties - white and red, but they always use the red variety in medicine
bark, bark (decoction) (PT)

khai nao ไข่เน่า
Vitex glabrata R. Br. Verbenaceae
bark, wood (VJ); *HE*, p.19; *LB*, p.496
The bark is used as an anthelmintic; the root as a tonic, and to treat diarrhoea
HE

kham คำ
1. Mineral: Gold
2. Plant: Safflower see *kham foi*

kham foi (*dok*) ดอกคำฝอย sweet flowers
kham (dok) ดอกคำ
Carthamus tinctorius L. Compositae (VJ)
Safflower
flower see Minerals: *kham*

kham ngoh คำเงาะ
kham chaat คำชาด
kham saet คำแสด see *kham Thai*

kham Thai คำไทย sweet flowers
kham ngoh คำเงาะ (VJ)
kham chaat คำชาด
kham saet คำแสด *HE*, p.4
Bixa orellana L. Bixaceae (VJ)
Annatto tree; Arnotto tree
flowers
The seeds are used as a laxative and febrifuge; the flowers, as a tonic, and for dysentery and to treat kidney trouble *HE*
The seed-coat yields an edible colour - Annatto.

khamao lek เขม่าเหล็ก
1. Mineral: Iron oxide Leguminosae
2. Plant: *Dendrobium thorelii* Schindl. (Papilionaceae) (VJ)

khamin ขมิ้น
khamin hua ขมิ้นหัว
Curcuma longa L. Zingiberaceae
Turmeric (VJ)
rhizome, powdered rhizome, root sap

khamin chan ขมิ้นชัน
C. longa L. *Mc* p.141
Turmeric (Long Turmeric) see *khamin kaeng*

khamin kaeng ขมิ้นแกง
khamin chan ขมิ้นชัน
Curcuma longa L. Zingiberaceae
(*C. domestica* Valeton) (VJ); *LB*, p.66

khamin khruea ขมิ้นเครือ toxic
kamphaeng chet chan กำแพงเจ็ดชั้น
Fibraurea tinctoria Lour. Menispermaceae *HE*, p.10; (VJ)
Combretum spp. Combretaceae (VJ)
The stem is used to treat jaundice, and as a carminative; the root, as a carminative, an antiseptic, and in the treatment of eye disease; the leaves are used as an emmenagogue *HE*
F. tinctoria contains berberine (VJ).

khamin oi ขมิ้นอ้อย
Curcuma zedoaria Rosc. Zingiberaceae

(*C. Zerumbet* Roxb.)		(VJ); *LB*, p.9;
Zedoary		*WW*, p.99
rhizome, dried rhizome, long rhizome		

khamot โขมด
taan ตาล
tanot โตนด
taan tanot ตาลโตนด

Nymphaea lotus L.		Nymphaeaceae (PT)
pod		

khan sung คันชุง
khan song คันทรง[misprint]
khan seung คันซึง[misprint]

1.*Colubrina asiatica* Brogn.		Rhamnaceae
C. longipes Back.		
2. *Ancistrocladus cochinchinensis* Gagnep.		Ancistrocladaceae
(*A. tectorius* Merr.)		(VJ)
root		

khanaak ขนาก

Juncellus inundatus C.B. Clarke		Cyperaceae
A kind of sedge plant		(VJ)
root		

khanthatsakon ขันทศกร, ขัญฑสกร		sweet
khanthatsakaraa ขันฑศรรกรา		
Concrete saccharine exudate		(VJ)
Syrup used as medicine; rock sugar, rock candy; thick molasses		*Mc*, p.150

khanun ขนุน	sweet	wood
	oily	seeds
Artocarpus heterophyllus Lamk.		Moraceae
Jackfruit tree		(VJ); *LB*, p.11
root, leaves, ripe and unripe fruit		

khanun lamut ขนุนละมุด	astringent	
	oily	seeds
Artocarpus heterophyllus Lamk.		Moraceae
A tender variety of Jackfruit		(VJ)
kernel, leaves		

khat mon ขัดมอน
Sida rhombifolia L. Malvaceae
Common sida (VJ), *LB*, p.232
root, bark, leaves

khat mon thang 2 ขัดมอนทั้ง๒
1. *Sida corylifolia* Wall. Malvaceae
2. *Sida rhombifolia* L.
Common sida
root

khee aai ขี้อ้าย
Terminalia triptera Stapf. Combretaceae
Walsura villosa Wall.
Walsura robusta Roxb.
W. trichostemon Meg. Meliaceae (VJ)
bark

khee kaa ขี้กา
muun kaa มูลกา
Can be either the white or red variety (*khaao* or *daeng*).
Khee khaa or *muun kaa* has white or red fruit the size of a small apple or large guava; comparable to the Arabian colocynth (VJ)

khee kaa daeng ขี้กาแดง bitter fruit
muun kaa daeng มูลกาแดง
Trichosanthes bracteata Voigt. Cucurbitaceae
T. tricuspidata Lour.
(*T. palmata* Roxb.)
(*T. integrifolia* Kurz)
red variety
fruit, leaves, stem, root
The fruit is a drastic purgative and is also used to treat asthma by smoking; the stem is an expectorant and the root, a febrifuge *HE*, p.18

khee kaa khaao ขี้กาขาว bitter fruit
muun kaa khaao มูลกาขาว
Trichosanthes cordata Roxb. Cucurbitaceae
white variety (VJ); *WW*, p.118
leaves, fruit

khee kaa liam ขี้กาเหลี่ยม	see *kradom*	
khee kaa thang 2 ขี้กาทั้ง๒	bitter	stem
1. *khee kaa khaao* ขี้กาขาว		
2. *khee kaa daeng* ขี้กาแดง		
white and red varieties		
roots, fruit		

*khee kaa thet** ขี้กาเทศ
Citrullus colocynthis (L.) Schrader — Cucurbitaceae
Colocynth; Bitter apple — (VJ)

khee lek ขี้เหล็ก	bitter	heartwood
khee lek baan ขี้เหล็กบ้าน		Leguminosae
Cassia simea Lamk.		(Caesalpiniaceae)
(*C. florida* Vahl.)		*HE*,p.5; *WW*,p.125
Siamese cassia		
heartwood, young leafy shoots, leaves		

The wood is used as a laxative, and for skin diseases; the flowers and young leaves are edible, and are also mildly laxative *HE*

(*bencha*) *khee lek* เบญจขี้เหล็ก
the whole plant. the five parts of the plant. i.e. stem, root, leaves, flowers and fruit
The flowers and young leaves are edible

khee lek paa ขี้เหล็กป่า
Cassia, siamea Lamk. — Leguminosae
Khee lek saan — (Caesalpiniaceae) (VJ)
samae saan — Leguminosae
Cassia garrettiana Craib. — (Caesalpiniaceae) (VJ)

khem daeng เข็มแดง		
1. *Ixora coccinea* L.		Rubiaceae
(*I. grandiflora* Ker.)		
(*I. bandhuca* Roxb.)		(VJ); *LB*, p.554
2. *Rauwolfia serpentina* Benth. ex Kurz	see *rayom*	Apocynaceae (VJ)
root, flowers		

khem lueang เข็มเหลือง
Ixora spp. — Rubiaceae
root — (VJ)

khing ขิง
Zingiber officinalis Roscoe — Zingiberaceae
Ginger — (VJ); *WW*, p.116
rhizome, fresh rhizome, dried rhizome

khing khraeng ขิงแครง
?

khlaa คล้า
Schumannianthus dichotomus Gagnep.
(*Donax arundastrum* Lour.) — Marantaceae
The rhizome is used as a febrifuge, and as an antimalarial — *HE*, p.16

khlai phrachedee ไคลพระเจดีย์
Moss attached to a pagoda.

khlai samao chai ไคลเสมาไชย
Moss attached to a stone tablet, such as a monastery stone mark

khoei taai เขยตาย
Glycosmis cochinchinensis Pierre — Rutaceae (VJ)
fruit

*khoi** ข่อย — astringent and toxic — bark
Streblus asper Lour. — Moraceae *WW*, p.102, *HE*, p.17
Bark-paper tree — Gerini, p.264
Siamese rough bush — *TS*, p.317
An infusion of the roasted leaf is taken to relieve pain during menstruation. The seed is used as a carminative, tonic and stomachic; the root bark as a cardiotonic. The bark is antimicrobial. — *HE*

khok kra-om โคกกระออม — bitter — stem
luup leep khuea [khruea] ลูปลีปเคือ (เครือ)
phot om โพธิ์ออม — *LB*, p.56
Cardiospermum halicacabum L. — Sapindaceae *LB*; *WW*, p.191
Balloon vine; Heart pea — *LB*
leaves, root

khok krasun โคกกระสุน
Tribulus terrestris L. — Zygophyllaceae
Small caltrops; Ground bur-nut — (PT)

khon thaa คนทา
mai see fan ไม้สีฟัน
Harrisonia perforata Merr. Simarubaceae
(*H. benneti* A.W.) (VJ); *LB*, p.297; *HE*, p.11
leaves, bark, root
The root is used as an antipyretic and to treat malaria, diarrhoea and dysentery *HE*
Small branches are used as tooth brushes (VJ)

khon thee khamao คนทีเขมา
Vitex negundo L. Verbenaceae (VJ); *LB*, p.497
leaves, root, flowers, fruit

khon thee so คนทีสอ
Vitex trifolia L. Verbenaceae
fruit, leaves, root (VJ); *LB*, p.499
The root is used as a diuretic, diaphoretic, antipyretic and stomachic, as well as being used in the treatment of liver and eye diseases *HE*, p.19

khondok ขอนดอก bland
1. *ton tabaek* ต้นตะแบก astringent bark
2. *phikun* พิกุล cool and fragrant flowers
1. *Lagerstroemia floribunda* Jack. Lythraceae
2. *Mimusops elengi* L. Sapotaceae
flowers, bark,wood
The wood of old trees infested by fungi is called *khondok* (VJ); *LB*, pp.59, 413

khong khaa dueat คงคาเดือด
talai khong khaa ตะไลคงคา
Arfeuillea arborescens Pierre Sapindaceae
bark, root (VJ); *LB*, p.339; *TS*

khong saam yaan ฆ้องสามย่าน
Kalanchoe lanciniata DC. Crassulaceae
leaves (VJ); *LB*, p.101

khop chanaang ขอบชะนาง toxic
Pouzolzia pentandra Benn. (VJ) *LB*, p.14; *HE*,p.15
P. indica (L.) Gaud. Urticaceae *LB;* (VJ)
leaves
The aerial parts are used as an anthelmintic, insecticide, emmenagogue and for leucorrhoea *HE*

khop chanaang thang 2 ขอบชะนางทั้ง๒ toxic
1. *khop chanaang khaao* ขอบชะนางขาว
2. *khop chanaang daeng* ขอบชะนางแดง
The white variety and the red variety of *khop chanaang* leaves, of which there are 2 species. The colour of the leaves of the same species is due to the location of the plant - whether in the open or in the shade. (VJ)

khraam คราม Leguminosae
Indigofera tinctoria L., and (Papilionaceae)
other *Indigofera* spp.
Indigo (VJ); *LB*, p.172
root

khraam dee ครามดี Leguminosae
Indigofera tinctoria L. (Papilionaceae) (VJ)
root

khraam thang 3 ครามทั้ง๓ Leguminosae
1. *Indigofera hirsuta* L. (Papilionaceae)
2. *I. suffruticosa* Mill.
3. *I. tinctoria* L. (VJ)
leaves

khrai bok ไคร้บก
?

khrai haang naat ไคร้หางนาค
1. *Phyllanthus taxodiifolius* Beille Euphorbiaceae (PT)
2. *Rotula aquatica* Lour. Ehretiaceae (VJ)

khrai hom ไคร้หอม
takhrai hom ตะไคร้หอม *TS*
Cympogonon nardus Rendle (VJ)
Citronella grass *TS*
leaves

khrai khruea ไคร้เครือ bitter root
Jasminum sp. Oleaceae
root (VJ)
Not to be confused with *khrai khruea ton* or *khrai ton*

khrai nam ไคร้น้ำ
Homonoia riparia Lour. Euphorbiaceae (PT)
root, leaf cell sap

khrai ton ไคร้ต้น
khaa ton ข่าต้น
khrai khruea ton ไคร้เครือต้น[misprint]
thep thaaro เทพทาโร
takrai ton ตะไคร้ต้น
Cinnamomum ilicioides Cheval
C. siamense Craib
C. porrectum Kostern
(*C. parthenoxylon* Nees) Lauraceae (VJ)
root

khrop chakrawaan ครอบจักรวาฬ
Abutilon graveolens W. et A. Malvaceae (VJ); *LB*, p.39
Abutilon hirtum Sweet *TS*, p.1
bark, root

khukha คุคะ
Smilax sp. Smilacaceae (PT)

khuun คูน
ton khuun ต้นคูน Leguminosae
1. *Cassia fistula* L. (Caesalpiniaceae)
(*Cathartocarpus fistula* Pers.) (VJ); *HE*
2. *Colocasia gigantea* Hook. f. Araceae (VJ)
Golden shower tree; Purging cassia; Indian laburnam
root
All parts are used as a purgative *HE*

*klaam maphraao** กล้ามมะพร้าว
The shiny white surface of coconut meat (VJ)

klinchong กลินจง[misprint] see *linchong*

kloi กลอย
Dioscorea hispida Dennst. Dioscoreaceae *WW*, p.13
(*D. triphylla* L.) (VJ)
Wild yam

tuber

kluai mai กล้วยไม้
orchid (VJ)

(mai) kluai ไม้กล้วย
Musa spp.
Usually *Musa sapientum* L. Musaceae (VJ)
Edible banana
fruit, root

kluai taanee กล้วยตานี
Musa balbisiana Colla Musaceae (VJ)
cell sap, decayed rootstock

kluai teep กล้วยตีบ
Musa sapientum L. Musaceae
(a variety with fruit with angular fingers and very astringent cell sap) (VJ)
root, sap

kot chadaa mangsee โกฏฐ์ชดามังสี, โกฏฐ์ชฎามังสี
Nardostachys jatamansi DC. Valeriaceae
Nard

kot chiang โกฏฐ์เชียง sweet root
Levisticum officinale Koch Umbelliferae (VJ)
Lovage
root and rhizome

kot chulaa lamphaa โกฏฐ์จุฬาลัมพา
Artemisia vulgaris L. Compositae (VJ); *FT*, p.1187
Mugwort; Wormwood; Motherwort
leaves

kot hua bua โกฏฐ์หัวบัว oily
Angelica archangelica L. Umbelliferae (VJ)
root

kot kaan phraao โกฏฐ์ก้านพร้าว bitter
Picrorhiza kurroa Benth. exotic Scrophulariaceae
(VJ); *LB*, p.82

kot kakling โกฏฐ์กะกลิ้ง	toxic	seeds
tumkaa daeng [*tuumkaa daeng*] ตุมกาแดง (ตูมกาแดง)		*LB*, p.67; *WW*, p.347
salaeng chai แสลงใจ		*LB*; *HE*, p.17
salaeng thon แสลงโทน		*LB*
Strychnos nux-vomica L.		(VJ); *LB*; *HE*; *WW*
S. nux blanda A.W. Hill		(PT)
Contains strychnine		Strychnaeaceae (Loganiaceae)
Nux-vomica tree; Dog button; Quaker button; Poison nut seeds		*LB*

The dry, ripe seed of *S. nux-vomica* (that is, nux-vomica) is called *kot kakling*.
The seeds are used as a tonic, diuretic, spinal cord stimulant, and as a dog and rat poison.
HE

kot kakraa โกฏฐ์กักรา		
kot kakkraa โกฏฐ์กักกรา		
Anacyclus pyrethrum (L.) DC.		Compositae
Pellitory		(VJ)
root		

kot khamao โกฏฐ์เขมา		
Atractyloides lyrata Lieb. et Zucc.		Compositae
Atractylis		(VJ); *TPS2*, p.26

kot kraduuk โกฏฐ์กระดูก	oily	
Saussurea lappa Clarke		Compositae
Costus		(VJ); *TPS2*, p.19
rhizome		

kot nam tao โกฏฐ์น้ำเต้า	astringent	
Rheum officinale Baillon		
Rheum palmatum L.		Polygonaceae (VJ)
Medicinal rhubarb		
rootstock		
Laxative		

kot phung plaa โกฏฐ์พุงปลา	astringent	
Terminalia chebula Retz.		Combretaceae
Black myrobalans		(VJ); *TPS2*, p.85
Galls from leaves or twigs		

kot so โกฏฐ์สอ	bitter	

kot so thet โกฏฐ์สอเทศ
Angelica sylvestris L. Umbelliferae (VJ)

kot thang 5 โกฏฐ์ทั้ง๕
1. *kot chiang* โกฏฐ์เชียง
2. *kot so* โกฏฐ์สอ
3. *kot hua bua* โกฏฐ์หัวบัว
4. *kot khamao* โกฏฐ์เขมา
5. *kot chulaa lamphaa* โกฏฐ์จุฬาลัมพา (VJ); *KSY*, p.301

The 5 *kot*.

kot thang 7 โกฏฐ์ทั้ง๗
The 5 *kot*, plus
6. *kot kraduuk* โกฏฐ์กระดูก
7. *kot kaan phraao* โกฏฐ์ก้านพร้าว (VJ); *KSY*, p.301

The 7 *kot*.

kot thang 9 โกฏฐ์ทั้ง๙
The 7 *kot*, plus
8. *kot phung plaa* โกฏฐ์พุงปลา
9. *kot chadaa mangsee* โกฏฐ์ชฎามังสี (VJ); *KSY*, p.301

The 9 *kot*.

kraai กราย astringent fruit; bark
praai ปราย[misprint]
plaai ปลาย
1. Fish
2. Plant:

Xylopia malayana Hook. f. et Thom. Annonaceae (VJ)
fruit

kraam chaang กรามช้าง
1. Molar tooth of an elephant. see *chaang* (animal)
2. Plant: *kraam chaang* (*kluai*) กล้วยกรามช้าง

A species of banana *Mc*, p.51
root

kraam daeng กรามแดง
khraam daeng ครามแดง

possibly *khrang daeng* ครางแดง
Albizia odoratissima Benth. — Mimosaceae
Black siris, Ceylon rosewood — FT, p.606
root

kraam raet (*ton*) ต้นกรามแรด
Aralia armata Seem. (Chumpon) — Araliaceae (VJ); *WW*, p.7

krabao กระเบา — toxic — seeds
kabao กะเบา
krabao nam กระเบาน้ำ(female plant)
kaeo kaa long แก้วกาหลง (male plant only)
Hydnocarpus anthelmintica Pierre (female plant only) — (VJ); *LB*, p.37
(*Gynocardia odorata* Pierre) (male plant)
Hydnocarpus kurzii Warb.(both male and female plants)
Chaulmoogra — Flacourtiaceae
roasted seeds, bark
The pulp contains cyanogenetic glycosides. Oil from the seeds is used to treat leprosy by injection; formerly leprosy was treated by fumigation by burning the seeds. (VJ)

krabian กระเบียน — toxic — seeds
Gardenia turgida Roxb. — Rubiaceae
bark, seeds — (VJ); *TS*, p.160

krabue chet tua กระบือเจ็ดตัว
Excoecaria bicolor Hassk. — Euphorbiaceae (VJ)
Excoecaria cochinchinensis Lour. var. *viridis* Merr.
leaves
The twigs are used as an abortifacient and uterine stimulant — *HE*, p.9

krachaai กระชาย — hot-and-spicy — root
krasaai กระชาย[misprint] — salty — leaf
Boesenbergia pandurata Holt. — Zingiberaceae (VJ)
(*Gastrochilus panduratus* Ridl.) — *LB* 70; *HE*, p.10
rhizome, root, dried root
diuretic, tonic, for dysentery — *HE*, p.10

krachaai thang 2 กระชายทั้ง๒
yellow variety and purple (dark) variety — (VJ); *LB* 70; *HE*, p.10

krachao daeng กระเช้าแดง

Holoptelea integrifolia Planch. Ulmaceae (VJ)
red variety

krachao khaao กระเช้าขาว
Holoptelea integrifolia Planch. Ulmaceae (VJ)
white variety
leaf cell sap, root

krachao thang 2 กระเช้าทั้ง๒
krachao khaao and *krachao daeng* กระเช้าขาว,กระเช้าแดง
Holoptelea integrifolia Planch. Ulmaceae (VJ)
white and red varieties
leaf cell sap

krachap กระจับ
Trapa bicornis L. Trapaceae (VJ)
T. bispinosa Roxb. *LB* p.395
Water chestnut
raw kernel, fruit, root
cf. *haeo sot*

krachap bok กระจับบก
a woody vine, with flat triangular fruit (VJ)
root

kradaan phon กระดานพน
Gardenia turgida Roxb. Rubiaceae (VJ)
root

kradaat กระดาด

kradaat khaao กระดาดขาว
Alocasia indica (Roxb.) Schott Araceae (VJ); *TS*, p.16; (PT)

kradaat daeng กระดาดแดง
Alocasia indica (Roxb.) Schott var. *metallica* Schott (VJ); (PT)

kradaat thang 2 กระดาดทั้ง๒
kradaat khaao and *kradaat daeng* กระดาดขาว,กระดาดแดง

kradang ngaa กระดังงา cool and fragrant flowers
kradang ngaa Thai กระดังงาไทย

kradang ngaa yai กระดังงาใหญ่
Canangrum odoratum Baill. — Annonaceae
(*Canangium odorata* Hook. f. et Th.) — (VJ); *LB*, p.55
Ylang-ylang; Ilang-ilang
leaves, flowers
Oil of ylang-ylang is used in perfumery

kradom กระดอม — bitter — fruit
kadom กะดอม
khee kaa liam ขี้กาเหลี่ยม — (VJ)
Gymnopetalum cochinchinense Kurz — Cucurbitaceae
flowers, fruit, whole plant — (VJ); *HE*, p.10; *WW*, p.285
The fruit is used as a tonic; cholagogue; and antidote for poisoning

kradom thang 5 กระดอมทั้ง๕
bencha kradom เบญจกระดอม
Gymnopetalum cochinchinense
whole plant, i.e. stem, leaves, roots, flowers and fruit

kradong daeng กระโดงแดง — see *fin ton*

krak khee กรักขี
krak chee กรัชี[misprint]
sak khee สักขี — (PT)
Dalbergia or *Cudranea* — (VJ)
Prismatomeris malayana Ridl. — Rubiaceae (VJ); (PT)
Dalbergia candenatensis Prain — Papilionaceae
Maclura cochinchinensis Corner — Moraceae
(*Cudranea*) — (PT); *TS* pp.106,216
P. malayana is *krak* or *krak phee* — *TS*, p.275

kralam phak กระลำพัก — bitter
1. *ton taa tum* ต้นตาตุ่ม — hot-and-spicy — latex
taa tum thale ตาตุ่มทะเล — *PB*, p.68; *WW*, p.325
2. *salat dai* สลัดได — *HE*, p.9
salat dai paa สลัดไดป่า — *LB*, p.45
1. *Excoecaria agallocha* — Euphorbiaceae *WW*, p.325
2. *Euphorbia antiquorum* L. — *HE*, p.9; *PB*, p.68; *WW*, p.679
1. Blind your eyes — *PB*, p.68
2. Triangular spurge — *LB*, p.45
heartwood of either 1 or 2, woodsap of 2

krameng กระเม็ง toxic
kameng กะเม็ง
Eclipta alba (L.) Hassk. Compositae
(*E. erecta* L.) (VJ); *LB*, p.589
Eclipta prostrata L.
(*E. alba* Hassk.)
(*E. erecta* Hassk.)
leaves
The cell sap is used to relieve the pain of toothache, as an antibacterial for wounds, and as a hair dye *HE*, p.9

kraphang hom กระพังโหม
kaphang hom กะพังโหม
phak mai ผักไหม *HE*, p.15
Oxystelma esculentum (L. f.) R. Br. Asclepiadaceae
root (VJ); *HE*
The aerial parts are used as a laxative for infants; and as an antimicrobial *HE*

kraphang hom thang 2 กระพังโหมทั้ง๒ - incorrectly named should be
yaan phaa hom ย่านพาโหม or
ton tot muu kap ton tot maa ต้นตดหมูกับต้นตดหมา
Paederia foetida L.
P. linearis Hook. f.
P. pilifera Hook. f.
P. pilosa Craib
P. tomentosa Blume. (VJ)

kraphang hom thang 5 กระพังโหมทั้ง๕
the whole plant of *kraphang hom* (*Oxystelma esculentum*)

kraphrao กระเพรา hot-and-spicy leaf; root
kaphrao กะเพรา
Ocimum sanctum L. Labiatae
Sacred basil (VJ)
leaves, root, seeds

kraphrao thang 2 กระเพราทั้ง๒
both the white and red varieties (VJ)

kraphrao thang 5 กระเพราทั้ง๕ *LB*, p.511

the whole plant, i.e. the stem, leaves, root, flowers and fruit

krasaai กระชาย [as an ingredient is a misprint] see *krachaai*

krasaai กระชาย or *nam krasaai* น้ำกระชาย means (medicinal) vehicle or excipient

krathiam กระเทียม
Allium sativum L. Alliaceae
Garlic cloves (Amaryllidaceae)
bulb, dried, cooked or crisp (PT); *TS*, p.15; (VJ)

krathin กระถิน
kathin กะถิน
Leucaena glauca Leguminosae (PT); *Mc*, p.32
The wild or horse tamarind

krathin daeng กระถินแดง
krathin wimaan กระถินวิมาน
Dichrostachys cinerea Wight et Arn. Leguminosae
The bark is used to treat diarrhoea

krathin thet กระถินเทศ
krathin hom กระถินหอม
Acacia farnesina Willd. Leguminosae (PT; (VJ)
(Mimosaceae) *HE*; *TS*, p.2
The gum is used as a demulcent and as an emulsifying agent *HE*
The bark is astringent, and the pods contain a balsamic liquid used medicinally *Mc*, p.32

krathing กระทิง
1. Animal
2. Fish
3. Plant:
krathing (*ton*) ต้นกระทิง
kathing กะทิง
kaa kathing กากะทิง
Calophyllum inophyllum L. Guttiferae (VJ); *HE*
Borneo mahogany
Alexandrian laurel *LB*, p.199
root, leaves and bark
The flowers are used as an ingredient in aromatic powder, the leaf juice in eye drops for conjunctivitis, and the seed oil is applied to joints to relieve pain *HE*

krathue กระทือ hot-and-spicy rhizome
kathue กะทือ
Zingiber zerumbet Smith Zingiberaceae
(*Zingiber aromaticum* Val.) (VJ); *TS*, p.355; HE, p.19
Wild ginger
rhizome, dried or fresh
nam kathue mok fai น้ำกะทือหมกไฟ- the cell sap squeezed from the rhizome after it has been covered with ash and heated under a stove VJ
The rhizome is used as a galactogogue, carminative, diuretic and tonic *HE*

krathuep yop กระทืบยอบ
krathuep yot กระทืบยอด[misprint]
1. *Biophytum sensitivum* DC. Oxalidaceae
(*Biophytum apodiscias* Edgew. et Hook f.)
2. *B. petersianum* Klotzsch
3. *B. adiantoides* Wight ex Edgew. et Hook. f. (VJ)
the whole plant

krathum khee muu กระทุ่มขี้หมู toxic leaves
astringent bark
Mitragyna brunonis Craib Rubiaceae (VJ); *WW*, p.378
leaves, bark

krathum naa กระทุ่มนา
kathom khee muu กะท่อมขี้หมู
Mitragyna javanica Koord. et Val. var. *microphylla* Craib Rubiaceae (VJ)
leaves

krathung maa baa กระทุงหมาบ้า toxic root
nguan muu ง้วนหมู (VJ)
huan muu ฮ้วนหมู (VJ)
Wattakaka volubilis (L. f.) Stapf. *WW*, p.378; *HE*, p.19
(*Dregea volubilis* Benth.) Asclepiadaceae *HE*
leaves, root
The root is used as a diuretic and as an antimicrobial *HE*

krawaan กระวาน hot-and-spicy fruit
krawaan khaao กระวานขาว
Amomum krervanh Pierre Zingiberaceae
Siam cardamon; Camphor seed (VJ); *LB*, p.8

seeds, fruit
The seeds are used as a carminative, expectorant, and stomachic *HE*

krisanaa กฤษณา   toxic   seed oil
cool and fragrant   wood
1. *A. crassna* Pierre ex H. Lee.   Thymelaeaceae(VJ)
2. *A. malaccensis* Lamk.   (VJ); *HE*, p.2
(*Aquilaria agallocha* Roxb.)   (VJ)
Eagle wood; Aloes wood; Agaric wood
The wood is used as a heart stimulant   *HE*

krop kraep กรอบแกรบ
a succulent-leafed vine   Vitidaceae (VJ)

krot กรด   astringent   root
Combretum tetralophum C.B. Clarke   Combretaceae
C. trifoliatum Vent.   (VJ)
root

*krot** กรอด
Bird   see *nok krot*

krung khamao กรุงเขมา
Cissampelos pareira L.   Menispermaceae
root, leaves   (VJ); *LB*, p.76
The roots are used as a febrifuge, to treat jaundice, and to treat eye diseases *HE*

kua kai กั่วไก่misprint] see *thua kai*
root

kulaap กุลาบ
Rosa damescena Miller   Rosaceae
Rosa chinensis Jacq.   (VJ), *LB*, p.63
Rose; Damask rose (*kulaap mon*)
kulaap is an Iranian word for rose water, called in Thai, *nam dok mai thet* น้ำดอกไม้เทศ(aromatic water made from exotic flowers)   (VJ)

kum thang 2 กุ่มทั้ง๒   hot-and-spicy   bark
1. *kum nam* กุ่มน้ำ
2. *kum bok* กุ่มบก
1. *Crataeva magna* DC.   Capparidaceae
(*C. nurvale* Ham.)   (VJ), *LB*, p.93

Crataeva adansonii DC. subsp. *trifoliata* Jacobs — *HE*, p.6
(*C. erythrocarpa* Gagnep.) — (VJ); *LB*, p.94
2. *Crataeva religiosa* Ham.
The heartwood is used as a diuretic; the leaves as a diaphoretic; the bark as a carminative, as a diaphoretic, and to treat hiccoughs; and the root as an antibiotic and stomachic *HE*

laan ลาน
Corypha umbraculifera L. — Palmae (PT); *TS*, p.94
Fan palm; Talipot palm; Lontar palm
leaves

lahung daeng ละหุ่งแดง
Ricinus communis L. — Euphorbiaceae (VJ)
Castor oil plant
root

lam chiak ลำเจียก (male plant) — cool and fragrant — flowers
toei เตย (female plant) — (VJ)
Pandanus tectorius Sol. — Pandanaceae (PT)
flowers, young twigs

lamduan ลำดวน — cool and fragrant — flowers
Sphaerocoryne claviceps Craib — Annonaceae
(*Polyalthia aberrans* Maingay)
Melodorum fructicosum Lour. — (VJ)
root, flowers

*lamphan** ลำพัน
a tree which is not used in medicine — (VJ)
Perhaps a misprint for *amphan*, or an abbreviation of *lamphan haang muu*

lamphan haang muu ลำพันหางหมู
Enhalus aconoides Rich. et Stered. — Hydrocharitaceae
The dugong likes to eat *lamphan haang muu.* It is sometimes called *hua ngo thale* sea sweet flag, which is a different plant from sweet flag. — (VJ)

lamphan thong ลำพันทอง
misprint for *amphan thong*

lamphong ลำโพง — toxic — seeds, root, flowers
Datura alba L. — Solanaceae *HE*, p.8; *TS*, p.108
D. metel L. — *WW*, p.680

Thorn apple
leaves, fruit juice

(*bencha*) *lamphong* เบญจลำโพง
the whole plant of *lamphong*

lamphong kaa salak ลำโพงกาสลัก
D. fastuosa L. Solanaceae *HE*, p.8
Dark violet double-flowered variety *WW*
Black thorn apple *HE*
flowers
The flowers are used for smoking to relieve asthma; the seeds for skin diseases; and the powdered root is applied to relieve inflammation *HE*

lamut ละมุด
1. *lamut farang* ละมุดฝรั่ง
2. *lamut seedaa* ละมุดสีดา
1. *Achras zapota* L. Sapotaceae (PT)
2. *Madhuca esculenta* Fletcher Sapotaceae (PT)
1. Sapodilla; Chiku tree *Mc*, p.733
1. kernel
2. young twigs

lan thom ลั่นทม
Plumeria acuminata Ait. Apocynaceae *HE*, p.15
P. acutifolia Poir.
Frangipanni
root
The heartwood is used as an alterative for women *HE*

lao เหล้า see *suraa*

lao lak เหลาหลัก
fruit
A species of areca nut having soft rind *Mc*, p.944

la-ong phra krit ละอองพระกฤษ
leaves

lep mue naang (ton mai) เล็บมือนางต้นไม้ toxic root
Quisqualis indica L. *HE*, p.15; (VJ); *WW*, p.696
Q. densiflora Wall. (VJ); *WW*

(*Q. conferta* Excell.) (VJ)
Rangoon creeper Combretaceae
root
The kernel is used as an anthelmintic for roundworm and threadworm *HE*
If used as an anthelmintic, it is *Quisqualis.*
There is also a shrub by this name. The bark is used as a fish poison, and contains a large number of saponins. In Hong Kong it is called Goat's horn. This is *Aegiceras corniculatum* Blanco (A. majus Gaertn.) Aegicerandaceae, but this has not been used in medicine as far as can be ascertained. (VJ)

lian เลี่ยน bitter leaves
Melia azedarach L. Meliaceae
Persian lilac; Chinaberry tree (VJ); *HE*, p.12; *WW*, p.698
leaf sap, bark, bark sap

liang paa เลียงผา
Captricornis sumatraensis (VJ)

lin chong ลินจง
len chong เลนจง(*Khmer*)
klin chong กลินจง[misprint]
Nymphaea cyanea L. Nymphaeaceae (VJ)
flowers, pollen see *bua phan*

lot โลด
1. *Aporusa villosa* Baill. Euphorbiaceae (PT); *TS*, p.28
2. Symplocos racemosa Roxb. Symplocaceae (VJ)
2. Lodh tree
This yields Lotur or Lodh bark (VJ)
bark

lot thanong โลดทนง
Trigonostemon reidiides Craib Euphorbiaceae *HE*, p.18; (PT)
The root causes nausea and vomiting *HE*

lueat raet เลือดแรด
1. Rhinoceros blood
2. Plant: *lueat raet (ton)* เลือดแรดต้น oily
?

luuk ลูก
In botanical terms, fruit or seed

maa mieo ม่าเมียว
1. A superior kind of *Eugenia malaccensis* L. Myrtaceae (VJ)
2. An animal

maak หมาก astringent root
Areca catechu Palmae (VJ)
Areca nut; Betel nut; Areca palm; Betel palm
seeds (nuts), ripe areca nut (*maak song*), juice, fruit, rind juice
The seeds are used as a taeniafuge (VJ)

maak khaao nieo หมากข้าวเหนียว
The almost ripe seed of the areca nut (VJ)

*(nam chaan) maak** น้ำชานหมาก
The juice of a chewed quid of betel leaf and areca nut see *phluu*

(*nam*) *maak dip* น้ำหมากดิบ
fresh unripe areca nut sap

(thalaai) maak dip ทลายหมากดิบ
A bunch of areca fruit when still green and soft

(nam thalaai) maak dip น้ำทลายหมากดิบ
Decoction of the still green and fresh rachis of the bunch of unripe areca fruit. The fruit is removed and the remaining rachis is used.
Thalaai has two meanings. The rachis is called *thalaai*, but with the fruit it is called *thalaai maak*, meaning a bunch of fruit. (VJ)

1. *maak phuu* หมากผู้ bland leaf
2. *maak mia* หมากเมีย astringent root
1. male plant
2. female plant
   Cordyline fruiticosa Goeppert Liliaceae
   (*C. terminalis* Kunth.)
   Dracaena palm (but this is not a palm)
   Ti plant (Hawaii)

leaves, root
Both male and female leaves can occur on the same species. The leaves can be green and pink. The male leaf is narrow, the female leaf, large. Hawaiian skirts are made from the Ti leaf blade, which resembles strips of banana leaf blade. Thai people put the leaf of *Cordyline fruiticosa* into water and use the water to bathe to relieve skin inflammation.

(VJ)

*maak mok** หมากหมก see *mok*

(*bencha*) *maatsalaa* เบญจมาศลา
?

madan มะดัน
Garcinia schomburgkiana Pierre Guttiferae (PT)

(*bencha*) *madan* เบญจมะดัน
the five parts of the plant: stem, leaves, root, flowers and fruit

maduea มะเดื่อ
madue มะดือ[misprint]
Ficus spp. *WW*, p.303
leaves, bark, young twigs

maduea din มะเดื่อดิน
Aganosma marginata G. Don. (PT); *FT*, p.1022
root sap

maeng lak แมงลัก hot-and-spicy leaf
Ocimum canum Sims Labiatae (PT)
(*O. americanum* L.)
Hoary basil
root, leaves

maeng lak thang 2 มแงลักทั้ง๒
stem and leaves of *maeng lak* (PT)

mafai มะไฟ sour fruit
Baccaurea sapida Muell.-Arg. Euphorbiaceae
leaves, root (VJ); *WW*, p.570,
The fruit looks like a langsat *Lansium domesticum* Corr. Meliaceae (VJ)

(*bencha*) *mafai* เบญจมะไฟ
the five parts of the plant: stem, leaves, root, flowers and fruit

mafai duean haa มะไฟเดือนห้า
Scoparia dulcis L. Scrophulariaceae (PT)

mafo มะฝ่อ
Trewia nudiflora L. Euphorbiaceae (PT)
root

mafueang มะเฟือง
mafueang prieo มะเฟืองเปรี้ยว sour fruit
mafueang waan มะเฟืองหวาน sweet fruit
Averrhoa carambola L. Averrhoaceae (PT)
leaves, fruit

mahaa kaan มหากาฬ,
waan mahaa kaan ว่านมหากาฬ
Gynura pseudo-china DC. Compositae (VJ)
rhizome

mahaa lalaai มหาละลาย
Gynura procumbens Lour. Compositae (VJ)
leaves

mahaa hing มหาหิงคุ์
hing yaang pho หิงคุ์ยางโพ
hingu Pāli and Skt
Ferula foetida Regel Umbelliferae
F. assa-foetida L.
Ferula spp.
Asafoetida
gum
hing yaang pho (sticky asafoetida) is a kind of asafoetida which looks like the concentrated latex of the Bo tree. The edition of *KPC* of B.E.2495 (A.D. 1952) uses *mahaa hing* for *hing* . (VJ)

mahaat มะหาด
haat nun หาดหนุน
Artocarpus lakoocha Roxb. Moraceae (PT)
heartwood, bark
Heartwood chips are boiled and the floating matter is dried. This is called *puak haat.* (VJ)

mahaatsadam มหาสดำ
Alsophila laterosa Hook. Cyatheaceae

Alsophila glabra Hook. *PB*, p.3
A tree fern.
rhizome and stipes (VJ)

mai ไม้
ton mai ต้นไม้
tree

mai bong ไม้บง
Dendrocalamus brandisii Kurz Gramineae
Ternstroemia sp. Theaceae (VJ)
The sawdust of *Ternstroemia* sp. is used to make joss sticks (PT)

mai daeng ไม้แดง
Xylia kerrii Craib et Hutch. Leguminosae (PT)
bark

*mai kluai** ไม้กล้วย
katthalee กัทลี
Musa spp.
Usually *Musa sapientum* L. Musaceae (VJ)
Edible banana
root, fruit

*mai phai** ไม้ไผ่
mai wen ไม้เวฬุ see *phai mai*

mai ruak ไม้รวก
ruak รวก
phai ruak ไผ่รวก
Thyrostachys siamensis Gumble Gramineae (VJ); TS, p.331
Called Feathery bamboo, but it is not the same genus
outer covering, enamelled rind (*phiu* ผิว)

mai thao yaai mom ไม้เท้ายายม่อม see *thao yaai mom*

makaa มะกา bitter leaves
Bridelia burmanica Hook. f. Euphorbiaceae *HE*, p.4
leaves
The leaves are used as a purgative and emmenagogue and to treat dysentery *HE*

makhaam มะขาม		astringent	bark, seeds, pod
makhaam khop มะขามขบ		oily	roasted seeds
makhaam kradaan มะขามกระดาน		sour	fruit juice
makhaam khee maeo มะขามขี้แมว		sweet	Leguminosae

Tamarindus indica L. (Caesalpiniaceae)
Tamarind (VJ); (PT); *HE*, p.17
m. kradaan has a large pod with sour pulp
m. khee maeo has a small pod with sweet pulp
bark, the ripe fruit pulp (*makhaam piak*), flowers, roasted seed shells, leaves, root
The pulp is used as a mild laxative, and refrigerant; the heartwood is used as an expectorant *HE*

(*nam*) *makhaam piak* น้ำมะขามเปียก
nam som makhaam piak น้ำส้มมะขามเปียก
A triturate of ripe sour fruit pulp of the tamarind in water

makhaam pom มะขามป้อม
Phyllanthus emblica L. Euphorbiaceae
Malacca tree; Emblic myrobalans; Indian gooseberry (VJ); *HE*, p.13; *WW*, p.110
The fruit is an anti-scorbutic see *tree phalaa* *HE*

makham dee khwaai มะคำดีควาย see *prakham dee khwaai*

makham kai มะคำไก่ see *prakham kai*
leaves

makhuea มะเขือ
Solanum melongena L. Solanaceae
Egg plant; Aubergine
seeds
There are many kinds, shapes and sizes of egg plant, all edible (VJ)

makhuea khuen มะเขือขื่น
Solanum xanthocarpum Schrad. et Wendl. Solanaceae
(*S. aculeatissimum* Jacq.) (PT)
root, fruit

makhuea thang 2 มะเขือทั้ง๒
1. *makhuea* มะเขือ
2. *makhuea proh* มะเขือเปราะ
2. *Solanum melongena* L. Solanaceae (VJ)

Green egg plant
root

makhwit มะขวิด astringent sap
Feronia limonia Swing. Rutaceae
(*Feronia elephantum* Corr.) (VJ)
Elephant apple
leaves, bark, sap from the bark, young twigs

maklam dam มะกล่ำดำ Leguminosae
Abrus fruticulosus Wall. ex Wight et Arn. (Papilionaceae) (VJ)

maklam ton มะกล่ำต้น
1. *Adenanthera pavonina* L. Leguminosae
2. *Adenanthera microsperma* Teyson et Binn. (Mimosaceae (VJ))
fruit

maklam khaao มะกล่ำขาว
maklam phueak มะกล่ำเผือก
Abrus cantoniensis Hance var. *bossel* Craib Leguminosae (PT) (VJ)
fruit (Papilionaceae)

maklam khruea มะกล่ำเครือ Leguminosae
Abrus praecatorius L. (Papilionaceae) (VJ)
Indian liquorice
leaves

maklam taa chaang มะกล่ำตาช้าง Leguminosae
Adenanthera pavonina L. (Mimosaceae)
Sandalwood tree; Fake red sandal (PT)
fruit

maklam taa nuu มะกล่ำตาหนู Leguminosae
Abrus praecatorius (Papilionaceae) (VJ)

maklam thang 2 มะกล่ำทั้ง๒
maklam ton มะกล่ำตน
maklam khruea มะกล่ำเขรือ
root

makluea มะเกลือ toxic root and fruit

Diospyros mollis Griff. salty bark of the trunk or stem
bark, root, fruit, seeds, fruit juice Ebenaceae *HE*, p.8; *WW*, p.80
The pulp juice of fresh, unripe fruit is used as an anthelmintic for all kinds of intestinal worms *HE*

makluea lueat มะเกลือเลือด
1. *Terminalia corticosa* Pierre ex Laness Combretaceae (PT); *TS*, p.327
bark
2. *Terminalia mucronata* Craig et Hutch. (VJ)

makok มะกอก astringent leaf
Spondias pinnata Kurz Anacardiaceae
bark, seeds, root sap, fruit

makok bok มะกอกบก
root
possibly synonym for *makok nam* q.v.

makok nam มะกอกน้ำ
Elaeocarpus huygrophilus Kurz Elaeocarpaceae (VJ)
(E. madopetalus Pierre)
root

makok thet มะกอกเทศ
makok farang มะกอกฝรั่ง
Spondias dulcis Forst. f. Anacardiaceae
(*S. cythera* Sonn.)
fruit

makruut มะกรูด
makruut yai มะกรูดใหญ่
Citrus hystrix DC. Rutaceae (VJ); *HE*
Porcupine orange; Leech lime; Kaffir lime.
fruit rind, seeds, bark
makruut yai is just a healthy plant which gives large fruit; some special varieties are sweet, but the ordinary fruit is sour. The fruit pulp is an antiscorbutic; the fruit rind and leaves are used to season food *HE*

malako มะละกอ
1. *malako tua phuu* มะละกอตัวผู้
2. *malako tua mia* มะละกอตัวเมีย
1. male tree

2. female tree
Carica papaya L. (PT)
Papaya
root

malet เมล็ด
seeds

malet khaao mao เมล็ดข้าวเม่า see *khaao mao*

mali มะลิ cool and fragrant flowers
mali son มะลิซ้อน
mali laa มะลิลา
Jasminum sambac, Ait. Oleaceae (PT); *TS*, p.194
mali son is the double variety
mali laa is the single variety
Jasmine
flowers, root, flower water

mali wan มะลิวัลย์ cool and fragrant flowers
Jasminum anastemosans Wall. Oleaceae (PT)
root, flowers, flower water, leaf sap

mamia มะเมีย see *maphuu*

mamuang มะม่วง astringent seed
mamuang kalon มะม่วงกะล่อน (PT)
chok ช้อก *Mc*, p.283
Mangifera indica L. Anacardiaceae (VJ)
Mango
cell sap, seed

mamuang khan มะม่วงคัน
Mangifera quadrifida Jack. Anacardiaceae (PT)
bark, bark sap

mamuang phruan มะม่วงพรวน
A species of mango *Mc*, p.565
bark sap

manaao มะนาว exotic bitter fruit kernel

Citrus aurantifolia Swing. bland root
Lime; Sour lime sour fruit juice
fruit juice, fruit kernel, leaves, leaf sap, root, flowers Rutaceae (VJ); *LB*, p.52
There are four kinds of lime grown in Thailand

manaao prieo มะนาวเปรี้ยว
Citrus aurantifolia Swing. Rutaceae
Lime, a species which is not sweet.

manaao waan มะนาวหวาน
Citrus mitis Blanco Rutacea
Sweet lime (VJ)

mangkhut มังคุด
Garcinia mangostana L. Guttiferae (PT)
Mangosteen
root

mangua มะงั่ว sour fruit
Citrus medica L. Rutaceae (VJ)
Citron
kernel, root, leaves, juice

maphlap cheen มะพลับจีน
Diospyros kaki L. Ebenaceae (PT)
Japanese persimmon; Chinese date plum; Persimmon
fruit

maphraao มะพร้าว astringent root and bark
maphraao fai มะพร้าวไฟ oily meat
maphraao naalike มะพร้าวนาฬิเก sweet; cool and fragrant flower
Cocos nucifera L. Palmae (VJ); (PT)
Coconut
oil, meat, milk, cream, fruits (coconuts), root

maphraao kathi มะพร้าวกะทิ
A very soft, oily coconut meat, obtained from coconuts from particular coconut trees, especially from branches on the east side of the tree only

maphuu มะผู้
maphuu mamia มะผู้มะเมีย
Cordyline fruiticosa Goeppert Liliaceae

(*C. terminalis* Kunth.) (VJ)
Dracaena palm; Ti plant
leaves

mara มะระ bitter leaves
mara khee nok มะระขี้นก
phak hai ผักไห่
Momordica charantia L. Cucurbitaceae (VJ)
Bitter gourd; African cucumber; Balsam pear; Balsam apple (PT); *LB*, p.89
leaves, root

marum มะรุม oily seed
marum baan มะรุมบ้าน hot-and-spicy bark
Moringa oleifera Lamk. Moringaceae (PT)
root, bark

masaang มะซาง
Madhuca pierrei Lam. Sapotaceae (VJ)
heartwood, bark

mataat มะตาด
Dillenia indica L. Dillenaceae (PT)
fruit

matuum มะตูม
tuum ตูม
Aegle marmelos Corr. Rutaceae (VJ); *TS*, p. 8
Bael tree
root, leaves, fruit, fruit rind, bark
The root is used to treat asthma and coughs, and as a febrifuge, carminative and antimicrobial; the young fruit are used as a carminative, stomachic, digestant and expectorant *HE*, p.3

ma-uek มะอึก
ma-ik มะอิก[misprint]
Solanum ferox L. Solanaceae (PT)
root sap

mawaeng มะแว้ง bitter fruit
could refer to either
1. *mawaeng ton* มะแว้งต้น

2. *mawaeng khruea* มะแว้งเครือ
1. *Solanum indicum* L. and	Solanaceae (PT); *WW*, p.719
Solanum sanitwongsei Craib	(VJ)
2. *Solanum trilobatum* L.	Solanaceae
fruit juice, fruit, root	(PT); *HE*, p.16
2. The whole plant is used as a diuretic, diaphoretic, anti-tussive and anti-asthmatic; the root is used as an anti-tussive, diuretic and expectorant; and the fruit are used to treat diabetes	*HE*

mawaeng thang 2 มะแว้งทั้ง๒
1. *mawaeng ton* มะแว้งต้น
2. *mawaeng khruea* มะแว้งเครือ
1. *S. indicum* L. and
S. sanitwongsei Craib
2. *Solanum trilotabum* L.	Solanaceae (PT)
fruit, root

mayom มะยม	sour	leaves
mayom tua phuu มะยมตัวผู้
mayom prieo มะยมเปรี้ยว
mayom mia มะยมเมีย
mayom waan มะยมหวาน
Phyllanthus acidus Skeels	Euphorbiaceae (VJ)
(*P. distichus* Meull. Arg.)
Star gooseberry
root, fruit, leaves

mayong paa มะยงป่า
Bouea oppositifolia Meissn.	Anacardiaceae (VJ)
root

(dee) mee ดีหมี	see *dee mee (ton)*

mo noi หมอน้อย
samo noi สมอน้อย
1. *Vernonia cinerea* Less.	Compositae (PT)
Probably not this because the fruit is so small
2. A species of	Malvaceae (VJ)
fruit, root

mo sai ม่อไส้	bland	root

Allophylus cobbe Blume var. *glaber* Hiern
A. sootepensis Craib — Sapindaceae (PT)
root

mok luang โมกหลวง
mok yai โมกใหญ่ — see *muuk luang*

mok man โมกมัน — see *muuk man*

mok หมก
maak mok หมากหมก
Adenia penangiana Wilde. — Passifloraceae *TS*, p.6
This is not areca (see *maak*), although '*penang*' means 'areca nut palm'
flowers
maak mok yields a cyanogenetic glycoside from all parts of the plant. It must be pickled first before eating, to drive off the hydrocyanic acid. The flower is eaten. (VJ)

mong โมง
Ternstroemia gymnanthera Bedd. — Theaceae (VJ)
root, fruit

mon ko มอลกอ — see *malako*

mot yop มดยอบ
Commiphora mukul Engl.
Commiphora myrrha (Nees) Engl. — Burseraceae *TE*, p.463
Myrrh — (PT)

mue fak มือฟัก — see *fak*
Tendrils of the gourd

mue nam tao มือน้ำเต้า — see *nam tao*
Tendrils of the calabash plant — (VJ)

mueat khon เหมือดคน — bitter — root
Scleropyrum wallichiarum Arn. — Santalaceae
root — (PT); *TS*, p.302; *WW* p.617

muuk luang มูกหลวง
mok luang โมกหลวง
mok yai โมกใหญ่

Holarrhena antidysenterica (L.) Wall. Apocynaceae
(*Wrightia antidysenterica* J. Grah.) (PT)
Kurchi; Conessi
fruit, bark
The stem and root bark (Kurchi bark) is used to treat dysentery and diarrhoea *HE*, p.11

muuk man มูกมัน
mok man โมกมัน
Wrightia tomentosa Roem. et Schult. Apocynaceae (PT); *LP*, p.144
bark, fruit

muun kaa มูลกา see *khee kaa*

muun kaa daeng มูลกาแดง see *khee kaa daeng*

muun kaa khaao มูลกาขาว see *khee kaa khaao*

muun kaa thang 2 มูลกาทั้ง๒ see *khee kaa thang* 2

muun lek มูลเหล็ก see *khee lek*

naam waai khom หนามหวายขม see *waai khom*

naang dam นางดำ
raang dam รางดำ
possibly *Dialium cochinchinense* Pierre. Leguminosae *FT*, p. 646
or *Diospyros bracteata* Fletcher
Diospyros castanea Fletcher Ebenaceae *FT*, p. 998; (VJ)

naang nuun นางนูน
1. *Adenia pierrei* Gagnep. Passifloraceae *TS*, p.6
2. *A. viridiflora* Craib (VJ)
root

naat หนาด
naat luang หนาดหลวง (PT)
Blumea balsamifera (L.) DC. Compositae (VJ); *HE*
Ngai camphor plant (from Chinese *ngai phiang*)
leaves (*bai*), root
The leaves are used as a diaphoretic; expectorant; carminative; and stomachic *HE*
The plant contains borneol (ngai camphor) (VJ)

nam น้ำ
Water, liquid, juice, sap. Prefix for any fluid.

nam chaa น้ำชา
Tea (PT)

nam chaan maak น้ำชานหมาก see *phluu*
The juice of a chewed quid of betel leaf and areca nut

nam chai khrai น้ำใจใคร่
Solanum nigrum L. Solanaceae (PT)

nam chan น้ำจันทน์ see *chan*

nam chan thang 2 น้ำจันทน์ทั้ง๒ see *chan thang* 2
A watery paste made from powdered Dracaena and Sandalwood. To make this, the upturned lid of a rough surfaced earthenware pot is used as a funnel-shaped container. Water is poured in, and the wood is rubbed against the rough surface inside the lid, in the water. (VJ)

nam dap fai น้ำดับไฟ

yaa nam dap fai หญ้าน้ำดับไฟ

Lindenbergia philippensis Benth. Scrophulariaceae (PT)
leaf sap

nam dok mai น้ำดอกไม้
nam dok mai Thai น้ำดอกไม้ไทย
rot sukhon dok mai รสสุคนธ์ดอกไม้
thao arakhon/ankhon เถาอรคนธ์
Aromatic water, flower water; usually prepared from Jasmine flowers (see *mali*) or the flowers of
Cananga odorata Hook. f. et Th. Annonaceae
Tetracera indica Merr. Dilleniaceae
(*T. assa* DC.) etc.
Tetracera indica has a reddish flower. The leaf of another species, *Tetracera scandens*, is used instead of sandpaper (VJ)

nam dok mai thet น้ำดอกไม้เทศ cool and fragrant

nam kulaap น้ำกุหลาบ
Rose water see *kulaap*

nam het muun kho น้ำเห็ดมูลโค see *het mun kho*

nam kathue mok fai น้ำกะทือหมกไฟ see *krathue*

nam klaep น้ำแกลบ see *kaeo klaep*

nam krisanaa น้ำกฤษณา see *krisanaa*
A triturate of eagle wood in water

nam kulaap น้ำกุหลาบ see *nam dok mai thet*

nam lao น้ำเหล้า see *suraa*

nam luuk chaak น้ำลูกจาก see *chaak*

nam man dip น้ำมันดิบ
Fresh vegetable or animal oil

nam man ngaa น้ำมันงา see *ngaa*
Sesame oil

nam maphraao naalike น้ำมะพร้าวนาลิเก see *maphraao*
Coconut milk

nam nom raatchasee น้ำนมราชสีห์
nam nom raatchasee khruea น้ำนมราชสีห์เครือ
Euphorbia hirta L. Euphorbiaceae
(*E. pilulifera* L.) (PT)

nam nom raatchasee ton น้ำนมราชสีห์ต้น bitter
Anotis trimera Craib Rubiaceae (PT)
root

nam nong น้ำนอง
1. Nest of a particular kind of termite
2. Plant:
Cissus pedata Lamk. Vitidaceae (VJ)
root

nam oi ngop น้ำอ้อยงบ
Raw sugar cane juice
ngop nam oi งบน้ำอ้อยis a slice of raw sugar cane (VJ)

nam phrik Thai น้ำพริกไทย see *phrik Thai*

*nam rak an piak** น้ำรักอันเปียก see *rak*
The resin from the sap of the Burmese lacquer tree obtained by making a hole in the trunk through the bark, but not as far as the heartwood (PT)

nam saao khaao น้ำซาวข้าว
Water which has been used to wash rice.
This probably contains a small amount of starch and minerals from the rice particles, and particles of bran (VJ)

nam som น้ำส้ม
1. Vinegar (*nam som saai chuu*)
2. Any tangerine fruit juice

nam taan น้ำตาล
1. Palm sugar
2. Sucrose

nam tao น้ำเต้า bitter root
nam tao khom น้ำเต้าขม
nam tao taek น้ำเต้าแตก
Lagenaria siceraria Standl.
(*Lagenaria leucantha* Rusby) Cucurbitaceae (VJ)
(*L. vulgaris* Ser.) (PT); *Mc*, p.454
Calabash cucumber; Bottle gourd; Trumpet gourd
leaves, tendrils (*mue* มือ), skin

nam thalaai maak dip น้ำทลายหมากดิบ see *maak*
Decoction of the still green and fresh rachis of the bunch of unripe areca fruit. The fruit is removed, and the remaining rachis is used.
(*Thalaai* has two meanings. The rachis is called *thalaai*, but with the fruit it is called *thalaai maak*, meaning a bunch of fruit). (VJ)

nam thao tamlueng น้ำเถาตำลึง see *tamlueng*

nam tum kaa daeng น้ำตุมกาแดง see *kot kakling*

nam yaa fin น้ำยาฝิ่น see *fin*
1. A residual deposit in the pipe after smoking opium. This is scraped out and put in water to wash it and make it liquid for use as a very potent method of stopping the diarrhoea of cholera.
2. Raw opium boiled with water to improve the otherwise foetid odour of the crude opium. (VJ)

nam yat [yaat] lao น้ำหยัด(หยาด)เหล้า see *suraa yat [yaat]*

neraphuusee เนระพูสี,เนียรภูสี astringent wood
Microlepia speluncae Moore Dennstaedtiaceae
(VJ); *Ts*, p.227; *WW*, p.423
Pteridrys syrmatica C. Chr. Filicales
(*Dryopteris syrmatica* O. Kuntze) *Mc*, p.463; *FT*, p.235
A fern
rhizome and stipe

*neraphuusee daeng*เ นระพูสีแดง
possibly synonym for *neraphuusee*

neraphuusee khaao เนระพูสีขาว
possibly synonym for *neraphuusee Thai*

neraphuusee Thai เนระพูสีไทย
Tacca chantrieri Andre. Taccaceae *FT* p.247
Black lily

neraphuusee thang 2 เนระพูสีทั้ง๒
?

neraphuusee thet เนระพูสีเทศ
Pteridys syrmatica Willd. C. Chr. et Ching
(*Aspidium syrmaticum* Willd.) Dryopteridaceae (VJ)

ngaa งา oily seed
Sessamum indicum L. Pedaliaceae
(*S. orientale* L.) *HE*, p.16; *WW*, p.202
Sesame
seed
The seeds are edible; the seed oil is used as a nutrient, emollient and demulcent

ngap phit งับฟิษ see *rangap phit*

ngiu งิ้ว astringent leaf
Bombax ceiba L.
(*Bombax malabaricum* DC.) Bombacaceae (VJ)
(*Salmalia malabarica* Schott & Endlich) *WW*, p.I
Silk cotton tree; Red cotton tree; Cotton tree (VJ)
Shaving brush *TS*, p.50
root, wood sap

ngoh เงาะ
Nephelium lappaceum L. Sapindaceae
Rambutan (VJ); *TS*, p.240
The exocarp of the fruit [*plueak* เปลือก]

nguan muu ง้วนหมู
huan muu ฮ้วนหมู
root see *krathung maa baa*

no mai หน่อไม้
There are many kinds, but it is usually
Bambusa blumeana Schult. Gramineae
B. arundinacea Willd. or
B. flexuosa Munro or it could be
Thyrostachys siamensis Gamble Gramineae (VJ)
Bamboo sprouts see *ruak*

no mai dong หน่อไม้ดอง
Pickled bamboo sprouts (VJ)

no mai nam หน่อไม้น้ำ
Zizania latifolia Turcz. Gramineae
Truffle (obtained after the stem has been infested by fungus) (VJ)

nom maeo นมแมว
nom maeo noi นมแมวน้อย
Rauwenhoffia siamensis Scheff. Annonaceae (PT)
root

nom maeo thang 2 นมแมวทั้ง๒

leaves and roots of *nom maeo* (PT)

nom phichit นมพิจิตร
Trichosanthes anguina L. Cucurbitaceae (VJ)
leaves

nom sawan นมสวรรค์ bitter root
phanom sawan พนมสวรรค์
phuu mak
Clerodendron paniculatum L. var. *diversifolium* C.B. Clarke Verbenaceae
Pagoda flower (PT); *FE*; p.109; *LE*, p.77
root
nom tamria นมตำเรีย
Hoya ovalifolia W. A. Asclepiadaceae (PT)
Hoya parasitica (VJ)

nun นุ่น
1. *Bombax ceiba* L. Bombacaceae
(*Bombax malabricum* DC.) (VJ)
2. *Ceiba pentandra* Gaertn. Bombaceae
Floss
1. The seed of the White silk cotton tree or Kapok tree *nun*, which looks like velvet, means the hairy part of the inside of the pod
2. The seed of the Red cotton tree
C. pentandra is considered to be inferior to *B. ceiba*, which is very soft and lasts longer. Kapok fibres break after five years. The pod of *C. pentandra* is about 8"-12" long; that of *B. ceiba*, about 6"-7". *Nun* นุ่น(floss) is used for mattresses and for padding, e.g. quilting. (*faai* ฝ้ายcotton, the same part of *Gossypium*, is used to make cloth). (VJ)

oi อ้อย sweet fresh juice
Saccharum officinarum L. (PT)
Sugar cane
cane juice

oi daeng อ้อยแดง sweet
Saccharum sinense Roxb. Gramineae
Black sugar cane
cane juice, buds (*taa* ตา), root
The culm is used as a diuretic; the buds are used as an ingredient in an antipyretic formula *HE*, p.15

opchoei อบเชย

Cinnamomum inners		Lauraceae (VJ)
Cinnamon		
opchoei thang 2 อบเชยทั้ง๒		
1. *opchoei thet* อบเชยเทศ		
2. *opchoei yuan* อบเชยญวน		
1. *Cinnamomum zeylanicum* Nees		Lauraceae
2. *C. loureirii* Nees		
1. Ceylon cinnamon		
2. Saigon cinnamon		(VJ)
opchoei thet อบเชยเทศ		
Cinnamomum zeylanicum Nees		Lauraceae
Ceylon cinnamon		
bark		
opchoei yuan โบเชยญวน		
Cinnamomum loureirii Nees		Lauraceae (VJ
Saigon cinnamon		
palong ปะโลง, โปลง		
Ceriops spp.	see below	Rhizophoraceae (VJ)
palong thang 2 ปะโลงทั้ง๒		
1. *Ceriops decandra* Ding Hou		Rhizophoraceae
C. roxburghiana Arn.)		
2. *C. tagal* C. B. Robinson		
1. White *palong*		
2. Red *palong*		(VJ)
peep ปีบ	fragrant	flowers
Millingtonia hortensis L.		Bignoniaceae *HE*, p.12
Indian cork tree		*Mc*, p.528
leaves, root		
The root is used to treat lung troubles		*HE*
phaat shon พาดโฉน	hot-and-spicy	root
Linostoma scandens Kurz		Thymelaeaceae (PT)
root		
phai mai ไผ่ไม้	salty	root
mai phai ไม้ไผ่		

mai wen ไม้เวฬุ
Bambusa arundinacea Willd. and other *Bambusa* spp. — Gramineae (VJ)
Bamboo
buds, outer part of trunk

(mai) phai paa ไม้ไผ่ป่า — Gramineae (VJ)
Bambusa arundinaceare Willd. — (Bambusaceae)

mai phai see suk ไม้ไผ่สีสุก — Gramineae (VJ)
Bambusa blumeana Scholt. — (Bambusaceae)

mai see suk ไม้สีสุก — Gramineae (VJ)
Bambusa flexuosa Munro — (Bambusaceae)

phak ผัก
vegetable

phak bung ผักบุ้ง — bland — leaf
phak bung Thai
Ipomoea aquatica Forsk. — Convolvulaceae *Mc*, p.484
(Ipomoea reptans Poir.) — *WW*, p.452

(bencha) phak bung เบญจผักบุ้ง
the whole plant of *phak bung*

phak bung khan ผักบุ้งขัน
Ipomoea asarifolia (Desr.) R. et Sch. — Convolvulaceae (VJ)

phak bung thet ผักบุ้งเทศ
possibly synonym for *phak bung farang* ผักบุ้งฝรั่ง
Ipomoea carnea Kerr — Convolvulaceae *FT* p.1049
Ipoemia [sic] *coccinea* L. — *FT* p.1054
Star ipoemia [sic]

phak chee ผักชี — hot-and-spicy — fruit
phak chee laa ผักชีลา
phak chee raa ผักชีรา[misprint]
(means 'infested by fungus')
Coriandrum sativum L. — Umbelliferae (VJ)
Coriander; Chinese parsley

fruit

phak chee thang 2 ผักชีทั้ง๒

1. *phak chee laa* ผักชีลา
2. *phak chee lom* ผักชีล้อม

1. *Coriandrum sativum* L. — Umbelliferae
2. *Oenanthe stolonifera* Wall. — Umbelliferae

1. Coriander; Chinese parsley
2. The Chinese *chang chueng chee* จั๋งชึ่งจี๋

fruit

phak eenuun ผักอีนูน — see *phak saap*

phak hai ผักไห่ — see *mara*

phak hom ผักโหม

phak hom hat ผักโหมหัด

1. Amaranthus gracilis Desf. — Amaranthaceae (VJ)
   (*A. viridis* L.)
2. *A. lividus* L.

root, leaves, leaf sap

phak hom hin ผักโหมหิน

Boerharvia diffusa L. — Nyctaginaceae (PT)

Spreading hog weed

root

phak hom naam ผักโหมหนาม

Amaranthus spinosus L. — Amaranthaceae

Thorny aramanth; Spiny pigweed; Careless weed — (PT)

aerial parts, root

phak kaat ผักกาด

phan phak kaat พรรณผักกาด (mustard seed)

suphan phak kaat สุพรรณผักกาด (white mustard seed)

Brassica hirta Moench. — Cruciferae

(*B. alba* Hook. f.)

1. (*Sinapis alba* L.)
2. *Brassica nigra* L. Koch (black mustard)
   Brassica juncea (L.) Coss. (India mustard) — (VJ)

1. Mustard seed (white or yellow)

2. Mustard seed (black brown, or red)
2. The seed contains sinigrin, which contains a sulphur compound
seed

phak khet ผักเค็ด
phak khlet ผักเคล็ด (PT)
Cassia sophora L. Caesalpiniaceae (VJ)
leaves

phak khraat ผักคราด hot-and-spicy
phak khraat hua waen ผักคราดหัวแวน
Spilanthes acmella Murr. Compositae (VJ)
Spilanthes oleracea (L.) Jacq. *HE*, p.17
leaves
The twigs are used in the treatment of tonsilitis *HE*

phak khuang ผักขวง bitter
Glinus oppositifolius A. DC. Aizoaceae (Ficoideae)
leaves, root (PT); *WW*, p.100

phak krashet ผักกระเฉด bland white flotation pads along the stems
Neptunia oleracea Lour. Mimosaceae (PT) (Leguminosae) (VJ)

phak nok ผักหนอก see *bua bok*

phak pet ผักเปิด
phak pet daeng ผักเปิดแดง
Alternanthera triandra Lamk. Amaranthaceae (VJ)
leaves

phak phaeo ผักแพว
phak phaeo daeng ผักแพวแดง
Polygonum odoratum Lour. Polygonaceae
P. chinense L. (VJ)
Contains a volatile oil

phak plaap ผักปลาบ
Commelina bengalensis L. Commelinaceae
leaves (PT)

phak plang ผักปลัง
phak plang khaao ผักปลังขาว
Basella rubra L. — Basellaceae *HE*, p.3; (VJ)
(*B. cordifolia*) Lamk.
Ceylon spinach; Malabar nightshade
leaves, root
The fruit is red.
The whole plant is used for ringworm, and the root for leucoderma of the extremities *HE*

phak saap ผักสาบ
phak eenuun ผักอีนูน
Adenia viridiflora Craib — Passifloraceae *HE* (VJ)
Contains a cyanogenic glycoside

phak sian phee ผักเสี้ยนผี
Cleome viscosa L. — Cleomaceae (PT); *TS*, p.86
leaves

phak top ผักตบ
Monochoria hastata Solms. - Laub. — Pontederiaceae (VJ)

phak waan ผักหวาน
phak waan baan ผักหวานบ้าน
Sauropus androgynous Merr. — Euphorbiaceae (VJ)
(*S. albicans* Blume)
leafy parts, root

phak waen ผักแว่น
Marsilea crenata Presl. — Marsileaceae (VJ)
leaves, root

phalaan sat ผลาญศัตุ
phalaan satruu ผลาญศัตรู
fruit

phan nguu พันงู
Achyranthes sp. — Amaranthaceae (PT)
Achyranthes aspera L. — *TS*, p.4
whole plant

phan nguu daeng พันงูแดง
Cyathula prostrata Bl. Amaranthaceae (VJ)

phan phak kaat พรรณผักกาด
suphan phak kaat สุพรรณผักกาด see *phak kaat*

phanom sawan พนมสวรรค์ see *nom sawan*

phayaa mue lek พญามือเหล็ก
phayaa muun lek พญามูลเหล็ก [misprint]
1. *Strychnos roborans* A. W. Hill Strychnaceae (VJ)
2. *Strychnos krabiensis* A.W. Hill
root leaves

phayaa raak dam พญารากดำ bitter resin
1. *Diospyros variegata* Kurz Ebenaceae (PT); *PB* p.95
2. *Diospyros rubra* Lec. (VJ)

resin

phayaa raak khaao พญารากขาว
possibly *Albizzia lucida* Craib Leguminosae FT p.605
(The plant thus distinguished in Uttaradit)

phayom พยอม
Shorea floribunda Kurz Dipterocarpaceae (PT)
bark

phayom saam bai to พยอมสามใบต่อ
?

phekaa เพกา astringent bark, root
Oroxylum indicum Vent. Bignoniaceae (VJ)
leaves, bark sap

phetsanukam เพ็ศณุกรรม์
phetshaluukan เพจฉลูกรร
perhaps *phitsanaat* พิษนาศน์
root

phikun พิกุล see *khondok*

phimsen พิมเสน
phumsen พุมเสน, ภุมเสน
bhimsaim Skt
Dryobalanops aromatica Gaertn. Dipterocarpaceae
(*D. camphora Colebr.*) (VJ); *LB*, p.37
Borneo camphor; Borneol; et al.
flakes, leaves
It is taken from the wood (VJ)
There are other kinds of camphor see *kaarabuun*

phinlangkaasaa พิลังกาสา hot-and-spicy leaves
Ardisia colorata Roxb. Myrsinaceae
fruit, root

phitsanaat พิษนาศน์
Artemisa indica Willd. var. *heyneana* Pampan. Compositae (PT); *TS*, p.34
root

phlai ไพล
phrai ไพร [misprint]
phlai lueang ไพลเหลือง
Zingiber cassumunar Roxb. Zingiberaceae *WW*, p.564
rhizome only
The rhizome has cardiac depressant properties. In liquor, it used to be applied to the abdomen to warm it to counteract flatulence, just as asafoetida was used to smear over a baby's abdomen. It is also used to make a tincture for application as a mosquito repellant. (VJ)

phlai dam ไพลดำ
phlai muang ไพลม่วง
Zingiber ottensii Valeton Zingiberaceae *HE*, p.19; *TS*, p.355
The rhizome is used as a tonic *HE*

phlai lueang ไพลเหลือง see *phlai*

phlap cheen พลับจีน
Diospyros kaki L. Ebenaceae (PT)
Japanese or Chinese persimmon
fruit juice

phlap phlueng พลับพลึง
Crinum asiaticum L. Amaryllidaceae
Crinum lily
The heated leaves are used to wrap inflamed areas to relieve pain *HE*, p.6

phlee kam พลีกรรม see *khrueang phlee kam*

phluang พลวง
1. Metal
2. Plant:
Dipterocarpus tuberculatus Roxb. Dipterocarpaceae (PT)
leaves

phluu พลู
phluu kin kap maak พลูกินกับหมาก
Piper betle L. Piperaceae
Betel vine (VJ); *HE*, p.14
leaves, root
The leaves are used in an application to treat urticaria *HE*
The leaves contain a phenolic compound, chavicol, which is used mixed with liquor on inflamed areas, such as occur with herpes and skin diseases. Betel leaf in the mouth gives a burning sensation because of the phenols.

The main ingredients used by Thais in chewing betel are:
Betel leaf: containing a phenolic compound, chavicol. The leaf is smeared with a paste of slaked lime mixed with turmeric (see *puun*).
Areca nut: containing the alkaloid arecoline, a tranquilizer and vermifuge, as well as tannins, which are astringent to the mucus membrane. Young areca nut is milder than the older.
(The Indians use also sweet fennel.)
Mild, fine cut tobacco, i.e. very young leaf.
Sometimes alum is used to work out some alkali.
Astringent bark of certain plants, e.g. cutch.
Sometimes freshly prepared coconut oil in beeswax to smear on the lips to prevent burning. (VJ)

phluu kae พลูแก toxic whole plant
Piper sp. Piperaceae (VJ)
leaves

pho baai โพบาย
Sappium baccatum Roxb. Euphorbiaceae

young twigs, bark (VJ); *TS*, p.295

phok phaai โพกพาย bland stem
Pachygone dasycarpa Kurz Menispermaceae (VJ); *HE*, p.13
leaves
The stem is used as an antidote for poison, as a diuretic and in the treatment of kidney disorders and arthritis *HE*

phot โพธิ์
pho โพ
ton see mahaa phot ต้นสรีมหาโพธิ์
Ficus religiosa L. Moraceae
Sacred fig tree; Bo tree; (VJ);
Pipal tree; Bodh tree *Mc*, p.609
thickened latex

phraamon พร้ามอญ
san phraamon สันพร้ามอญ
Justica gendarussa L. Acanthaceae
(*Gendarussa vulgaris* Nees) (PT)
leaves

phrai ไพร[misprint] see *phlai*

*phrik khee** พริกขี้
phrik khee nok พริกขี้นก
Pepper seed from bird droppings. This is the most potent. Birds eat only the red fruit, which has the most important piperine content, but cannot digest the seed. The growers collect these seeds and use them, regarding them as a superior grade of white pepper. (VJ)

phrik haang พริกหาง
Piper cubeba L. Piperaceae (PT)
Tailed pepper

phrik hom พริกหอม
Zanthoxylum limonella Alston Rutaceae *TS*, p.334
(*Z. rhetsa* DC.)
(*Z. budrunga* Wall. ex Hook. f.) (VJ)

phrik Thai พริกไทย hot-and-spicy seeds (peppercorns)
phrik พริก

Piper nigrum L. — Piperaceae
Black pepper (whole ripe and unripe fruit)
White pepper (seed of the ripe fruit) — (VJ); *HE*, p.14; *WW*, p.531
The rind or shell of the pepper seed becomes black. This is mixed with the white pepper of the shelled seed to make a milder and better product, which is more fragrant, due to the oil from the shell rind. (VJ)
The fruit or seeds are used as a stomachic, carminative, stimulant, febrifuge, tonic, and irritant. *HE*

(nam) phrik Thai น้ำพริกไทย
1. Infusion of the fruit or seed powder of *Piper nigrum* L. (VJ)
2. A Thai hot sauce

phrik Thai lon พริกไทยล่อน
White pepper; the seed or fruit of just ripened pepper. The fruit goes green, then yellow, then red. The riper it is, the more important is the piperine. (VJ)

phrommi พรหมมี
Brahmi Skt
Bacopa monniera (L.) Wettst. — Scrophulariaceae (VJ)
(*Bacopa monniera* Pennel) — *HE* p.3
Thyme-leaved Geratiola — *LB* p.82
leaves
The whole plant is used as an alterative, febrifuge, expectorant and cardiotonic *HE*

phum riang baan พุมเรียงบ้าน — exotic
phum riang พุมเรียง
chammariang ชำมะเรียง — *WW*, p.255
Otophora cambodiana Pierre — Sapindaceae
Domestic variety — (VJ); *WW*, pp.255, 556
root

phum riang paa พุมเรียงป่า
Aphania viridis Pierre — Sapindaceae
Wild variety — (VJ); *HE*, p.2
root
Antimalarial — *HE*

phum riang thang 2 พุมเรียงทั้ง๒ — toxic — roots
1. *phum riang baan* พุมเรียงบ้าน
2. *phum riang paa* พุมเรียงป่า — (VJ)
roots

phung do พุงดอ sour root
Azima sarmentosa Benth. Salvadoraceae (VJ)
leaves, root

phut son พุดซ้อน
Gardenia jasminoides Ellis Rubiaceae (VJ)
root, leaves

phutsaa พุทรา
Zizyphus jujuber Mill. astringent leaf; underripe fruit
Indian jujube; Chinese date Rhamnaceae (VJ)
The leaf is oval shaped, and about 1" across; the wild fruit is the size of a cherry, the cultivated fruit is egg sized (VJ)

phutta raksaa พุทธรักษา
Canna indica L. Cannaceae
Canna; Indian shot (PT)
flowers

plaa lai phueak ปลาไหลเผือก bitter root
plaa laai phueak ปลาหลายเผือก
plaa lai (laai) ปลาไหล (หลาย)
Eurycoma longifolia Jack. Simaroubaceae
root *LB*, p.49; *WW*, p.471

plaai ปลาย [misprint] see *kraai*
praai ปราย [misprint]

plaai khaao saan ปลายข้าวสาร see *khaao*
Broken rice, broken, not whole grain, used for making flour (PT)

plao noi เปล้าน้อย
1. *Croton joufra* Roxb. Euphorbiaceae (VJ)
2. *Croton longissimus* Airy Shaw *HE*, p.7
3. *Croton lyratus* Kurz
root

plao thang 2 เปล้าทั้ง๒
1. *plao noi* เปล้าน้อย
2. *plao yai* เปล้าใหญ่

1. *Croton longissimus* Airy Shaw — Euphorbiaceae
2. *Croton oblongifolius* Roxb. — (PT)

plao yai เปล้าใหญ่
Croton oblongifolius Roxb. — Euphorbiaceae *HE*
The leaves are used as a stomachic; the root, for skin diseases; the heartwood is usaed as an emmenagogue, and as an anthelmintic for round worms; and the fruit are also used as an emmenagogue — *HE*, p.7
root

plueak เปลือก
bark, rind, shell, husk

praai ปราย[misprint] — see *kraai*

praduu ประดู่ — Leguminosae
Pterocarpus indicus Willd. — (Papilionacae) (PT)
leaves, wood, bark sap

prakham dee khwaai ประคำดีควาย — bitter — fruit [pulp]
Sapindus emarginatus Wall. — (VJ); *TS*, p.295
S. rarak A. DC. — Sapindaceae (VJ)
Some sources give *S. emarginatus* for *prakham dee khwaai*, and *S. rarak* for *makham dee khwaai*, but *'ma'* here means fruit, and both *S. emarginatus* and *S. rarak* fruit are *prakham dee khwaai* (VJ)
fruit pulp, leaves, root, fruit juice
The seeds are used to make a rosary of usually 108 beads — (VJ)

prakham kai ประคำไก่ — bitter — leaves
makham kai มะคำไก่
Putranjiva roxburghii Wall. — Euphorbiaceae
leaves, bark, fruit — (PT); *WW*, p.171

prayong ประยงค์
Aglaia odorata Lour. — Meliaceae *HE*
The flowers are used for perfuming tea and clothes. An infusion of the leaves is given as a tonic in excessive menses. — *HE*

prik ปริก
Asparagus sprengeri Regel. — Liliaceae (PT); *TS*, p.37
root

proh hom เปราะหอม hot-and-spicy rhizome
proh เปราะ
proh sot เปราะสด
waan proh ว่านเปราะ
Kaemferia galanga L. Zingiberaceae
(VJ); (PT); *HE*, p.11; *WW* p.504
The rhizome is used as an expectorant, carminative and diuretic *HE*

pruu ปรู astringent bark
puu ปู
Alangium salviifolium (L.f.) Wang Alangiaceae *HE*
(*A. lamarckii* Thw.)

puu chao loi thaa ปู่เจ้าลอยท่า
Hygroryza aristata Nees Gramineae (VJ)

puu chao phung kae ปู่เจ้าพุงแก
Capparis siamensis Kurz
(*C. winitii* Craib) Capparidaceae (VJ)

puu chao saming kui ปู่เจ้าสมิงกุย
?

raang daeng รางแดง
Ventilago calyculata Tul. Rhamnaceae
(*V. denticulata* Willd.) (PT)
root

raang dam รางดำ see *naang dam*

raatchadat ราชดัด bitter root
Brucea javanica L. Merr. Simarubiaceae
(*B. amarissima Desv.*) (PT); *HE*, p.4
(*B. sumatrana* Roxb.)
Macassar seeds
The kernel is used to treat amoebic dysentery *HE*
fruit

raatcha phrik ราชพฤกษ์
ton raatcha phrik ต้นราชพฤกษ์
Cassia javanica L. Caesalpiniaceae

C. nodosa Ham. (VJ); *TS*, p.71
pod, seeds, leaves, juice

(bencha) raatcha phrik เบญจราชพฤกษ์
the five parts - stem, root, leaves, flowers and fruit

*rak** รัก
Melanorrhoea usitata Wall. Anacardiaceae
Burmese lacquer tree (VJ); (PT); *Mc*, p.700

*(nam) rak an piak** น้ำรักอันเปียก
The resin from the sap of the Burmese lacquer tree obtained by making a hole in the trunk through the bark, but not as far as the heartwood (PT)
Wet Burmese lacquer see *rak* above (VJ)

rak khaao รักขาว
Cerbera manghas L. Apocynaceae
The plant contains a cardiotonic glycoside (VJ)
leaves

rak son รักซ้อน
Calotropis gigantea R. Br. Asclepiadaceae (VJ)
Double variety
root

ram khaao on รำข้าวอ่อน
Fine rice bran; Rice polishings (VJ)

rang(mai)* ไม้รัง
Shorea siamensis Miq.
Pentacme siamensis Kurz Dipterocarpaceae (VJ)
(*P. malayana* King)

rangap ระงับ Leguminosae
1. *Mimosa pudica* L. (Mimosaceae)
2. *Biophytum sensitivum* DC. Oxalidaceae (VJ)
leaves, root

rangap phit ระงับพิษ
Barleria siamensis Craib Acanthaceae (VJ)

rangap thang 2 ระงับทั้ง๒
?
leaves

rangap yai ระงับใหญ่
Breynia glauca Craib — Euphorbiaceae
Breynia glauca is the species used in medicine — (VJ)
leaves

rayom ระย่อม — bitter — root
rayom daeng ระย่อมแดง
yom teen maa ย่อมตีนหมา
Rauwolfia serpentina Benth. — Apocynaceae (VJ); *HE*, p.15
Insanity herb
root — see *khem daeng*

reesee prasom laeo ฤาษีประสมแล้ว
reesee phosom laeo ฤาษีผสมแล้ว
Coleus atropurpureus Benth. — Labiatae (VJ)
Coleus blumei Benth.

rong thong รงทอง — toxic — oleogum-resin
rong รง
Garcinia hanburyi Hook. f. — Guttiferae
Gamboge tree — (PT); *LB*, p.38; *WW*, p.652
oleogum-resin
The oleogum-resin is used as an antiseptic and cathartic — (VJ)

ruak รวก — see *mai ruak*
phai ruak ไผ่รวก

saam sip สามสิบ — sweet — root
raak saam sip รากสามสิบ
satta mun Skt (100 roots)
Asparagus racemosus Willd. — Liliaceae (VJ); *HE*; *TS*, p.37
The root is used as a nutrient helpful for the foetus in the expectant mother *HE*

saap raeng saap kaa สาบแร้งสาบกา
Ageratum conyzoides L. — Compositae (PT)

saaraek khaat สาแหรกขาด
Broken rattan carrying frame for a basket (VJ)

saaraphat phit สารพัดพิษ
Sophera tomentosa Papilionaceae (PT)
The seed has about seven alkaloids (Dept.of Medical Sciences)
seed, root

saaraphee สารภี cool and fragrant flowers
1. *Ochrocarpus siamensis* T. and Guttiferae (VJ)
2. *Ochrocarpus harmandii* Pierre
flowers, pollen

sabaa สะบ้า toxic fruit (perhaps, seeds)
sabaa yai สะบ้าใหญ่
sabaa mon สะบ้ามอญ Leguminoseae
Entada phaseoloides Merr. (Mimosaceae) *WW*, pp.443,444
(*E. scandens* Benth.)
St Thomas' bean; Sea bean *LB*, p.30
seeds

sabaa ling สะบ้าลิง
Entada glandulosa Pierre ex Gagnep. Leguminosae
seeds (Mimosaceae) (PT); *WW*, p.445

sabaa Thai สะบ้าไทย
might be *Entada* (PT)

sadao สะเดา bitter leaves
satao สะเตา[misprint]
Azadirachta indica A. Juss. var. *siamensis* Valeton Meliaceae (VJ); *HE*, p.2
leaf stems, heartwood, bark, leaves, flowers, seeds, leaf sap
The root is an expectorant; the rachis of the compound leaf is used as an antimalarial; the leaves as a stomachic; and the heartwood for checking nausea and vomiting *HE*

saen prasa khruea แสนประสะเครือ
?

saen prasa ton แสนประสะต้น
Isotoma longiflora L. Lobeliaceae (PT)

sahatsakhun สหัสคุณ
hatsakhun หัสคุณ see *salot*

sahatsakhun thang 2 สหัสคุณทั้ง๒ see *hatsakhun thang* 2

sahatsakhun thet สหัสคุณเทศ [correctly *hatsakhun thet* หัสคุณเทศ q.v.]

(ton) sai ต้นไทร
Ficus bengalensis L.
Banyan tree Moraceae (VJ)

sai yoi ไทรย้อย
Ficus benjamina L. Moraceae (VJ); *HE*, p.10
Ficus retusa L. (rotund leaf) (VJ)
Leaves, root
The adventitious root is used as a diuretic *HE*

sak สัก
Tectona grandis L. f. Verbenaceae
Teak (PT)
bark, charcoal from the wood

sak khee สักขี see *krak khee*

sakae สะแก toxic seeds
sakae naa สะแกนา
Combretum quadrangulare Kurz Combretaceae (VJ); *LB*, p.61
bark, young leafy shoots, fruit, leaf sap, seeds, root, wood, ash, leaves

sakhaan สะค้าน hot-and-spicy root and stem
Piper sp. Piperaceae
stem (VJ)

salat dai สลัดได toxic
Euphorbia antiquorum L. Euphorbiaceae *HE*, p.9
leaves
The latex is used for the removal of warts. Latex from the old wood is used as a purgative. *HE*

salat dai paa สลัดไดป่า see *kralam phak*

salit สลิด
Telosma pallida (Roxb.) Craib Asclepiadaceae (PT)
flowers, root

salot สลอด toxic, astringent, cool leaf
salot kin long สลอดกินลง hot-and-spicy root
hatsakhun หัสคุณ
sahatsakhun สหัสคุณ
Croton tiglium L. Euphorbiaceae
Croton
leaves, root, seed, fruit (VJ); (PT); *WW*, p.740
The dose of the oil is one drop, therefore one seed is a very drastic purgative. (VJ)
For the method of 'purifying' *salot*, see prescription No. 556.

salot nam สลอดน้ำ bland root
Ficus heterophylla L. Moraceae (VJ); *WW*, p.741
root

saluuk ชะลูก [misprint] see *chaluut*

samae saan แสมสาร see *khee lek phaa*

samae thale แสมทะเล salty
Avicenna officinalis L. Verbenaceae (PT)
sap, heartwood

samae thang 2 แสมทั้ง๒
1. *samae saan* แสมสาร
2. *samae thale* แสมทะเล Leguminosae
1. *Cassia garrettiana* Craib (Caesalpiniaceae)
2. *Avicennia officinalis* L. Verbenaceae (PT) (VJ)
heartwood

samee สมี Leguminosae
Sesbania sesban Merr. (Papilionaceae) (VJ)
(*S. aegyptiaca* Pers.)
leaves
The standard of the flower has brown spots
samee means a Buddhist priest in trouble - accused of breaking an important rule (VJ)

samo สมอ sour fruit

samo thai สมอไทย
Terminalia chebula Retz. Combretaceae
Chebulic myrobalans (PT); (VJ); *HE*, p.18;
fruit juice *WW*, p.737
The fruit are used as a febrifuge and carminative; the leaves yield 'Terminalia gall', an astringent product *HE*

samo faai thet สมอฝ้ายเทศ
fruit of *Gossypium brasiliense* see *faai thet*
samo here means 'fruit of the cotton plant'. It is never used for other fruit, just as 'hip' is used only for rose hip.

samo phiphek สมอพิเภก astringent fruit; leaf
Terminalia belerica Roxb. sour underripe fruit
Ink nut; Beleric myrobalans Combretaceae
fruit - ripe or young (VJ); *HE*, p.18; *WW*, p.737

(nam) samo phiphek น้ำสมอพิเภก
A decoction of the ripe fruit
The name 'Ink nut' is derived from the use of the fruit mixed with iron rust to make blue-black ink (VJ)
The young fruit are laxative; the ripe fruit are astringent *HE*

samo rong raeng สมอร่องแร่ง
Terminalia sp. (VJ)
Long stemmed myrobalans

samo Thai สมอไทย see *samo*

samo thale สมอทะเล
Sapium indicum Willd. Euphorbiaceae (PT)
leaves

samo thang 3 สมอทั้ง๓ sour fruit
1. *samo Thai* สมอไทย
2. *samo thet* สมอเทศ
3. *samo phiphek* สมอพิเภก
1. *Terminalia chebula* Retz. Combretaceae
2. *Terminalia* sp.
3. *Terminalia belerica* Roxb.
1. Chebulic myrobalans
2. ?

3. Beleric myrobalans; Ink nut
The three kinds of myrobalans

samo thet สมอเทศ sour fruit
Terminalia sp. Combretaceae (VJ)
fruit

samrong สำโรง
Sterculia foetida L. Sterculiaceae (PT)
bark, root

samun waeng สมุลแว้ง hot-and-spicy bark
samon waeng สมลแว้ง [misprint]
Temmodaphne thailandica Kosterm. Lauraceae (VJ)
bark

samut kluean สมุดเกลื่อน
?

san phraa hom สันพร้าหอม
Eupatorium stoechadosmum Hance. Compositae
leaves
The whole plant is used as an antipyretic and tonic; and in aromatic powder *HE*, p.9

san phraa mon สันพร้ามอญ
Justica gendarussa L.
(*Gendarussa vulgaris* Nees) (PT)
root

san phraa naang ae สันพร้านางแอ astringent bark
shiang phraa naang ae เฉียงพร้านางแอ
Carallia brachiata Merr. Rhizophoraceae
(*C. integerrima* DC.) (VJ); *WW*, p.752
bark

sang karanee สังกรณี
Barleria strigosa Willd. Acanthaceae *HE*, p.3; *WW*, p.750
The root is used to treat spasmodic cough *HE*

saniat เสนียด bitter leaves
bua haa khaao บัวฮาขาว

Adhatoda vasica Nees — Acanthaceae
leaves, root, leaf sap, fruit juice — (PT); *HE*, p.1; *WW*, p.775
It is used as an expectorant to treat asthma and bronchitis — *HE*

sanun สนุ่น
Salix tetrasperma Roxb. — Salicaceae
Willow; Thai willow; Indian willow; White willow — (VJ); *TS*, p.294
bark
The bark contains salicin. The weeping willow (Chinese) is *Salix babylonica.* (VJ)

sapparot สับปะรด
Ananas comosus Merr. — Bromeliaceae
Pineapple — (PT); *TS*, p.21
leaves
Pineapple is harmful to women who have colds just before menstruation; and also to women who have colds immediately following menstruation. The condition before menstruation is not considered to be the same as that after. (DT)

satao สะเตา[misprint] — see *sadao*
leaves

sattabongkot สัตตบงกช
Nelumbo nucifera Gaertn. — Nelumbonaceae
Sacred lotus - red double, short form — (VJ)
flowers, pollen

sattabut สัตตบุษย์, สัตตบุศย์
Nymphaea lotus L. — Nymphaeaceae
White lotus (large white flower) — (VJ); *FT*, p.525
flowers, pollen

sawaat สวาด — Leguminosae
Caesalpinia crista L. — (Caesalpiniaceae) (VJ)
Nickernut; Grey nickers
leaves
The seed is shiny and grey, about 1" in diameter — (VJ)

see huat สีหวด
see huat yai สีหวดใหญ่
Erioglossum rubiginosum Blume — Sapindaceae (VJ) FT p.785

see huat noi สีหวดน้อย

Erioglossum rubiginosum Blume var. — Sapindaceae (VJ)
root

see huat thang 2 สีหวดทั้ง๒
1. *see huat noi* สีหวดน้อย
2. *see huat yai* สีหวดใหญ่

see siat สีเสียด — Leguminosae
Acacia catechu Willd. — (Mimosaceae)
Cutch; Catechu tree — *TS*, p.2; (VJ)

see siat thang 2 สีเสียดทั้ง๒ — astringent — bark
1. *see siat* สีเสียด
2. *see siat thet* สีเสียดเทศ
1. *Acacia catechu* Willd. — Mimosaceae (Leguminosae)
2. *Uncaria gambir* (Hunter) Roxb. — Rubiaceae
1. Cutch; Catechu tree
2. Gambir; Gambier; Pale catechu — (VJ)

see siat thet สีเสียดเทศ
Uncaria gambir (Hunter) Roxb. — Rubiaceae
Gambier; Gambier; Pale catechu — (VJ)

see suk สีสุก — see *phai paa*

shat phra in ฉัตพระอินทร์
1. *Exacum bicolor* Roxb. — Getianaceae
2. *Leonotis nepetaefolia* R.Br. — Labiatae (VJ)

sian เสี่ยน [misprint] — see *lian*

som ส้ม
A generic name for all citrus fruits and almost invariably qualified by a term designating the variety meant — *Mc*, p.814.
An orange

(nam) som น้ำส้ม
1. Any fruit juice with a sour taste — (PT)
2. Vinegar

som kop ส้มกบ

Oxalis corniculata L. Oxalidaceae

(*O. repens* Thunb.) *HE*, p.13

root

The plant is used as an expectorant, antitussive, and emmenagogue *HE*

som kung ส้มกุ้ง

1. *Begonia inflata* C.B. Clarke Begoniaceae
2. *Ampelocissus martinii* Planch. Vitidaceae
3. *Rubus moluccanus* L. Rosaceae (VJ)

root

(yaa) som kung หญ้าส้มกุ้ง

Phyllanthus orientalis Airy Shaw Euphorbiaceae (VJ)

som kung noi ส้มกุ้งน้อย

Embelia ribes Burm. f. Myrsinaceae (VJ)

root

som kung yai ส้มกุ้งใหญ่

Ardisia siamensis Fletcher Myrsinaceae

Garcinia lanessanii Pierre Guttiferae (VJ)

som makhaam piak ส้มมะขามเปียก see *see makhaam piak*

som poi ส้มป่อย

Acacia rugata Merr. Leguminosae

(*A. concinna* DC.) (Mimosaceae) (VJ) *TS*, p.3

pods

(*nam*) *som poi* น้ำส้มป่อย

The pods are left in water until soft, then squeezed to produce *nam som poi* (VJ)

som saa ส้มซ่า sour fruit juice

A cultivated hybrid of *Citrus* spp.; it might be

Citrus webberi Wester

(*C. nobilis* Lour. x Hystrix Aug. DC.) Rutaceae (VJ)

kernel, juice, leaves, skin

som sieo (yaa) ส้มเสี้ยว sour pod

Bauhinia malabrica Roxb. Leguminosae

(*Piliostigma malabrica* Benth.) (Caesalpiniaceae) (VJ); *WW*, p.1

root, leaves, bark

son สน

son saam bai สนสามใบ

Pinus kesiya Royle ex Gordon — Pinaceae(PT); *TS*, p.264

wood, flowers

son song bai สนสองใบ

Pinus merkusii Jungh. — (PT); *TS*, p.264

son thet สนเทศ

son sek สนเสก[misprint]

Thuja orientalis L. — Cupressaceae

Chinese arbor-vitae — (VJ); *LB*, p.53

wood, root

song baadaan ทรงบาดาล — Leguminosae

C. surattensis Burm. f. — (Caesalpiniaceae)

(*Cassia glauca* Lamk.) — (PT) (VJ)

root, leaves

song maeo ซองแมว — bitter — root

yuang khanun

Gmelina phillipinensis Cham. — Verbenaceae

(*Gmelina hystrix* Kurz & Schultz) — (PT); *PB*, p.109

root

song salueng สองสลึง

(*Solenospermum duperreanum* Taid.)

Lophopetalum duperreanum Pierre — Celastraceae (VJ)

leaves

sueak khao fai เชือกเขาไฟ — see *chuak khao fai*

suraa สุรา

nam suraa น้ำสุรา

lao เหล้า

nam lao น้ำเหล้า

Spirituous liquor;Alcohol; Intoxicating liquor; Fermented Toddy, about 28-35 degrees Beaumé, Arrack — (VJ)

suraa yat [*yaat*] สุราหยัด(หยาด)
nam yat [*yaat*] *lao* น้ำหยัด(หยาด)เหล้า
Proof spirit, proof alcohol (not less than 81 degrees)

suraamrit สุรามฤตย์
Cocculus laurifolius DC. Menispermaceae
Cinnamomum iners Bl. Lauraceae (VJ)
root of *Cocculus laurifolius* (i.e. if it is the root, it is probably this plant)
bark of leaves of *C. iners* (i.e. if it is the bark or leaves, then it is probably this plant)
The fruit of *C. laurifolius* is called fish berry which is fish poison (VJ)

taa suea ตาเสือ toxic bark and fruit
Aphanamixis polystachya Parker Meliaceae
cell sap of the bark *TS*, p.27

taa tum ตาตุ่ม
taa tum thale ตาตุ่มทะเล Euphorbiaceae (VJ)
Excoecaria agallocha L. see *kralamphak*

taan ตาล astringent outer layer of leaf stalks
taan tonot ตาลตะโหนด, ตาลโตนด sweet inflorescence
Borassus flabellifer L. Palmae
Palmyra palm; Fan palm; Lontar palm; Brale palm *FT*, p.334; *WW*, p.334
Mc, p.364 differentiates between *taan*, *Borassus flabelliformis*, the palmyra tree or fan-palm, and *taan tanot*, *Borassus flabellifera*, which produces food and drink, including sugar

(nam) taan น้ำตาล
Palm sugar

taan dam ตานดำ or ตาลดำ toxic root and wood
Diospyros montana Roxb. (VJ); *WW*, p.332
Diospyros transitoria Bakh. (PT); *TS*, p.125
wood, root, *nam* (liquid) unspecified Ebenaceae

taan khamooi ตานขโมย toxic leaves and wood
1. *Allophylus montanus* Williams Sapindaceae
2. *Apostasia odorata* Bl.
3. *Apostasia wallichii* R. Br. Apostasiaceae
4. *Glossocarya longifora* Fletch. Verbenaceae
5. *Ophiopogon malayanum* Ridl. Liliaceae (VJ)
fruit, root, leaf sap, *nam* (unspecified)

taan mo ตาลหมอ
Sugar from the coconut of the Palmyra palm

taan mon ตานหม่อน | sweet | root
Vernonia elliptica DC. | Compositae
(*V. elaeagnifolia* DC.) | (VJ); *HE*, p.18; *WW*, p.333
Lee Gkwan Yew vine
leaves, root
The whole plant is used as a stomachic and tonic, and as an anthelmintic for round worms | *HE*

*taan saan** ตานซ่าน
Schizaea dichotoma Sw. | Schizaeaceae (VJ)

taan sian ตานเสี้น
1. *Filicium decipiens* (W. et A.) Thw. | Sapindaceae
2. *Ponteria burmanica* Bachni | Sapotaceae
3. *P. siamensis* Bachni | Sapotaceae
4. *Planchonella siamensis* Fletch. | Sapotaceae (VJ)
root

taan thang 5 ตานทั้ง๕
bencha taan เบญจตาน
1. *taan mon* ตาหม่อน
2. *taan sian* ตานเสียน
3. *taan dam* ตานดำ
4. *taan khamooi* ตานขโมย
5. *taan tanot* ตาลตะโหนด
The 5 *taan*
roots

taan tanot ตาลตะโหนด | see *taan*

*tabaek** ตะแบก
ton tabaek ต้นตะแบก | see *khondok*

tabuun ตะบูน
Xylocalrpus granatum Koen.
(*Xylocarpus obovatus* A. Juss.) | Meliaceae (VJ)
(*Carapa obovata* Blume-A.Juss.)

fruit

taeng cheen แตงจีน
Citrullus lanatus (Thunb.) Mansf. — Cucurbitaceae
Water melon
fruit

taeng kwaa แตงกวา
Cucumis sativus L. — Cucurbitaceae (PT)
Cucumber
juice, seeds, flowers

taeng mo แตงโม — sweet — fruit pulp
Citrulus vulgaris Schard. — Cucurbitaceae (PT)
Watermelon
seeds

taeng nuu แตงหนู
1. *Zehneria marginata* Keraud.-Aymo
Melothria affinis King. — Cucurbitaceae (PT)
2. *Mukia maderaspatana* Roem.
root

taeng thuean แตงเถือน
? *samut* สมุทร
Amalocalyx microlobus Pierre ex Spire — Apocynaceae (PT)
root

takhian ตะเคียน — see *chan takhian*

takhop ตับบ — astringent
takhop Thai ตับบไทย
Flacourtia rukam Zoll. et Mor. — Flacourtiaceae (VJ)
(*F. inermis* auct. Merr. non Roxb.

takhop khwaai ตับบควาย
Flacourtia jangomas Raeusch. — Flacourtiaceae
(*F. cataphracta* Roxb.)
East Indian plum — *TS*, p.156

takhop paa ตับบป่า
Flacourtia indica Merr

(*F. sepiaria* Roxb.)
(*F. thorelii* Gagnep.) Flacourtiaceae (VJ)
bark, root
Both have edible fruit and thorny stems

takhrai ตะไคร้
Cympogonon citratus Stapf Gramineae
The petiole is used as a carminative and flavouring agent *HE*, p.6

takhro ตะคร้อ
Schleichera oleosa Merr. Sapindaceae
(*S. trijuga* Willd.) (PT)
bark

takhrong * ตะครอง
Zizyphus cambodiana Pierre Rhamnaceae (PT); *TS*
bark
It has thorny branches and bears an astringent fruit which is chewed with betel nut
Mc, p.352

tako ตะโก astringent unripe fruit
takonaa ตะโกนา
Disopyros rhodocalyx Kurz Ebenaceae *HE*, p.8
root
The bark is used as an ingredient of a rejuvenating formula; the bark and the wood as an aphrodisiac, stomachic, antimicrobial and to treat leucorrhoea

takuu ตะกู
leaves
1. *Nauclea orientalia* L. var. *pubescens* Craib Rubiaceae
2. *Anthocephalus chinensis* Rich. ex Walp. Rubiaceae (VJ)

talum phuk ตะลุมพุก
Randia uliginosa Poir. Rubiaceae (VJ)
fruit

tamlueng ตำลึง bland leaf
thao tamlueng เถาตำลึง
Coccinia indica W. et A. Cucurbitaceae
leaves, root and stem sap (*nam thao*) (VJ); *HE*, p.7; *WW*, p.336
There are both male and female plants, but these have no special names, and are not to be confused with *tamlueng shaek*.

The young leaves contain an amylolytic enzyme and are used to treat skin inflammation. The stem is used as an ingredient in an asthma remedy. *HE*

tamleung laai ตำลึงลาย
?

tamlueng shaek ตำลึงแฉก bland leaf
tamlueng tua phuu ตำลึงตัวผู้
thao tamlueng tua phuu เถาตำลึงตัวผู้
Melothria leucocarpa Cogn. Cucurbitaceae
Melothria heterophylla (Lour.) Cogn. (VJ); *HE*, p.7
leaves, leaf sap

*tamlueng thong** ตำลึงทอง
Heterostemma wallichii Wight Asclepiadaceae (VJ)

tanot โตนด, ตะโหนด see *khamot*

tao rang เต่ารั้ง
Caryota mitis Lour. Palmae (VJ); (PT)
Fish-tail palm
young shoots

tap tao noi ตับเต่าน้อย
Nymphoides cristatum Ktze. Menyanthiaceae (PT)

tap tao yai ตับเต่าใหญ่
Nymphoides indicans Ktze. Menyanthiaceae (PT)

tap tao thang 2 ตับเต่าทั้ง๒
1. *tap tao noi* ตับเต่าน้อย
2. *tap tao yai* ตับเต่าใหญ่

teen pet khruea ตีนเป็ดเครือ
Cryptolepis buchanani Roem. et Sch. Periglocaceae (VJ)
bark

teen pet ton ตีนเป็ดต้น
sattaban สัตตบรรณ
Alstonia scholaris R. Br. Apocynaceae (PT)

bark

thaeng thuai แทงทวย
Mallotus philippensis Muell. Arg. Euphorbiaceae(VJ)
bark

thalaai maak dip ทะลายหมากดิบ see *maak*
A bunch of the edible areca fruit when still green and soft

(nam) thalaai maak dip น้ำทะลายหมากดิบ see *maak*

thao khan เถาคัน
thao khan daeng เถาคันแดง
Columella trifolia Merr. Ampetidaceae (PT); *Mc*, p.391
ripe fruit, rhizome

thao tamlueng เถาตำลึง see *tamlueng*

thao tamlueng tua phuu เถาตำลึงตัวผู้ see *tamlueng shaek*

thao wan priang เถาวัลย์เปรียง Leguminosae
Derris scandens (Roxb.) Benth. (Papilionaceae) (PT); *HE*, p.8
root
An infusion of the roasted stem is used to treat debility *HE*, p.8

thao yaa naang เถาหญ้านาง see *yaa naang* (stem)

thao yaai mom (mai) ไม้เท้ายายม่อม
Clerodendron siphonanthus R. Br. Verbenaceae *HE*, p.7
Clerodendron indicum Kuntze
(*C. siphonanthus* R.Br.) (PT)
Turk's turban
root, stem, leaves
The root is used as an expectorant, febrifuge, antibiotic, and to treat asthma, and to check nausea and vomiting *HE*

thap thim ทับทิม exotic toxic root
astringent leaves and fruit rind
Punica granatum L. Puniaceae
Pomegranate (VJ); *HE*, p.15; *WW*, p.373
leaves, leaf sap, fruit, fruit rind, flowers, young leafy shoots

The fruit rind and leaves are used as an astringent treatment for diarrhoea, the seeds for scurvy and the root bark to expel tape-worm (*HE*)

thap thim thang 5 ทับทิมทั้ง๕
bencha thap thim เบญจทับทิม
All five parts of the tree - stem, root, flowers, leaves and fruit

thep thaaro เทพทาโร see *khrai ton*

thian เทียน astringent
Lawsonia inermis L. Lythraceae
There are two varieties:
var. *alba* Hassk. (white flower)
var. *miniata* Hassk. (red flower) (VJ)
Henna; Tree Mignonette
leaves
Thian means 'burning candle', 'candle', or 'spice', (but not 'incense') which can be burnt. Such spices are usually inflammable because of the presence of volatile oils, and sometimes the name of the plant is related to this. This is not the case here, because Henna is not a spice; cf. Balsams. (VJ)

thian daeng เทยนแดง
Lepidium sativum L. Cruciferae (VJ)
Garden cress seed. This is not red, but bright orange (VJ)

thian dam เทียนดำ hot-and-spicy fruit
Nigella sativa L. Ranunculaceae (VJ)
Black cumin; Black cummin
fruit

thian khaao เตียนขาว hot-and-spicy seeds
Cuminum cyminum L. Umbelliferae (VJ)
Cumin; Cummin
fruit

thian khaao plueak เทียนข้าวเปลือก
Foeniculum vulgare Hill. var. *dulce* Alef.
F. dulce Mill.) Umbelliferae (VJ)
sweet fennel
cf. *thian taa tak taen* เทียนตาตักแตน

thian sattabut เทียนสัตตบุษย์ hot-and-spicy seeds

Pimpinella anisum L. — Umbelliferae (VJ)
Anise; Aniseed; Sweet cumin

thian taa kop เทียนตากบ
Carum carvi L. — Umbelliferae (VJ)
Caraway

thian taa tak taen เทียนตาตั๊กแตน
Anethum graveolens L., and
A. cowa Roxb. — Umbelliferae
(*Peucedanum graveolens* Benth. et Hook. f.) — (VJ)
feucedanum
Dill and Indian dill
cf. *thian khaao plueak* เทียนข้าวเปลือก

thian thang 5 เทียนทั้ง๕
1. *thian khaao* เทียนขาว
2. *thian khaao plueak* เทียนข้าวเปลือก
3. *thian dam* เทียนดำ
4. *thian daeng* เทียนแดง
5. *thian taa tak taen* เทียนตาตั๊กแตน

1. *Cuminum cyminum* L. — Umbelliferae
2. *Foeniculum vulgare* Hill. var. *dulce* Alef. — Umbelliferae
3. *Nigella sativa* L. — Ranunculaceae
4. *Lepidium sativum* L. — Cruciferae
5. *Anethum graveolens* L. — Umbelliferae
   (*Peucedanum graveolens* Benth. et Hook. f.)
   Anethum cowa Roxb.

1. Cumin
2. Sweet fennel
3. Black cumin
4. Garden cress seed
5. Dill and Indian dill

thian thet เทียนเทศ
?

thian yaowa phaanee เทียนเยาวภาณี hot-and-spicy — seeds
Petroselinum crispum (Mill.) Nyman — Umbelliferae
(*P. sativum* Hoffm.)

(*P. hortense* Hoffm.)
Parsley (VJ)
fruit and seeds

thon dee ทนดี see *tong taek*

thong ทอง see *bai ngoen bai thong* and *bai thong*

thong laang bai mon ทองหลางใบมน — Leguminosae
Erythrina suberosa Roxb. — (Papilionaceae) (PT)
Erythrina arborescens — Leguminosae
Tiger's claw; Indian coral tree — *Mc*, p.403
leaves, bark

thong laang naam ทองหลางหนาม — toxic — root; leaf
thong laang ทองหลาง — Leguminosae
Erythrina fusca Lour. — (Papilionaceae)
root, leaves, bark — (VJ); *WW*, p.369

thong phan chang ทองพันชั่ง — toxic — root, leaves
Rhinacanthus nasutus (L.) Kurz — exotic — Acanthaceae
leaves, root — *HE*, p.15; *WW*, p.369
The leaves and root are used for the treatment of skin diseases, especially ring-worm; also as a diuretic and laxative *HE*

thop thaep ถอบแถบ — toxic — stem
Derris trifoliata Lour. — Leguminosae
(bencha) thop thaep whole plant — (Papilionaceae) (PT)

thua ถั่ว
Can refer to cowpea, pea, bean, mung, bean, pulse, gram, vetch or lentil (VJ)

thua kai ถั่วไก่
root
?

thua khieo ถั่วเขียว — oily — seeds
Phaseolus aureus Roxb. — Leguminosae
(*P. mungo* Auct.) — (Papilionaceae) (PT)
Mung beans
seeds

thua phuu ถั่วพู sweet rhizome
Psophocarpus tetragonolobus DC. oily rhizome; seeds
seeds, root sap Papilionaceae (PT); *TS*, p.276
A four angled bean, about 6"-8" long and 3/4"-1" wide (PT)

thua rae ถั่วแระ Lebuminosae
1. *Glycine max* Merr. (Papilionaceae) (VJ)
(*G. hispida* Maxim.)
(*G. hispida* Maxim.)
(G. soja Sieb. et Zucc.)
2. *Cajanus cajan* Millsp.
3. (*C. indicus* Spreng)
Soy bean; Soja bean; Pigeon pea;
Angola pea; Congo pea
leaves

thum maraatchaa ทุมมะราชา
Clerodendron serratum perhaps (VJ)
leaves

thung theng ทุงเทง
thum theng ทุมเทง
Physalis minima L. Solanaceae (PT)
leaves, root

to sai ต่อไส้ bland root
Allophyllus cobbe Blume var. *glaber* Hook. Sapindaceae
S. sootepensis Craib (PT); *PB*, p.77; *TS*, p.16
root

*ton sai** ต้นไทร
Ficus bengalensis L. Moraceae
Banyan tree; Banian tree *Mc*, p.429; (VJ)

ton see mahaa pho ต้นสรีมหาโพธิ์ see *phot*

ton tot muu kap ton tot maa ต้นตดหมูกับต้นตดหมา see *kraphang hom thang* 2

tong taek ตองแตก
thon dee ทนดี
Baliospermum axillare Blume Euphorbiaceae(PT); (VJ)

(*B. montanum* Muell. Arg.)	(PT)
root	

tree katuk ตรีกฏุก
tree katuk saam ตรีกฏุกสาม
1. *khing* ขิง
2. *phrik Thai* พริกไทย
3. *dee plee* ดีปลี

1. *Zingiber officinale* Rosc.	Zingiberaceae (VJ); *LB*, p.73; *TS*, p.355
2. *Piper nigrum* L.	Piperaceae (VJ); *HE*, p.14
3. *Piper longum* L.	(VJ); (PT);
3. *Piper retrofactum* Vahl.	(VJ); (PT)
(*Piper chaba* Hunter)	*HE*; (PT)

1. Ginger
2. Black pepper or white pepper
3. Long pepper

The three hot-and-spicy substances.

tree phalaa ตรีผลา
tree phalaa hom ตรีผลาหอม
1. *samo phiphek* สมอพิเภก
2. *samo Thai* สมอไทย
3. *makhaam pom* มะขามป้อม

1. *Terminalia belerica* Roxb.	Combretaceae
2. *Terminalia chebula* Retz.	(VJ); *HE*, p.18
3. *Phyllanthus emblica* L.	Euphorbiaceae
1. Ink nut; Beleric myrobalans	(VJ); *HE*, p.13

2. Chebulic myrobalans
3. Emblic myrobalans; Malacca tree; Indian gooseberry

The three fruits.

tree saan ตรีสาร
1. *chetta muun phloeng* เจตมูลเพลิง
2. *sakhaan* สะค้าน
3. *chaa phluu* ช้าพลู

1. a. *Plumbago indica* L.	
(*Plumbago rosea* L.)	
b. *Plumbago zeylanica* L.	Plumbaginaceae
2. *Piper* sp.	Piperaceae
3. *Piper rostratum* Roxb.	

1. a. Rose coloured leadwort; (VJ)
   b. Ceylon leadwort; White leadwort
2. ?
3. ?

The three strong substances

tuum ตูม — see *matuum*

tumkaa ตุมกา

tumkaa daeng ตุมกาแดง — see *kot kakling*

tum kaa thang 2 ตุมกาทั้ง๒ — Strychnaeaceae (Loganiaceae) (PT)
Strychnos sp.

ubon อุบล — Nymphaeaceae (VJ)
Nymphaea spp.
Water lily
flowers

ueang phet maa เอื้องเพ็ดม้า — Polygonaceae (PT)
Polygonum chinense L.

ulok อุโลก — Rubiaceae (PT)
Hymenodictyon excelsum Wall.
(*H. thyrsiflorum* Wall.)
leaves

utta phit อุตพิด — Araceae (PT)
Typhonium trilobatum Schott.
rhizome

waa หว้า — astringent — leaf; fruit; seed
Eugenia cumini Druce — Myrtaceae (VJ)
Black plum; Jambolan — *TS*, p.143; *Mc*, p.924
bark, sap

*waai** หวาย — bitter — rootstock
Calamus sp. — Palmae (VJ)
Rattan

waai khom หวายขม — bitter — rootstock
Calamus viminalis Willd. — Palmae (VJ)

Bitter rattan
thorns (*naam*)

waai takhaa หวายตะค้า
Calamus tigrinus Kurz — Palmae
Rattan — (VJ); *WW*, p.713
stem

waai tamoi หวายตะมอย
Pothos scandens L. — Araceae *LP*, p.172

waan haang chaang ว่านหางช้าง
Belamcanda chinensis DC. — Iridaceae
Tiger lily
root, leaves
All parts contain an isoflavinoid compound. It is believed to be a cancer remedy — *HE*

waan haang chorake ว่านหางจรเข้ — Liliaceae (VJ)
Aloe vera L., and
Aloe spp.
leaves — see *yaa dam*

waan keep raet ว่านกีบแรด
waan keep maa ว่านกีบม้า — *HE*, p.2
keep maa lom กีบม้าลม — *HE*
Angiopteris evecta Hoffm. — Angiopteridaceae
rhizome — (VJ); *HE*; *TS*, p.2; *WW*, p.63
Used as a styptic — *HE*

waan lueang ว่านเหลือง
Curcuma longa — Cucurbitaceae
(*C. domestica* Valeton) — (PT)

waan naang kham ว่านนางคำ
1. *Curcuma aromatica* Salisb. — Zingiberaceae
2. *Anoectochilus geniculatus* Ridl. — Orchidaceae (VJ)

waan nam ว่านน้ำ — hot-and-spicy — rhizome
hua ngo หัวงอ — *HE*
Acorus calamus L. — Araceae
Acorus gramineus Soland. — (VJ); *HE*

Sweet flag
rhizome
Used as a carminative, expectorant, hypotensive, tranquillizer; the oil is used as an antifungal *HE*

waan nam daeng ว่านน้ำแดง see *lamphan haang muu*
Enhalus acoroides Rich. et Salisb. Hydrocharitaceae (VJ)

waan proh ว่านเปราะ see *proh hom*

waan ron thong ว่านร่อนทอง
Globba sp. Zingiberaceae
rhizome (PT); *WW*, p.654

waen แหวน
hua waen หัวแหวน see *phak khraat*

wan priang (thao) เถาวัลย์เปรียง see *thao wan priang*

(mai) wen ไม้เวฬุ see *phai mai*
mai phai ไม้ไผ่

yaa ยา
Medicine

yaa หญ้า
Grass or low growing herb.

yaa chan kaat หญ้าชันกาด
Panicum repens L. Gramineae (PT)
rhizome

yaa dam ยาดำ exotic toxic
Aloe perryi Baker (VJ); *TPS* 2
A. barbadensis Miller (VJ)
A. ferox Miller (VJ); *TPS* 2
A. vera and hybrids *TPS* 2
See also *waan haang chorakhe* Liliaceae
Aloes. Colloquial (smuggling) name, opium (VJ)
Leaf exudate
This is not to be confused with *yaa chue dam*

yaa dap fai หญ้าดับไฟ
Lindenbergia philippensis Benth. Scrophulariaceae (PT)

yaa faran หญ้าฝรั่น cool and fragrant
Crocus sativus L. Iridaceae (PT)
Saffron plant

yaa fin ยาฝิ่น see *fin*

yaa khaa หญ้าคา
Imperata cylindrica Beauv. Gramineae (PT)
root

yaa khaao yen ยาข้าวเย็น see *khukha*
Smilax glabra Roxb. Smilacaceae (VJ)

yaa khieo (*ton*) ยาเขียวต้น Thunbergiaceae (VJ)
1. Green medicine, composed mostly of the leaves of many medicinal plants
2. *Thunbergia laurifolia* Lindl

yaa klet hoi หญ้าเกล็ดหอย
Hydrocotyle sibthorpioides Lam. Umbelliferae(PT)

yaa klet hoi yai หญ้าเกล็ดหอยใหญ่
yaa kret hoi yai หญ้าเกร็ดหอยใหญ่ [misprint]
Desmodium triflorum DC. Leguminosae (VJ)

yaa luuk khlao หญ้าลูกเคล้า
?

yaa naang หญ้านาง
Tiliacora triandra Diels. Menispermaceae(VJ); (PT)
(*Limacia triandra* Miers) (PT)
root, leaves, stem (*thao*)

yaa nguang chaang หญ้างวงช้าง bland
yaa ngaang chaang หญ้างางช้าง [misprint]
yaa wong chaang หญ้าวงช้าง [misprint]
Heliotropium indicum L. Boraginaceae
Eye bright (PT); *Mc*, p.221
leaves, root

Widely used as a poultice for herpes and rheumatism *Mc*, p.221

(bencha) yaa nguang chaang เบญจหญ้างวงช้าง
the whole plant

yaa non taai หญ้าหนอนตาย see *khop chanaang*

yaa paak khwaai หญ้าปากควาย
Dactylotenium aegyptiacum Willd. Gramineae (PT)
root, sap

yaa peen to หญ้าปีนตอ sweet
Commelina sp. Commelinaceae (VJ)
The plant is cyanogenic

yaa phan nguu daeng หญ้าพันงูแดง
Cyathula prostrata Bl. Amaranthaceae (VJ)

yaa phraek หญ้าแพรก
Cynodon dactylon (L.) Pers. Gramineae (VJ)
Bermuda grass
leaves

yaa rang kaa หญ้ารังกา
Cyperus alternifolius L. Cyperaceae (PT)

yaa raak dam หญ้ารากดำ
Carex sp. Cyperaceae (VJ)

yaa raak khaao หญ้ารากขาว
Knoxia brachycarpa R. Br. Rubiaceae (VJ)
root

yaa sai หญ้าไซ
Leersia hexandra Sw. Gramineae (VJ)
leaves

yaa som kung หญ้าส้มกุ้ง
Phyllanthus orientalis Airy Shaw Euphorbiaceae (VJ)

yaa tai bai หญ้าใต้ใบ bitter

1. *Phyllanthus amarus* Schum. et Thonn. Euphorbiaceae *WW*, p.356
2. *P. urinaria* L. Euphorbiaceae *HE*, p.14

It is difficult to know which species is indicated in the old prescriptions. If it is for fever, then it should be *P. amarus,* if it is a diuretic, then it is *P. urinaria* . (VJ)
leaves, fruit

yaa tai bai khaao หญ้าใต้ใบขาว
P. amarus Schum. et Thonn. *HE*, p.13

yaa teen nok หญ้าตีนนก bitter
yaa teen kaa หญ้าตีนกา
Eleusine indica Gaertn. Gramineae
Goose grass; Yard grass; Wire grass (PT); *PB*, p.9; *WW*, p.341

yaa wong chaang หญ้าวงช้าง [misprint] *see yaa nguang chaang*

yaan phaa hom ย่านพาโหม see *kraphang hom thang* 2

yaang ยาง bitter resin
Dipterocarpus spp. Dipterocarpaceae
fruit (PT); *TS*, pp.126-128

yaang daeng ยางแดง
Dipterocarpus costatus Gaertn. f. Dipterocarpaceae (PT)
bark

yaang khaao ยางขาว
Dipterocarpus alatus Roxb. Dipterocarpaceae (PT)
bark

yaang pho ยางโพ see *phot*

yaang saai ย่างทราย
Tetracera hedecarpa Boul. Dilleniaceae (PT)
root

yat suraa หยัดสุรา see *suraa*

yo ยอ hot-and-spicy fruit

yo baan ยอบ้าน

Morinda citrifolia L. Rubiaceae
fruit juice (PT); *HE*, p.12
The fruit are used as an emmenagogue and to stop vomiting; the leaves are used as a tonic, febrifuge, to treat diarrhoea, and as an application to wounds and ulcers; the leaf sap is used to kill lice; and the root as a cathartic and as a dye *HE*

yo paa ยอป่า
Morinda elleptica Ridl. Rubiaceae (PT)

yo thakaa โยทะกา Leguminosae
Bauhinia monandra Kurz (Caesalpiniaceae) (PT)
flowers

yot ยอด
young leafy shoots

Appendix II

Glossary of some scientific terms used

Abortifacient	Inducing abortion.
Alteratives (obsolete term)	Medicines which produce certain ill-understood changes throughout the body.
Anodyne	Pain reliever.
Anthelmintic	A remedy for worms, usually present in the intestines.
Antibacterial	Suppressing the growth of bacteria and perhaps killing them.
Antibiotics	Chemical substances produced by various species of micro-organisms such as bacteria, fungi and actinomycetes that suppress the growth of other micro-organisms and may eventually destroy them.
Antimicrobial	Suppressing the growth of microbes (fungi, bacteria or viruses) and perhaps killing them.
Antipyretic	Fever-reducing.
Antiscorbutic	Medicine to treat scurvy.
Anti-tussive	Cough suppressant.
Aphrodisiac	A sexual stimulant.
Bitter	A bitter substance given to improve the appetite.

Calcined substances	Calcium bearing substances such as shells and bones which have been burnt to produce calcium or lime.
Cardiotonic	Heart stimulant.
Carminative	An aromatic substance which assists the eructation reflex.
Cholagogue	A medicine which increases the flow of bile, thus acting as a laxative.
Decoction	A liquid obtained by boiling drugs in water.
Diaphoretic	Inducing perspiration.
Diluent	A substance, liquid or solid, used to dilute another.
Diuretic	Increasing the quantity of urine.
Drug	A medicinal substance.
Emmenagogue	Stimulating menstruation.
Excipient	An ingredient of a medicine which makes it suitable for administration.
Expectorant	Promoting the removal of secretions from the bronchial tubes.
Febrifuge	Reducing the body temperature in a fever.
Fumigant medicines	Drugs which are administered as vapour by burning them and allowing the fumes to envelope the body or the affected part.
Galactagogue	Inducing a flow of milk.
Glycoside	A chemical compound which contains a saccharide unit attached to a non-carbohydrate moiety which is termed the aglycone.
Hallucinogenic	Causing hallucinations.
Infusion	A liquid obtained by steeping substances, usually plant material, in hot or cold water for a short time.
Mixture	(as a form of medicinal preparation) A liquid preparation to be taken by mouth.
Narcotic	A drug which relieves pain and induces deep sleep.

Oxytocic	Inducing labour.
Pharmacognosy	The name is derived from the Greek *pharmakon* a drug and *gignosco* to acquire a knowledge of. Pharmacognosy is mainly concerned with naturally occurring substances having a medicinal action.
Pharmacology	In broad terms, is mainly concerned with the action of drugs.
Poisonous	Potentially lethal.
Refrigerant (obsolete term)	An agent which cools the body or blood.
Saponin	A type of glycoside which produces a lasting froth when shaken with water.
Stomachic (obsolete term)	Aiding digestion or appetite.
Taeniafuge	An anthelmintic which expels tape-worms.
Toxic	Poisonous.
Tranquillizer	A drug that allays anxiety.
Trituration	Rubbing or grinding together two or more substances, usually solids, but sometimes a mixture of solids and liquids.
Vehicle	A medicinal vehicle is the diluent or medium by means of which drugs are made suitable for administration.

Bibliography

Sources written partly in English and partly in Thai are classed as Thai if they cannot be understood without a knowledge of the Thai script, for example *FT.* When the Thai names or words are transcribed into Roman script in a source otherwise written in English, that source is classed as English, for example *Mc.* When the distinction is doubtful the classification is Thai, for example *TS.*

Following the Thai custom of referring to people by their first names, the names of Thai authors are not reversed.

Thai sources are listed in English alphabetical order.

Thai Sources

Bradley, D. B. *Dictionary of the Siamese Language, 1873.* Bangkok: Kurusapha, BE 2514 (AD 1971).

Chote Suvatti. *Fauna of Thailand.* Bangkok: Department of Fisheries, 1950.

Chote Suvatti. *Flora of Thailand.* 2 Vols. Bangkok: Royal Institute, BE 2521 (AD 1978).

Krom Paa Mai (Royal Forest Department). *Chue phan mai haeng prathet Thai. lem1. Chue phriksasaat - chue phuen mueang* (Siamese plant names. Part 1. Botanical names - local names). Bangkok: Royal Forest Department, BE 2491 (AD 1948).

Laddawan Boonyarattanakornkit and Thanomjit Supavita. *Chue phuet samun phrai lae prayot* (Names and uses of medicinal plants). Bangkok: Chulalongkorn University, n.d.

Leenaa Phuuphattanaaphong. ed. *Samun phrai Thai* (Thai medicinal plants). Vol. II. Bangkok: *Krom Paa Mai* (Royal Forest Department), BE 2522 (AD 1979).

Ngaan nithatsakaan samun phrai khrang thee 1 (The first exhibition of medicinal plants). Bangkok: *Samaakhom samun phrai haeng prathet Thai* (Thai Pharmacognosy Society), BE 2518 (AD 1975).

Ngaan nithatsakaan samun phrai khrang thee 2 (The second exhibition of medicinal plants). Bangkok: *Samaakhom samun phrai haeng prathet Thai* (Thai Pharmacognosy Society), BE 2519 (AD 1976).

Phaetthayasaat songkhroh (The study of medicine). Vol. I. Bangkok: BE 2495 (AD 1952).

Phaetthayasaat songkhroh (The study of medicine). 3 Vols. Bangkok: *Samaakhom rong rian phaet phaen boraan Wat Phrachettuphon* (The Wat Pho Traditional Medical College Association). Vol. I, BE 2504 (AD 1961); Vol. II, BE 2513 (AD 1970); Vol. III, BE 2519 (AD 1976).

Pharmaceutical Botany. Bangkok: Faculty of Pharmaceutical Sciences, Chulalongkorn University. n.d.

Phitsanuprasaatwet, *Phrayaa.* ed. *Phaetthayasaat songkhroh* (The study of medicine). Vol. I. 2nd edn. Bangkok: Phritimaat, BE 2457 (AD 1914).

Phitsanuprasaatwet, *Phrayaa.* ed. *Wetchasueksaa phaetthayasaat sangkhep* (Manual for students of traditional medicine). 3 Vols. 2nd edn. Bangkok: Bangkok era 127 (AD 1909).

Photchanaanukrom phaet phesat Thai - chabap maattrathaan (Dictionary of Thai medicine and pharmacy, standard edn.). Bangkok: *Samaakhom phesat lae aayurawet boraan haeng prathet Thai* (Association of Traditional Pharmacy and *Āyurvedic* Medicine of Thailand), BE 2507 (AD 1964).

Photchanaanukrom sap phaet Angkrit pen Thai (English-Thai medical dictionary). Bangkok: Phrae Phitthayaa, BE 2520 (AD 1977).

Photchanaanukrom sap phaet Angkrit-Thai chabap raatchabanthitayasathaan (English-Thai medical dictionary of the Royal Institute). Bangkok: Royal Institute, BE 2508 (AD 1965).

Prasoet Phrommanee and Parinyaa Uthitchalaanon. eds. *Tamraa phesatchakam Thai phaen boraan* (Text-book of Thai traditional pharmacy). Bangkok: *Samnak phaet phaen boraan Wat Mahathat* (College of Traditional Medicine, Wat Mahathat), BE 2516 (AD 1973).

So Sethaputra. *New Model Thai-English Dictionary.* 2 Vols. 2nd edn. Bangkok: Thai Watana Panich Co Ltd, 1972.

Tamraa wetchasaat chabap luang r. 5 (The royal medical texts of the fifth reign). *Kamphee prathom chindaa (sangkhep). lem 1; lem 3-12* (book 1 and books 3-12). National Library, Bangkok. Formerly labelled 'case n, numbers 534-547, Department of Education Library' now labelled ' 6/ก,6/ข, 6/ค, 6/ง, 6/จ, 6/ฉ, 6/ช, 6/ซ, 6/ฌ, 6/ด'.

Tem Smitinand. ed. *Chue phan mai haeng prathet Thai: chue phriksasaat - chue phuen mueang* (Thai plant names: botanical names - vernacular names). Bangkok: *Krom Paa Mai* (Royal Forest Department), BE 2523 (AD 1980).

Winit Wanandorn, *Phya. Chue phan mai haeng prathet Thai: chabap chue phuen mueang - chue phriksasaat* (Thai plant names: vernacular names - botanical names). Thai Forest Record No. 1. Bangkok: *Krom Paa Mai* (Royal Forest Department), BE 2503 (AD 1960).

Other Sources

Bamber, Scott. *Lom: An examination of a term used in association with illness in traditional Thai medicine.* BA (Asian Studies) Honours sub thesis, Australian National University, 1982.

Fausböll, V. ed. *Buddhist Birth Stories; or Jātaka Tales.* trans. T W Rhys Davids. Vol. I. London: Trübner and Co, 1880.

Herbal Exhibition of the Fourth Asian Symposium on Medicinal Plants and Spices. Catalogue. Bangkok: 1980.

McFarland, George Bradley. *Thai-English Dictionary.* Stanford: Stanford University Press, 1944.

Maneepin Phromsuthirak. 'Hindu Brahmā in Thai Literature.' *JSS* , Vol. 69, January-July 1981, pp. 43-57.

Mulholland, Jean. *Medicine, Magic and Evil Spirits: Study of a text on Thai traditional paediatrics.* Faculty of Asian Studies Monographs: New Series No. 8. Canberra: Faculty of Asian Studies, Australian National University, 1987.

Mulholland, Jean. 'Thai Traditional Medicine: Ancient thought and practice in a Thai context.' *JSS* , Vol. 67, Part 2 (July 1979) pp. 80-115.

Mulholland, Jean. *Thai Traditional Medicine: A preliminary investigation.* BA (Asian Studies) Honours sub-thesis, Australian National University, 1977.

Mulholland, Jean. 'Thai Traditional Medicine: The treatment of diseases caused by the *tridoṣa,' South East Asian Review,* Vol. III, No. 2 (February 1979) pp. 29-38.

Mulholland, Jean. 'Traditional Medicine in Thailand' *Hemisphere,* Vol. 23, No. 4 (July/August 1979) pp. 224-229.

Needham, Rodney. ed. *Right and Left: Essays on dual symbolic classification.* Chicago: University of Chicago Press, 1973.

Nyānatiloka. *Buddhist Dictionary: Manual of Buddhist terms and doctrines,* 4th revised edn., ed. Nyanaponika. Kandy, Sri Langka: Buddhist Publication Society, 1980.

Phya Anuman Rajadhon. *Five Papers on Thai Custom.* Data Paper: No. 28. Southeast Asia Program. Cornell University. Ithaca, New York: 1958. pp. 5-8, 'The Expulsion of Evil Spirits.'

Reynolds, Frank E. and Reynolds, Mani B. trans. *Three Worlds According to King Ruang: A Thai Buddhist cosmology.* Berkeley Buddhist Studies Series 4. Berkeley, California: The Group in Buddhist Studies, University of California: 1982.

Rhys Davids, T. W. ed. *Dialogues of the Buddha.* Translated from the Pali of the Dīgha Nikāya, Part III, Sacred Books of the Buddhists. Vol. IV. T. W. and C. A. E. Rhys Davids. London: Luzac 1957.

Rhys Davids, T. W. and Stede, William. eds. *Pali-English Dictionary.* London: Luzac 1966.

Thomas, Edward J. *The Life of Buddha as Legend and History.* 3rd edn. (revised). London: Routledge and Kegan Paul, 1949, paperback 1975.

Index